Neuroendocrine Tumors

Jordan M. Cloyd · Timothy M. Pawlik
Editors

Neuroendocrine Tumors

Surgical Evaluation and Management

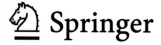 Springer

Editors
Jordan M. Cloyd
Division of Surgical Oncology
Department of Surgery
The Ohio State University
Wexner Medical Center
Columbus, OH
USA

Timothy M. Pawlik
Division of Surgical Oncology
Department of Surgery
The Ohio State University
Wexner Medical Center
Columbus, OH
USA

ISBN 978-3-030-62240-4   ISBN 978-3-030-62241-1   (eBook)
https://doi.org/10.1007/978-3-030-62241-1

This Springer imprint is published by the registered company Springer Nature Switzerland AG
The registered company address is: Gewerbestrasse 11, 6330 Cham, Switzerland

Foreword

Neuroendocrine tumors (NET) are tumors that arise from endocrine and nerve cells. They can occur anywhere in the body. While uncommon, their incidence is increasing. This may be because there is more awareness of these tumors than ever before. This book is totally about these tumors. It clearly gives the reader a complete understanding of all of the important aspects of these tumors. I have spent most of my surgical career working on these tumors. I want to share with you some important take-home messages of the book and controversies to think about as you read the various chapters.

NETs are ubiquitous. You need to know where a certain NET usually occurs and remember that it may still occur elsewhere. One example is gastrinoma. It usually occurs in the gastrinoma triangle which includes the head of the pancreas and the duodenum [1]. However, we have reported primary gastrinomas in the biliary system of the liver [2] and even the interventricular septum of the heart [3]. Even more confusing is that nodal primary gastrinomas have been described [4]. These ectopic sites were identified primarily by somatostatin receptor scintigraphy (SRS) which is an unbiased and accurate total body scan. Currently, we have the DOTATOC SRS scan that is even more sensitive and able to effectively identify these ectopic tumors (Chap. 2).

Rosalyn Yalow won the Nobel Prize in 1977 "for the development of radioimmunoassays (RIA) of peptide hormones." This was a major breakthrough for the field of NET surgery because it allowed precise diagnosis of hormonally functional NETs that are very well described in this book [5]. NETs secrete various hormones, which can be measured by RIA, and result in clinical syndromes that must be effectively managed before surgery. The hormone secreted also serves as a circulating marker of the tumor. For example, gastrinomas secrete gastrin that can result in severe peptic ulcer disease and diarrhea that is managed by proton pump inhibitors [6]. Ileal NETs secrete serotonin that may cause the life-threatening Carcinoid Syndrome that must be controlled before and during surgery [7]. Patients with VIPomas have severe diarrhea that results in dehydration and hypokalemia that also must be controlled prior to surgery [8]. The rash with glucagonoma is called necrolytic migratory erythema and patients with this have severe malnutrition and hypoaminoacidemia that needs to be managed [9]. The hormone excesses of serotonin, VIP, and glucagon are most effectively controlled with the inhibitory somatostatin analogues.

The next major problem with NETs is recognizing a familial syndrome. These occur and can alter management significantly. One example is the management of medullary thyroid carcinoma (MTC) in MEN-2. This is an excellent example of how research has changed care. MEN-2 was first described as Sipple's syndrome. It is the presence of unexpected pheochromocytomas in patients with thyroid cancer that affects the management. Failure to diagnose pheochromocytoma may be disastrous if an unprepared patient with a pheochromocytoma undergoes thyroid surgery. The diagnosis of MTC is done with assays. Initially, serum calcitonin levels, both basal and stimulated, were used as a circulating marker for MTC. Subsequently, RET gene mutations were identified and patients with normal serum calcitonin levels have undergone total thyroidectomy and a curative small focus of MTC can be excised [10]. So, the surgery was initially based on physical examination, then elevated blood hormone levels, and finally genetic changes. Another common familial genetic change that alters the surgical management of NETs is MEN-1 and paragangliomas/pheochromocytomas. Germline mutations of the succinate dehydrogenase genes SDHA, SDHB, SDHC, SDHD, and SDHAF2 are also present in 30–40% of patients with paragangliomas/pheochromocytoma [11]. NETs are multiple in MEN-1, so the surgery is seldom curative, but the goal of surgery is to remove potentially malignant tumors. In MEN-1, NETs are most commonly found in the pancreas where large tumors are removed because they are more probability malignant. Moreover in MEN-1, any NET within the thymus is malignant and should be excised [12].

Another difficult area is determining the malignant potential of NETs. Initially, most pathologists felt that all these tumors were benign. Then it became clear that a certain proportion of tumors develop distant metastases, so they can be malignant. In fact, most NETs are malignant, but some are clearly less aggressive than others. Malignant potential is best determined by the presence of metastases and Ki67 level [13]. Ki67 differentiates between NETs that can be treated surgically or primarily with chemotherapy [14]. Tumor size has importance in pancreatic NETs where tumors >2 cm are more clinically significant, but this size rule doesn't apply to ileal NETs that are usually small 2–3 mm but still can develop lymph node and liver metastases. Recent studies suggest that small pancreatic NETs in older individuals should be followed on imaging instead of surgery.

This book provides critical insight into each of these issues and other controversial areas in the management of NETs so that as you read the book you will become an expert and find answers to these and other questions. It is an essential read.

Jeffrey A. Norton
Stanford University School of Medicine
Stanford, CA, USA

References

1. Passaro E Jr, Howard TJ, Sawicki MP, Watt PC, Stabile BE. The origin of sporadic gastrinomas within the gastrinoma triangle: a theory. Arch Surg. 1998;133:13–6.
2. Norton JAFD, Blumgart LH, Poultsides GA, Visser BC, Fraker DL, Alexander HR, Jensen RT. Incidence and prognosis of primary gastrinomas in the hepatobiliary tract. JAMA Surg. 2018;153(3):e175083. https://doi.org/10.1001/jamasurg.2017.5033.
3. Noda S, Norton JA, Jensen RT, Gay WA Jr. Surgical resection of intracardiac gastrinoma. Diseases Pancreas. 1999;67:532–3.
4. Herrmann ME, Clesla MC, Chejfec G, DeJong SA, Yong SL. Primary nodal gastrinomas. Arch Pathol Lab Med. 2000;124:832–5.
5. Yalow RS. Radioimmunoassay: a probe for the fine structure of biologic systems. Science. 1978;200:1236–45.
6. Riff BP, Leiman DA, Bennett B, Fraker DL, Metz DC. Weight gain in Zollinger-Ellison syndrome after acid suppression. Pancreas. 2016;45:193–7.
7. Ito T, Lee L, Jensen RT. Carcinoid-syndrome: recent advances, current status and controversies. Curr Opin Endocrinol Diabetes Obes. 2018;25:22–35.
8. Mishra BM. VIPoma. N Engl J Med. 2004;351:2558. https://doi.org/10.1056/NEJM200412093512421.
9. Norton JA Kahn CR, Schiebinger R, Gorschboth C, Brennan MF. Amino acid deficiency and the skin rash associated with glucagonoma. Ann Intern Med. 1979;91:213–5.
10. Skinner MA DeBenedetti M, Moley JF, Norton JA, Wells SA Jr. Medullary thyroid carcinoma in children with multiple endocrine neoplasia types 2A and 2B. J Pediatr Surg. 1996;31:177–81.
11. Turchini J, Cheung VKY, Tischler AS, De Krijger RR, Gill AJ. Pathology and genetics of phaeochromocytoma and paraganglioma. Histopathology. 2018;72:97–105.
12. Norton JA, Zemek A, Longacre T, Jensen RT. Better survival but changing causes of death in patients with multiple endocrine neoplasia type 1. Ann Surg. 2015;261:e147–8. https://doi.org/10.1097/SLA.0000000000001211.
13. Genç CG, Falconi M, Partelli S, Muffatti F, van Eeden S, Doglioni C, Klümpen HJ, van Eijck CHJ, Nieveen van Dijkum EJM. Recurrence of pancreatic neuroendocrine tumors and survival predicted by Ki67. Ann Surg Oncol. 2018;25:2467–74.
14. Rinke A, Gress TM. Neuroendocrine cancer, therapeutic strategies in G3 cancers. Digestion. 2017;95:109–14.

Preface

Neuroendocrine tumors (NETs) are a diverse set of neoplasms that have heterogeneous clinical presentation, management, and prognosis. NETs are increasing in incidence worldwide and can occur nearly anywhere in the body. Over the last several decades, there has been a wealth of new information about the molecular characteristics and pathophysiology, novel diagnostic tools, and innovations in targeted therapies for NETs. The mainstay of treatment for most patients with NETs remains, however, surgical resection. Thus, a comprehensive textbook that addresses the contemporary surgical management of all NETs written by an international team of experts would be a valuable resource for practicing general, hepatopancreatobiliary, gastrointestinal, thoracic, and endocrine surgeons.

This textbook represents a comprehensive, state-of-the art, definitive reference for the surgical management of NETs. The book provides a practical, clinically useful guide that prioritizes the diagnostic work-up, indications for surgery, surgical principles, and perioperative care of patients with NETs in the context of multidisciplinary care. Most textbooks on NETs have traditionally focused on patients with advanced disease, highlighting systemic therapies and emerging treatment options. In contrast, this textbook provides a concise yet comprehensive summary of the surgical management of NETs. We hope that it serves as an invaluable resource for physicians, fellows, and residents who treat this difficult disease by providing helpful guidelines and up-to-date information on clinical management.

The textbook is comprised of four parts. In Part I, an overview of the diagnostic and perioperative considerations for NETs is provided, with a special chapter on carcinoid crisis pathophysiology. Part II focuses on the contemporary surgical management of gastroenteropancreatic NETs. In Part III, other primary NETs that commonly comprise a busy endocrine surgeon's practice are discussed. Finally, the management of advanced, metastatic NETs including liver and peritoneal metastases is discussed in Part IV. Throughout the textbook, all chapters are written by experts in the field and include the most up-to-date clinical information from national and international leaders in their respective disciplines.

Our sincere appreciation is owed to the authors for their contributions not only to this textbook but also to the science, research advances, and improvement in clinical care of patients with this fascinating malignancy. We hope that this textbook is not only an invaluable resource for many as they seek to provide the best possible surgical and multidisciplinary cancer care, but also an opportunity to identify new avenues of scientific discovery that may lead to significant advances in the diagnosis and management of NETs.

Columbus, OH, USA   Jordan M. Cloyd
                                                               Timothy M. Pawlik

Contents

Contributors

Valentina Andreasi Pancreas Translational & Clinical Research Center, Pancreatic Surgery IRRCS San Raffaele Hospital Vita-Salute San Raffaele University, Milan, Italy

Angela Assal, MD, MHSc, FRCPC Susan Leslie Clinic for Neuroendocrine Tumors, Sunnybrook Health Sciences Centre, Toronto, ON, Canada

Department of Medicine, University of Toronto, Toronto, ON, Canada

Sean Alexander Bennett, MD, MSc, FRCSC Department of Surgery, University of Toronto, Toronto, ON, Canada

Thomas E. Clancy, MD Department of Surgery, Brigham and Women's Hospital, Boston, MA, USA

Ashley Kieran Clift Department of Surgery & Cancer, Imperial College London, London, UK

Satya Das, MD, MSCI Vanderbilt University Medical Center, Department of Medicine, Division of Hematology and Oncology, Nashville, TN, USA

Arvind Dasari, MD, MS The University of Texas MD Anderson Cancer Center, Department of Gastrointestinal Medical Oncology, Division of Cancer Medicine, Houston, TX, USA

Bridget N. Fahy, MD Department of Surgery, Division of Surgical Oncology, University of New Mexico, Albuquerque, NM, USA

Massimo Falconi Pancreas Translational & Clinical Research Center, Pancreatic Surgery IRRCS San Raffaele Hospital Vita-Salute San Raffaele University, Milan, Italy

Adam C. Fields, MD Department of Surgery, Division of Gastrointestinal Surgery, Brigham and Women's Hospital, Harvard Medical School, Boston, MA, USA

Pier Luigi Filosso, MD University of Torino, Department of Surgical Sciences, Unit of General Thoracic Surgery, Torino, Italy

Elisa Carla Fontana, MD University of Torino, Department of Surgical Sciences, Unit of General Thoracic Surgery, Torino, Italy

Andrea Frilling Department of Surgery & Cancer, Imperial College London, London, UK

Victor A. Gall, MD Rutgers Cancer Institute of New Jersey, New Brunswick, NJ, USA

Maryam Ghadimi, MD Department of Radiology, Johns Hopkins University, Baltimore, MD, USA

Travis E. Grotz, MD Hepatobiliary and Pancreatic Surgery, Mayo Clinic, Rochester, MN, USA

Medhavi Gupta, MD Roswell Park Comprehensive Cancer Center, Buffalo, NY, USA

Julie Hallet, MD, MSc, FRCSC Department of Surgery, University of Toronto, Toronto, ON, Canada

Susan Leslie Clinic for Neuroendocrine Tumors, Sunnybrook Health Sciences Centre, Toronto, ON, Canada

Caitlin Hodge, MD, MPH Department of Surgery, Abington Hospital-Jefferson Health, Abington, PA, USA

James R. Howe, MD Department of Surgery, Division of Surgical Oncology and Endocrine Surgery, University of Iowa Carver College of Medicine, Iowa City, IA, USA

Julie Howle Department of Surgery, Westmead Hospital, Sydney, NSW, Australia

Maurizio Iacobone, MD Endocrine Surgery Unit, Department of Surgery, Oncology and Gastroenterology, University of Padua, Padua, Italy

Renuka Iyer, MD Roswell Park Comprehensive Cancer Center, Buffalo, NY, USA

Ihab R. Kamel, MD, PhD Department of Radiology, Johns Hopkins University, Baltimore, MD, USA

Xavier M. Keutgen Department of Surgery, Endocrine Research Program, University of Chicago Medical Center, Chicago, IL, USA

Bhavana Konda, MD, MPH Ohio State University Wexner Medical Center, Columbus, OH, USA

Amanda M. Laird, MD, FACS Rutgers Cancer Institute of New Jersey, Rutgers Robert Wood Johnson Medical School, New Brunswick, NJ, USA

Calvin How Lim Law, MD, MPH, FRCSC Department of Surgery, University of Toronto, Toronto, ON, Canada

Susan Leslie Clinic for Neuroendocrine Tumors, Sunnybrook Health Sciences Centre, Toronto, ON, Canada

Jennifer L. Leiting, MD Hepatobiliary and Pancreatic Surgery, Mayo Clinic, Rochester, MN, USA

Pamela W. Lu, MD Department of Surgery, Division of Gastrointestinal Surgery, Brigham and Women's Hospital, Harvard Medical School, Boston, MA, USA

David A. Mahvi, MD Department of Surgery, Brigham and Women's Hospital, Boston, MA, USA

Nelya Melnitchouk, MD, MSc Department of Surgery, Division of Gastrointestinal Surgery, Brigham and Women's Hospital, Harvard Medical School, Boston, MA, USA

Sahar Mirpour, MD Department of Radiology, Johns Hopkins University, Baltimore, MD, USA

Francesca Muffatti Pancreas Translational & Clinical Research Center, Pancreatic Surgery IRRCS San Raffaele Hospital Vita-Salute San Raffaele University, Milan, Italy

Sten Myrehaug, MD, FRCPC Susan Leslie Clinic for Neuroendocrine Tumors, Sunnybrook Health Sciences Centre, Toronto, ON, Canada

Department of Radiation Oncology, University of Toronto, Toronto, ON, Canada

Stefano Partelli Pancreas Translational & Clinical Research Center, Pancreatic Surgery IRRCS San Raffaele Hospital Vita-Salute San Raffaele University, Milan, Italy

Timothy M. Pawlik, MD, MPH, PhD, FACS, FRACS (Hon.) Department of Surgery, The Ohio State University, Wexner Medical Center, Columbus, OH, USA

Rodney F. Pommier, MD Division of Surgical Oncology, Department of Surgery, Oregon Health & Science University, Portland, OR, USA

Gillian Prinzing, BS Roswell Park Comprehensive Cancer Center, Buffalo, NY, USA

Matteo Roffinella, MD University of Torino, Department of Surgical Sciences, Unit of General Thoracic Surgery, Torino, Italy

J. Bart Rose Division of Surgical Oncology, University of Alabama Birmingham, Birmingham, AL, USA

Scott K. Sherman, MD Department of Surgery, Division of Surgical Oncology and Endocrine Surgery, University of Iowa Carver College of Medicine, Iowa City, IA, USA

Heloisa Soares, MD, PhD Huntsman Cancer Institute at University of Utah, Division of Oncology, Salt Lake City, UT, USA

Vineeth Sukrithan, MD Montefiore Medical Center/Albert Einstein College of Medicine, The Bronx, NY, USA

Francesca Torresan, MD Endocrine Surgery Unit, Department of Surgery, Oncology and Gastroenterology, University of Padua, Padua, Italy

Tanaz M. Vaghaiwalla Department of Surgery, Endocrine Research Program, University of Chicago Medical Center, Chicago, IL, USA

Michael Veness Department of Radiation Oncology, Westmead Hospital, Sydney, NSW, Australia

Sarah M. Wonn, MD Department of Surgery, Oregon Health & Science University, Portland, OR, USA

Zhaohai Yang, MD, PhD Department of Pathology and Laboratory Medicine, University of Pennsylvania Perelman School of Medicine, Hospital the University of Pennsylvania, Philadelphia, PA, USA

Rui Zheng-Pywell Department of General Surgery, University of Alabama Birmingham, Birmingham, AL, USA

Part I

General Considerations

Epidemiology and Diagnosis of Neuroendocrine Tumors

1

Vineeth Sukrithan and Bhavana Konda

Epidemiology of Neuroendocrine Tumors

Neuroendocrine tumors (NETs) constitute a group of malignancies arising from neuroendocrine precursor cells that can arise anywhere in the body (Fig. 1.1). The incidence and prevalence of NETs have steadily increased over the past four decades, and it is estimated that there were 170,000 patients with a diagnosis of NET in 2012 [1].

Incidence and Prevalence of Gastroenteropancreatic Neuroendocrine Tumors

In the Surveillance, Epidemiology, and End Results (SEER) database analysis from 2012 by Dasari et al., gastroenteropancreatic (GEP) neuroendocrine tumors (NETs) had an incidence of 3.6/100,000 persons in GEP sites (1.05/100,000 in the small intestine, 1.04/100,000 in the rectum, and 0.48/100,000 in the pancreas). It was therefore estimated that there were 170,000 patients with a diagnosis of NET in 2012. Rectal NETs have the highest prevalence among GEP NETs followed by small intestine, pancreas, and stomach NETs.

The incidence of NETs has increased approximately 7-fold since 1973, with site-specific increases ranging from 15-fold in the stomach to 2-fold in the cecum. This increase in incidence has been most prominent in localized, Grade 1 (G1) tumors. For example, when stratified by stage, there has been a 15-fold increase

V. Sukrithan (✉) · B. Konda
Ohio State University Wexner Medical Center, Columbus, OH, USA
e-mail: vineeth.sukrithan@osumc.edu; Bhavana.Konda@osumc.edu

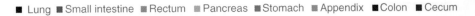

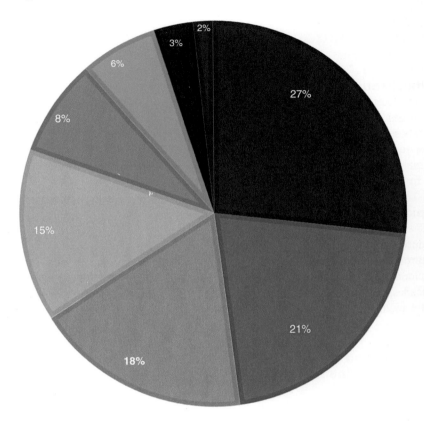

Fig. 1.1 Incidence of neuroendocrine tumors by site

in the incidence of localized NETs (0.21/100,000 in 1973 to 3.15/100,000 in 2012). Localized NETs now constitute close to half of all newly diagnosed NETs. Remarkably, there has been a 253-fold increase in the incidence of G1 NETs (0.01/100,000 in 1973 to 2.53/100,000 in 2012). G1 NETs now comprise nearly two-thirds of all newly diagnosed NETs. While the reasons for this increase are unclear, contributing factors likely include increased utilization of endoscopic procedures for screening and a widespread availability of sensitive imaging modalities, such as MRIs, beginning in the 1990s. Also, with Ga 68 DOTATATE PET scans gaining approval in 2016, a further increase in incidence may be expected.

An analysis of the National Comprehensive Cancer Network (NCCN) NET Outcome Database indicated that 22% of pancreatic NETs (pNETs) were functional, of which up to 70% were insulinomas, followed by glucagonomas (15%), gastrinomas and somatostatinomas (10%), and NETs secreting vasoactive intestinal peptide (VIP) and cholecystokinin (5%) [2].

Incidence and Prevalence of Lung NET

A population-based study by Dasari et al. of the SEER program showed an incidence rate of 1.49/100,000 in 2012 compared to 0.3/100,000 in 1973. Lung NETs comprise the fastest-growing subset of NETs and constitute close to a quarter of all incident NETs [1]. Subsequently, the prevalence of lung NETs has also increased from approximately 0.0015% in 1993 to around 0.0095% in 2012, constituting a sixfold increase.

A descriptive epidemiological study that used data from a US commercial claims database between 2009 and 2014 showed a 7.4% (p = 0.027) annual increase in the age-adjusted incidence of lung NETs for males and a 6.8% increase for (p = 0.052) females [3]. The age-adjusted prevalence also registered an annual increase of 9.9% in males and 16.2% in females.

The increasing incidence of NETs in the general population has become a cause of concern. It is likely that with the increasing use of imaging modalities, such as CT and MRI, in the general population over time, many localized NETs are being detected incidentally [4]. The greatest rise in incidence was seen in the stomach (fifteenfold) and rectum (ninefold), indicating that increased use of endoscopic screening procedures may underlie the rise of the incidence of these subtypes of NETs. It is unclear if the true rate of development of NET has increased, since causative biologic and environmental factors behind most non-genetically linked NETs are still unknown.

Survival

Survival in NETs varies widely based on site, stage, and grade making prognostication challenging (Fig. 1.2). The median overall survival (OS) for localized NETs ranged between 13.3 years for small intestinal NETs and >30 years for rectal and appendiceal NETs in the SEER study by Dasari et al. The overall 5-year survival was 68.1%, with the best survival seen in rectal NETs, followed by appendix, small intestine, stomach, colon, and pancreatic NET being the worst. The median OS for distant NETs, however, is only around 12 months with a wide range. Survival is around 5.8 years for metastatic small intestine NETs but only 4 and 6 months for distant colon and lung NETs, respectively [1].

Dasari et al. used the SEER histologic grade information to classify cases as grade (G)1, well differentiated; G2, moderately differentiated; G3, poorly differentiated; and G4, undifferentiated or anaplastic. Higher grades of differentiation portend worse survival ranging from 16.2 years in G1 NETs to 10 months in G3/4 NETs. Patients with G3/4 NETs had OS ranging from 30 and 33 months for the small intestine and appendix, respectively, to 8 months for the cecum and colon. After adjusting for age, stage, grade, race, and cohort year, lung and colon NETs were found to have similar survival, while appendix and small intestine NETs had better survival (HR = 0.53), followed by rectal, cecal, and pancreatic NETs. On the other hand, stomach NETs had worse survival compared to lung and colon NETs.

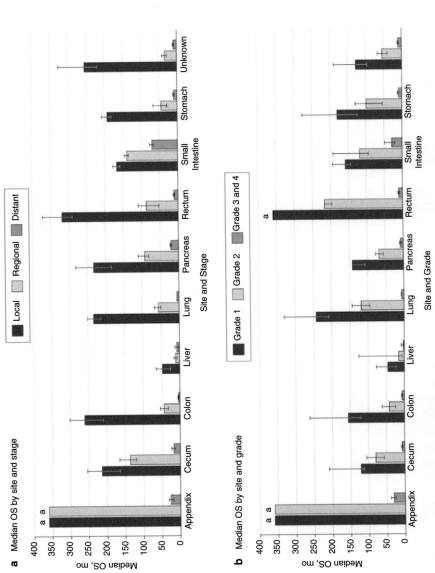

Fig. 1.2 Median overall survival of neuroendocrine tumors by site, stage, and grade (Adapted from Dasari et al [1], with permission)

Patients with metastatic G1/2 NETs that are metastatic at presentation constitute a group with worse prognosis than localized G1/2 NETs. On one end of the spectrum, median survival in this group was 14 months and 24 months for colon and lung NETs, respectively, whereas survival was 5 years and 8.6 years for pancreatic and small intestinal (SI) NETs [1].

There is evidence of racial disparity in the incidence and survival among Black patients with NET when compared to non-Hispanic Whites. Based on a SEER and SEER-Medicare database analysis by Shen et al., Blacks tended to have higher incidence of distant disease than non-Hispanic Whites (OR = 1.12), younger age of diagnosis, more distal colorectal disease (OR = 1.78), and a trend toward worse OS (HR = 1.2, p = 0.056) after adjusting for age, sex, site, comorbidity, carcinoid syndrome, stage, income, poverty, education, geographic region, and treatment status [5]. Whether this is due to tangible biological differences or residual unmeasured confounding is unclear.

Diagnosis of NETs

It has been recognized from the early twentieth century onward that some NETs have a unique ability to secrete peptide hormones leading to the use of the word "karzinoide" to describe this phenomenon by Oberndorfer in 1907 [6]. A SEER-Medicare analysis by Halperin et al. revealed that 19% of US patients with NETs had carcinoid syndrome. Based on their ability to secrete hormones, NETs may be classified as "nonfunctioning" or "functioning." Even within the functioning subset, the presence of carcinoid signs and symptoms may vary depending on the site and size of the tumor. Unfortunately, due to the rarity of the disease and general lack of sensitivity and specificity of the clinical symptoms, a prompt diagnosis of NETs is an exception rather than the rule. A prospective database study of 900 patients with NETs found that 1 in 4 patients reported symptoms for more than 1 year prior to diagnosis, underlining the necessity of a high index of suspicion to diagnose the disease [7]. Approximately two-thirds of carcinoid tumors originate from the gastrointestinal tract, and another 25% arise in the bronchopulmonary tract [8].

Clinical Signs and Symptoms

While the majority of patients with functioning NETs are asymptomatic, between 8% and 28% of patients have symptoms that are classic for carcinoid syndrome. This is usually seen in patients with liver metastases or retroperitoneal disease whereby secreted vasoactive amines gain direct access to systemic circulation [9]. The majority of serotonin made by the gut is metabolized by the liver and lungs to 5-hydroxy-indoleacetic acid (5-HIAA) via first-pass metabolism prior to entering the general circulation. In patients with liver metastases, retroperitoneal disease, and rarely lung carcinoid, serotonin bypasses first-pass metabolism and enters systemic circulation directly leading to symptoms that are consistent with "carcinoid syndrome."

The symptoms include the following:

1. Flushing involving the head, neck, and upper chest, associated with a sensation of warmth and sometimes pruritus. These episodes may be triggered by stress, exercise, or the consumption of certain foods.
2. Diarrhea.
3. Symptoms of right heart failure secondary to tricuspid and pulmonic valvular defects and endocardial fibrosis. Cardiac manifestations are seen in up to two-thirds of patients with carcinoid syndrome [10].
4. Skin rash due to pellagra from niacin deficiency. Excessive serotonin production from the utilization of precursor tryptophan leads to a relative deficiency of other products of tryptophan metabolism. Prominent among these is vitamin B3 (niacin), which is a product of the oxidation of tryptophan by indole 2,3-dioxygenase via the kynurenine pathway.

Carcinoid syndrome is most commonly associated with midgut carcinoid tumors with liver metastases. Serotonin secretion in the gut causes an increase in gastrointestinal blood flow, motility, and fluid secretion. The paracrine effect of increased serotonin in the midgut intestine can cause diarrhea and tumor mass producing discomfort. Postprandial abdominal pain in the setting of fibrosis of the mesentery or intestinal obstruction is also reported. Foregut carcinoids may present with atypical signs and symptoms including bronchoconstriction (bradykinins and tachykinins), rhinorrhea, lacrimation, telangiectasia (serotonin), acromegaly (ectopic growth hormone-releasing hormone), and Cushing's disease (ectopic adrenocorticotropic hormone).

Biochemical Tests for the Diagnosis of Functioning NETs

The 24-hour urinary 5-HIAA is considered the gold standard for the diagnosis of functioning NETs, but may not be universally performed due to the onerous nature of the sample collection. Urine 5-HIAA has a sensitivity of 73% and specificity of 100% for diagnosing well-differentiated functional gastroenterohepatic NETs [11]. Foods rich in serotonin are generally to be avoided for 48 hours prior to urine collection to reduce the risk of false positives. This includes but is not limited to avocados, bananas, pineapples, plums, cantaloupes, grapefruits, plantains, melons, dates, honeydew, kiwis, walnuts, hickory nuts, butternuts, pecans, tomatoes, and eggplants. Drugs that must also be held for 48 hours include acetaminophen, ephedrine, nicotine, glyceryl guaiacolate, phenobarbital, anti-histaminics, benzodiazepines, cyclobenzaprine, and monoamine oxidase inhibitors. A single fasting plasma 5-HIAA assay has high correlation ($R^2=0.74$) with 24-hour urinary 5-HIAA. Plasma 5-HIAA testing has a sensitivity of 89%, a specificity of 97%, and a test efficiency of 93%, making it an acceptable alternative to 24-hour urine testing [12, 13].

Chromogranin A has a sensitivity and specificity of 73% and 95% for the diagnosis of NETs [14]. Interpretation of chromogranin A levels must be performed with caution as they may be spuriously elevated in patients taking proton pump inhibitors or with renal or hepatic impairment. Chromogranin A levels may also have prognostic value in addition to being a tool for diagnosis. A study of a prospective database showed that chromogranin A levels elevated to more than twice normal levels were an independent factor for poor prognosis in metastatic NETs irrespective of tumor subtype (HR = 2.8, $p < 0.001$) [7].

In the appropriate clinical scenarios, it is recommended to test for additional hormones that are associated with specific NETs, as detailed in the following section.

Biochemical Testing for Peptide Hormones in Functional NETs

Functioning pNETs secrete peptides such as insulin, glucagon, gastrin, etc. which lead to associated symptoms that point toward underlying functioning pancreatic NETs.

Gastrinoma

Gastrinomas are gastrin-secreting tumors which occur most commonly as multiple lesions in the duodenum and less commonly as a solitary lesion in the pancreas. The latter has more malignant potential, most commonly to the regional lymph nodes and the liver. Zollinger-Ellison syndrome (ZES) is a triad of non-beta islet cell tumors of the pancreas, gastric acid hypersecretion, and mucosal ulcerations in the distal duodenum or proximal jejunum that was first described in 1956 by Drs. Robert Zollinger and Edwin Ellison. Most patients with ZES have the sporadic form (75–80%), whereas the remainder (20–25%) have it as part of multiple endocrine neoplasia type 1 syndrome (MEN1). It is worth noting that the majority (60–90%) of gastrinomas are malignant in nature with up to 53% of patients having liver metastases at diagnosis [15, 16]. The most common symptoms in patients with ZES are abdominal pain and upper gastrointestinal bleeding, with associated complications such as perforation and fistulization. The diagnostic criteria include a >10-fold elevation in fasting serum gastrin levels (serum gastrin levels >1000 pg/ml, with normal being <100 pg/ml) and a gastric pH of ≤2 when measured off anti-secretory therapy. Gastrin levels may be elevated in other conditions such as atrophic gastritis, *H. pylori* infections, or PPI use. Therefore, testing for inappropriately elevated gastrin should be done in the right clinical setting. It is generally inadvisable to stop antiacid therapy in patients with ZES; therefore, an alternative strategy may be to switch to an H2 blocker for 1 week and to replace the H2 blocker with liberal use of antacids for 24 hours prior to testing [17]. A secretin stimulation test may be required if gastrin levels are more than the upper limit of normal but less than 1000 pg/ml. However, this test should be avoided in patients with severe symptoms of ZES, given the risk of potentially fatal complications off adequate acid suppression therapy. Gastrin-secreting G cells have calcium-sensing receptors (CaR) that respond to extracellular Ca^{2+} levels to cause proliferation, gastrin secretion, and acid production [18]. In the case of suspected gastrinomas, which are almost invariably associated with hyperparathyroidism and hypercalcemia, the successful treatment of hyperparathyroidism can reduce fasting serum gastrin levels and even reverse a previously positive secretin test [19].

Glucagonoma

Glucagonomas are islet cell carcinomas of alpha cells of the pancreas. In a review of 1310 cases of pancreatic NETs assessed over a 28-year period, they had an incidence of 2% [20]. The majority are located in the tail or body of the pancreas [21]. Most glucagonomas are sporadic, but, when inherited, they are typically nonfunctional and associated with MEN1 syndrome or von Hippel-Lindau (VHL) syndrome [22, 23]. Necrolytic migratory erythema is a pruritic painful rash that appears as erythematous vesicles and bullae, later evolving into patches or plaques with irregular borders, crusting, ulcerations, and scaling [24]. Intertriginous areas and pressure points are commonly affected and may also form in areas of trauma (koebnerization). Other systemic symptoms include diabetes mellitus, weight loss, and diarrhea. Fasting glucagon levels >500 pg/ml are usually diagnostic (normal 70–160 pg/ml) [25]. False positives may occur in cirrhosis, chronic renal failure, pancreatitis, trauma, stress, or burns. Glucagonomas grow relatively slowly and metastasize late; therefore, early resection may prevent metastasis.

Insulinoma

Insulinomas are a rare variant of functioning pNETs. They are usually benign solitary tumors that are <2 cm in size. Most insulinomas are located in the pancreas or in the duodenal wall. Only 10% of insulinomas are malignant [26], and they are associated with a 10-year survival of around 30% [27]. Patients with insulinomas present with episodic hypoglycemic episodes characterized by diaphoresis, tremors, palpitations, confusion, personality changes, visual disturbances, seizures, and coma. The classic diagnostic criteria (Whipple's triad) are comprised of hypoglycemia (plasma glucose <50 mg/dL), neurologic symptoms of hypoglycemia, and prompt relief following the administration of glucose. Confirmatory biochemical testing involves documenting inappropriately high insulin ($\geq$5 mIU/L (36 pmol/L)), C-peptide ($\geq$0.6 ng/mL (0.2 nmol/L)), pro-insulin ($\geq$20 pmol/L), or insulin/c-peptide ratio < 1 after a 72-hour fast.

Calcitonin Levels and Pancreatic Polypeptide Levels

Calcitonin is a derivative of procalcitonin, a product of the Calc-1 gene, which also codes for calcitonin gene-related peptide (CGRP) in neuronal cells. Procalcitonin is mainly expressed in thyroidal C cells, where it is enzymatically cleaved to produce calcitonin. C cells, while predominantly present in the thyroid, are also present in the parathyroid glands, thymus, lungs, small intestine, liver, and bladder. Although elevated calcitonin levels are classically seen in medullary thyroid cancers, they are also encountered in GEP NETs. In a review of 176 NETs, high serum calcitonin (>100 ng/L) was found in 12% of cases, predominantly in foregut NETs of bronchial or pancreatic origin. There was also an association with higher-grade NETs and a trend toward poor prognosis in these patients [28].

Pancreatic polypeptide is a hormone of undetermined function that is expressed in the cells located within the head and uncinate process of the pancreas. One retrospective study in patients with pNET reported that serum levels of pancreatic polypeptide were elevated in 45% of patients [29]. Other large series reported a diagnostic sensitivity of pancreatic polypeptide between 41% and 63% for pNET [30, 31].

Clinical Approach to a Known or Suspected NET

The clinical approach to a patient with known or suspected NET begins with a thorough history and physical examination which should focus on relevant signs, symptoms, and relevant procedures and diagnostic work-up to date (Fig. 1.3). A thorough family history is also important to screen for potential germline mutations such as MEN1 and MEN2 especially relevant in NETs. Initial evaluation must include triple-phase CT imaging of the liver since vascular liver metastases, which are isodense with liver parenchyma, may be missed with routine modalities. Ga-68 DOTATATE PET/CT has been shown to be superior to In-111 DTPA scintigraphy and is considered standard of care for all patients with lesions harboring a suspicion of a NET diagnosis [32].

Somatostatin receptor (SSTR) imaging guidelines recommend the withdrawal of octreotide therapy before imaging, because of the possibility of interference of octreotide with tracer uptake in tumor cells due to competition for receptor occupancy as well as SSTR blockade [33]. Therefore, the current standard is to schedule SSTR imaging immediately prior to the administration of long-acting somatostatin analogs (SSA), though this is an area of debate [34]. Additional imaging may include colonoscopy, esophagogastroduodenoscopy, endoscopic ultrasound, endorectal ultrasound, capsule endoscopy, and bronchoscopy as appropriate. A 24-hour urine or plasma 5-HIAA is recommended in patients with carcinoid syndrome in addition to chromogranin A.

In patients with metastatic NET with carcinoid syndrome, performing a baseline echocardiogram and co-management with a cardiologist may be indicated in select patients, given that up to two-thirds of patients with carcinoid syndrome also develop cardiac manifestations during the course of their disease [10]. N-terminal (NT) pro-BNP, a neurohormone released by the atria and ventricles in response to wall stress, has been studied as a biomarker to screen for carcinoid heart disease. NT pro-BNP levels >260 pg/ml (31 pmol/L) have been shown to have high sensitivity and specificity (92% and 91%, respectively) for the detection of carcinoid heart disease along with negative and positive predictive values of 98% and 71%, respectively. A 24-hour urinary 5-HIAA of >300 μmol is associated with a threefold increase in development or diagnosis of carcinoid heart disease and is also a useful screening marker [35]. A high chromogranin level (>120 ug/L) has almost 100% sensitivity but only 30% specificity, so normal levels of chromogranin may help rule out carcinoid heart syndrome [36].

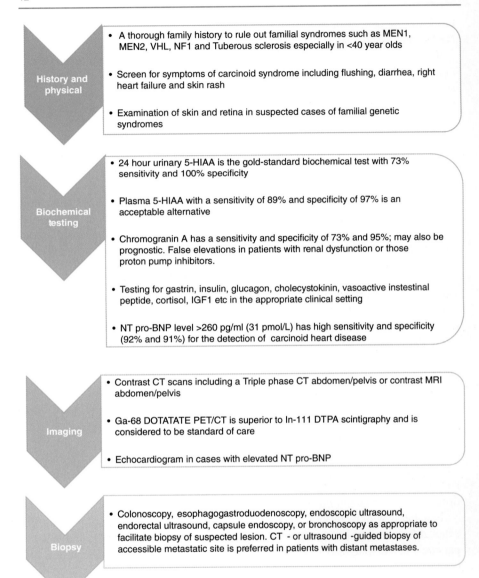

Fig. 1.3 Clinical approach to suspected neuroendocrine tumor

Biochemical testing for functioning tumors of the pancreas requires special care to prevent false-positive results. Similarly, in patients with suspected insulinomas, other causes of hypoglycemia, including iatrogenic insulin use and adrenal insufficiency, need to be ruled out first before performing a 72-hour fasting test of insulin, pro-insulin, and c-peptide levels. Insulinomas are also known to be less octreotide-avid and may be missed on somatostatin receptor-based imaging.

Elevated gastrin levels may be seen in any condition causing achlorhydria, including PPI, and the safe management of antiacid therapy in anticipation of testing for gastrin levels has been covered previously. Other biochemical markers to be tested in the appropriate clinical settings include serum VIP, glucagon, and pancreatic polypeptide.

Up to 10% of GEP NETs are estimated to have a hereditary background. Syndromes associated with these include MEN1, VHL, neurofibromatosis type 1 (NF1), and tuberous sclerosis (TS) [37]. In pNETs, preceding history of renal stones, hypercalcemia, or pituitary adenomas may indicate underlying MEN1. In any patient presenting with a pNET at a young age (<40 years old) or with multiple pancreatic microadenomas, a diagnosis of an inherited syndrome should be considered [38]. This is especially true for gastrinomas in which 25% of all patients have underlying MEN1. When associated with MEN1, the duodenal gastrinomas are usually small and multiple and frequently metastasize to local lymph nodes, which is in contrast to sporadic tumors which are more frequently pancreatic and consist of a single large adenoma [39]. A thorough physical examination, including the skin and retina, along with a family history is the cornerstone of the approach to a patient with a suspected hereditary syndromic predisposition to NET.

References

1. Dasari A, Shen C, Halperin D, et al. Trends in the incidence, prevalence, and survival outcomes in patients with neuroendocrine tumors in the United States. JAMA Oncol. 2017;3(10):1335–42.
2. Choti MA, Bobiak S, Strosberg JR, et al. Prevalence of functional tumors in neuroendocrine carcinoma: an analysis from the NCCN NET database. J Clin Oncol. 2012;30(15_suppl):4126.
3. Broder MS, Cai B, Chang E, Neary MP. Incidence and prevalence of neuroendocrine tumors of the lung: analysis of a US commercial insurance claims database. BMC Pulm Med. 2018;18(1):135.
4. Smith-Bindman R, Kwan ML, Marlow EC, et al. Trends in use of medical imaging in US health care systems and in Ontario, Canada, 2000-2016. JAMA. 2019;322(9):843–56.
5. Shen C, Gu D, Zhou S, et al. Racial differences in the incidence and survival of patients with neuroendocrine tumors. Pancreas. 2019;48(10):1373–9.
6. Obendorfer. Karzinoide tumoren des dunndarms. Frankf Z Pathol. 1907;1:425–9.
7. Ter-Minassian M, Chan JA, Hooshmand SM, et al. Clinical presentation, recurrence, and survival in patients with neuroendocrine tumors: results from a prospective institutional database. Endocr Relat Cancer. 2013;20(2):187–96.
8. Verbeek WH, Korse CM, Tesselaar ME. GEP-NETs UPDATE: secreting gastroenteropancreatic neuroendocrine tumours and biomarkers. Eur J Endocrinol. 2016;174(1):R1–7.
9. Soga J, Yakuwa Y, Osaka M. Carcinoid syndrome: a statistical evaluation of 748 reported cases. J Exp Clin Cancer Res. 1999;18(2):133–41.
10. Palaniswamy C, Frishman WH, Aronow WS. Carcinoid heart disease. Cardiol Rev. 2012;20(4):167–76.
11. Feldman JM, O'Dorisio TM. Role of neuropeptides and serotonin in the diagnosis of carcinoid tumors. Am J Med. 1986;81(6B):41–8.
12. Tellez MR, Mamikunian G, O'Dorisio TM, Vinik AI, Woltering EA. A single fasting plasma 5-HIAA value correlates with 24-hour urinary 5-HIAA values and other biomarkers in midgut neuroendocrine tumors (NETs). Pancreas. 2013;42(3):405–10.

13. Carling RS, Degg TJ, Allen KR, Bax ND, Barth JH. Evaluation of whole blood serotonin and plasma and urine 5-hydroxyindole acetic acid in diagnosis of carcinoid disease. Ann Clin Biochem 2002;39(Pt 6):577–582.

14. Yang X, Yang Y, Li Z, et al. Diagnostic value of circulating chromogranin a for neuroendocrine tumors: a systematic review and meta-analysis. PLoS One. 2015;10(4):e0124884.

15. Metz DC, Jensen RT. Gastrointestinal neuroendocrine tumors: pancreatic endocrine tumors. Gastroenterology. 2008;135(5):1469–92.

16. Yu F, Venzon DJ, Serrano J, et al. Prospective study of the clinical course, prognostic factors, causes of death, and survival in patients with long-standing Zollinger-Ellison syndrome. J Clin Oncol. 1999;17(2):615–30.

17. Ito T, Cadiot G, Jensen RT. Diagnosis of Zollinger-Ellison syndrome: increasingly difficult. World J Gastroenterol. 2012;18(39):5495–503.

18. Feng J, Petersen CD, Coy DH, et al. Calcium-sensing receptor is a physiologic multimodal chemosensor regulating gastric G-cell growth and gastrin secretion. Proc Natl Acad Sci U S A. 2010;107(41):17791–6.

19. Poitras P, Gingras MH, Rehfeld JF. Secretin stimulation test for gastrin release in Zollinger-Ellison syndrome: to do or not to do? Pancreas. 2013;42(6):903–4.

20. Yao JC, Eisner MP, Leary C, et al. Population-based study of islet cell carcinoma. Ann Surg Oncol. 2007;14(12):3492–500.

21. Wu SL, Bai JG, Xu J, Ma QY, Wu Z. Necrolytic migratory erythema as the first manifestation of pancreatic neuroendocrine tumor. World J Surg Oncol. 2014;12:220.

22. Castro PG, de Leon AM, Trancon JG, et al. Glucagonoma syndrome: a case report. J Med Case Rep. 2011;5:402.

23. Eldor R, Glaser B, Fraenkel M, Doviner V, Salmon A, Gross DJ. Glucagonoma and the glucagonoma syndrome – cumulative experience with an elusive endocrine tumour. Clin Endocrinol. 2011;74(5):593–8.

24. Kimbara S, Fujiwara Y, Toyoda M, et al. Rapid improvement of glucagonoma-related necrolytic migratory erythema with octreotide. Clin J Gastroenterol. 2014;7(3):255–9.

25. Kanakis G, Kaltsas G. Biochemical markers for gastroenteropancreatic neuroendocrine tumours (GEP-NETs). Best Pract Res Clin Gastroenterol. 2012;26(6):791–802.

26. La Rosa S, Klersy C, Uccella S, et al. Improved histologic and clinicopathologic criteria for prognostic evaluation of pancreatic endocrine tumors. Hum Pathol. 2009;40(1):30–40.

27. Service FJ, McMahon MM, O'Brien PC, Ballard DJ. Functioning insulinoma – incidence, recurrence, and long-term survival of patients: a 60-year study. Mayo Clin Proc. 1991;66(7):711–9.

28. Nozieres C, Chardon L, Goichot B, et al. Neuroendocrine tumors producing calcitonin: characteristics, prognosis and potential interest of calcitonin monitoring during follow-up. Eur J Endocrinol. 2016;174(3):335–41.

29. Adrian TE, Uttenthal LO, Williams SJ, Bloom SR. Secretion of pancreatic polypeptide in patients with pancreatic endocrine tumors. N Engl J Med. 1986;315(5):287–91.

30. Panzuto F, Severi C, Cannizzaro R, et al. Utility of combined use of plasma levels of chromogranin A and pancreatic polypeptide in the diagnosis of gastrointestinal and pancreatic endocrine tumors. J Endocrinol Investig. 2004;27(1):6–11.

31. Walter T, Chardon L, Chopin-laly X, et al. Is the combination of chromogranin A and pancreatic polypeptide serum determinations of interest in the diagnosis and follow-up of gastroentero-pancreatic neuroendocrine tumours? Eur J Cancer. 2012;48(12):1766–73.

32. Deppen SA, Liu E, Blume JD, et al. Safety and efficacy of 68Ga-DOTATATE PET/CT for diagnosis, staging, and treatment management of neuroendocrine tumors. J Nucl Med. 2016;57(5):708–14.

33. Sundin A, Arnold R, Baudin E, et al. ENETS consensus guidelines for the standards of care in neuroendocrine tumors: radiological, nuclear medicine & hybrid imaging. Neuroendocrinology. 2017;105(3):212–44.

34. Ayati N, Lee ST, Zakavi R, et al. Long-acting somatostatin analog therapy differentially alters (68)Ga-DOTATATE uptake in normal tissues compared with primary tumors and metastatic lesions. J Nucl Med. 2018;59(2):223–7.

35. Bhattacharyya S, Toumpanakis C, Chilkunda D, Caplin ME, Davar J. Risk factors for the development and progression of carcinoid heart disease. Am J Cardiol. 2011;107(8):1221–6.
36. Korse CM, Taal BG, de Groot CA, Bakker RH, Bonfrer JM. Chromogranin-A and N-terminal pro-brain natriuretic peptide: an excellent pair of biomarkers for diagnostics in patients with neuroendocrine tumor. J Clin Oncol. 2009;27(26):4293–9.
37. Anlauf M, Garbrecht N, Bauersfeld J, et al. Hereditary neuroendocrine tumors of the gastroenteropancreatic system. Virchows Arch. 2007;451(Suppl 1):S29–38.
38. Thakker RV, Newey PJ, Walls GV, et al. Clinical practice guidelines for multiple endocrine neoplasia type 1 (MEN1). J Clin Endocrinol Metab. 2012;97(9):2990–3011.
39. Anlauf M, Schlenger R, Perren A, et al. Microadenomatosis of the endocrine pancreas in patients with and without the multiple endocrine neoplasia type 1 syndrome. Am J Surg Pathol. 2006;30(5):560–74.

Imaging of Neuroendocrine Tumors

Sahar Mirpour, Maryam Ghadimi, Timothy M. Pawlik,
and Ihab R. Kamel

Introduction

Neuroendocrine tumors (NETs) are rare tumors arising from embryonic neural crest tissue and represent a wide spectrum of disease. NETs are clinically classified as functioning tumors when the tumor induces symptoms caused by hormonal hypersecretion and results in a clinical syndrome; in contrast, nonfunctioning tumors demonstrate no signs of hypersecretion and no recognizable clinical syndrome [1]. Functioning tumors present relatively early due to the associated clinical syndrome and may be a challenge for the radiologist to localize as these tumors are often small. Nonfunctioning tumors generally go unrecognized for many years and present much later with a large lesion and possible mass effect [2].

Imaging of functioning tumors is indicated to localize and stage these tumors, as well as to assist in surgical planning and facilitate potential surgical resection. In addition, imaging is valuable in the follow-up of recurrent or metastatic disease. In this chapter, the clinical and imaging features of NETs and the role of the different imaging and radionuclide techniques are discussed.

Role of Imaging in Diagnosis and Management

Imaging plays an essential role in the diagnosis, staging, treatment selection, and follow-up of NETs. The diagnosis of NETs relies on the combination of

S. Mirpour · M. Ghadimi · I. R. Kamel (✉)
Department of Radiology, Johns Hopkins University, Baltimore, MD, USA
e-mail: smirpou1@jhmi.edu; mghadim1@jhmi.edu; ikamel@jhmi.edu

T. M. Pawlik
Department of Surgery, The Ohio State University, Wexner Medical Center,
Columbus, OH, USA
e-mail: Tim.Pawlik@osumc.edu

© Springer Nature Switzerland AG 2021
J. M. Cloyd, T. M. Pawlik (eds.), *Neuroendocrine Tumors*,
https://doi.org/10.1007/978-3-030-62241-1_2

morphological and functional techniques, which provide complementary information [3]. Current morphologic modalities include computed tomography (CT), magnetic resonance imaging (MRI), transabdominal ultrasound (US), endoscopic US (EUS), and intraoperative US (IOUS). Functional imaging consists of scintigraphy including single photon emission computed tomography (SPECT) with ^{111}In-pentetreotide or, more recently, positron emission tomography (PET) with ^{68}Ga-labeled somatostatin analogs (SSA), ^{18}F-DOPA, and ^{11}C-5-HTP [4].

Hybrid nuclear medicine and morphological imaging such as PET/CT, PET/MRI, and SPECT/CT that are currently available with modern scanners generally achieve a better imaging yield compared with separate or combined morphological and functional techniques [5].

Imaging Modalities

A wide variety of imaging modalities are used for the localization of the primary tumor and for the detection of metastases. The choice of imaging depends on patient presentation and specific circumstances. For example, a functioning pancreatic NET may produce pronounced hormonal symptoms and be very small. For preoperative localization of such lesions, several morphological and functional imaging techniques, as well as endoscopy, may be required. Other patients may present with disseminated NET or bulky metastases for whom the imaging workup is straightforward and usually includes tumor staging with CT scanning or MRI and somatostatin receptor imaging by PET or SPECT. The choice of imaging modality also depends on the indication, whether imaging is performed for primary tumor detection, tumor staging of the primary tumor and regional and distant metastases, surveillance and detection of recurrent disease after surgery with curative intent, or therapeutic monitoring of locoregional and systemic therapies.

Imaging the Primary Tumor: Pancreatic NETs

Ultrasound (US)

Transabdominal US

Transabdominal US is a noninvasive and widely available imaging method, but has a relatively low sensitivity for localizing small primary tumors, ranging between 20% and 86% [[6], [7]]. Recent techniques such as contrast-enhanced US (CEUS) have, however, improved the diagnostic sensitivity of US. US is noninvasive, is inexpensive, and has a high specificity; thus, it continues to be considered in the available armamentarium of imaging techniques [2].

The scanning technique should be optimized for visualization of the pancreas. Drinking water prior to scanning allows the stomach to be used as an acoustic window; positioning the patient in both the upright position and lying in the left posterior oblique may help for better visualization of the pancreas [2]. NET appearance on US is typically a well-defined homogeneously hypoechoic lesion relative to the pancreas with internal vascularity on color Doppler imaging [8].

Endoscopic US (EUS)

EUS allows close proximity of the transducer to the pancreas; thus, a high-frequency US probe can be used (7.5–10 mHz) resulting in improvement of image resolution and increased sensitivity for the detection of small tumors [[9], [10]]. The overall sensitivity of this technique is 79–100% [10]. EUS also has the advantage of allowing real-time tissue sampling.

Despite the advantages of EUS due to greater ability to localize small and multiple tumors or tumors that are located in the duodenal wall, this method is technically challenging because it requires specialized training. As such, EUS may not be widely available. Also, it may not be suitable for all patients (e.g., patients with duodenal scarring).

Computed Tomography (CT)

CT is the most common diagnostic modality for the localization and staging of pancreatic NETs. It has the advantage of being widely available and is not operator-dependent. For CT scanning of pancreatic NETs, the imaging technique should be optimized. The patient should be fasting to ensure that the stomach and duodenum are emptied; the stomach should be distended with water. Following intravenous administration of contrast medium, biphasic scanning (arterial and portal venous phases) is recommended. Arterial phase scanning is started after a delay of 25 sec and portal venous scanning after a delay of 60–70 sec. The scan is usually performed with 1.25-2 mm section thickness, and the entire liver should be included in all phases [11]. Multiplanar reconstructions may also help improve lesion assessment.

Functioning tumors are usually small and subtle, with low inherent contrast between the tumor and surrounding pancreas. The majority of islet cell tumors are hypervascular and are best seen on arterial phase [12–14] (Fig. 2.1). However, some prior investigations demonstrated that the portal venous phase is significantly more helpful in identifying islet cell tumors [15]. At present, therefore, biphasic imaging following contrast injection is recommended to optimize the sensitivity of this technique [2]. Rarely, insulinomas may be hypovascular or cystic and appear hypodense to the surrounding pancreas (Fig. 2.2). Cystic pancreatic NETs may represent up to 14% of all cystic pancreatic lesions identified over a 10-year period [16]. Cystic pancreatic NETs are usually nonfunctioning and cannot be reliably differentiated from other cystic pancreatic neoplastic lesions on imaging alone [17]. In patients with a suspected gastrinoma, particular attention should be given to the "gastrinoma triangle," which is the anatomical area in the abdomen from which the majority (90%) of gastrinomas are thought to arise. The triangle is formed by joining the three points including confluence of the cystic and common bile ducts (superiorly), junction of the second and third portions of the duodenum (inferiorly), and the junction of the neck and body of the pancreas (medially).

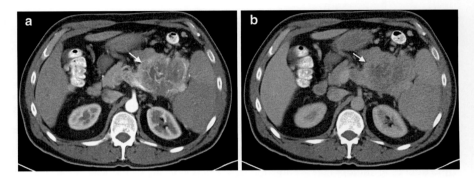

Fig. 2.1 Pancreatic neuroendocrine tumor in a 49-year-old male. A 10.5 × 7.4 cm, round, centrally necrotic mass (arrow) in the axial CT imaging. The mass was highly enhanced peripherally in the early arterial phase (**a**). Contrast was washed out in venous phase (**b**)

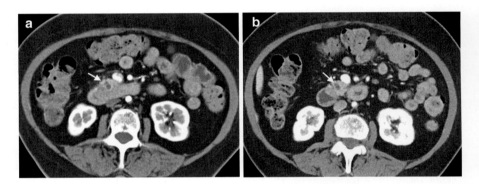

Fig. 2.2 Pancreatic neuroendocrine tumor with cystic degeneration in a 65-year-old female. A 1.7 × 1.3 cm cystic lesion in the pancreatic head with peripheral enhancement (arrow) in the axial CT imaging in arterial (**a**) and portal venous phases (**b**)

Lesion features that are generally associated with malignancy include large size, necrosis, as well as overt infiltration into the surrounding retroperitoneal structures such as vessels and calcification [18]. Detection of the primary tumor is directly related to tumor size, with no tumors identified under 1 cm. Tumor detection is reported to be 30% for tumors between 1 cm and 3 cm and 95% for tumors >3 cm [19, 20]. The location of the tumor also affects the ability of CT to detect the lesion. Prior studies have demonstrated that 68% of primary tumors and 86% of hepatic metastases were detected by CT scanning; in addition, 90% of pancreatic head tumors, 80% of pancreatic body tumors, and 45% of pancreatic tail tumors were diagnosed on CT exams [20, 21]. Small tumors <1 cm in the duodenum are often missed on CT, and CT sensitivity for the detection of extrahepatic and extra-pancreatic gastrinomas, which are often small at presentation, is only 30–50% [19, 22]. In general, helical CT has equal sensitivity, specificity, and accuracy to soma-tostatin receptor imaging in detecting primary neuroendocrine tumor and hepatic metastasis. However, helical CT appears to be more sensitive in detecting extrahe-patic metastasis from primary NETs [23].

MR Imaging

MR imaging had demonstrated lower sensitivity than CT for the detection of either the primary NETs or metastatic disease in early studies [15, 24]. However, with recent improvements in MR technology, the diagnostic performance of MR imaging has improved dramatically, and the sensitivity of MR imaging is now equal to or may even exceed that of CT in the diagnosis of NETs [15, 24, 25]. In fact, MR imaging sensitivity is 94% for pancreatic lesions, but may be less for extra-pancreatic lesions [24] [26].

As with the other cross-sectional imaging methods, tumor detection does depend on good quality images and tumor size. For example, image degradation due to motion artifact or poor signal-to-noise ratio in obese patients may reduce the sensitivity for tumor detection. The required imaging sequences include axial fat-suppressed T1-weighted spin-echo and gradient echo, axial fast spin-echo T2-weighted, and axial dynamic contrast-enhanced gradient echo sequence.

Pancreatic NETs usually appear as low signal intensity on T1-weighted and high signal intensity on T2-weighted sequences relative to the pancreas. The tumors are most conspicuous on the fat-suppressed T1-weighted image, whether spin echo or gradient recalled echo [24, 26]. Rarely, tumors contain a high collagen or fibrosis that causes a low signal on T2-weighted images [15]. Following intravenous gadolinium, there is a characteristic marked homogeneous enhancement in the arterial phase, reflecting the hypervascular nature of these tumors. In cystic lesions, rim enhancement may be seen [24] (Fig. 2.3).

Diffusion-weighted (DWI) MRI sequence is a rapid imaging technique, which reveals tissue contrast based on the difference in Brownian motion of water molecules within different tissues. Increased cellular density in tumors results in less extracellular space, thus reducing the mobility of water protons and resulting in restricted diffusion and high signal on DWI [27]. Associated low signal on the apparent diffusion coefficient (ADC) maps quantitatively measures the magnitude of diffusion (Fig. 2.4). DWI can be performed in breath-hold acquisitions and without the need for IV contrast. However, its main disadvantage is higher likelihood of artifact and distorted images. Furthermore diffusion-weighted imaging as a complementary with post-contrast images showed significant changes after transarterial chemoembolization (TACE) of neuroendocrine tumors and can be used to assess response of targeted tumors [28].

Imaging the Primary Tumor: Carcinoid Tumors

Localization

The diagnosis of primary carcinoid is mainly made by either endoscopy, particularly for gastric, duodenal, rectal, or colonic lesions, or bronchoscopy for endobronchial carcinoids [2]. Image-guided biopsy of a mass, liver lesions, or lymph nodes may help to establish the diagnosis. However, imaging is used extensively for the localization of primary carcinoid tumors, as well as tumor staging. The majority of

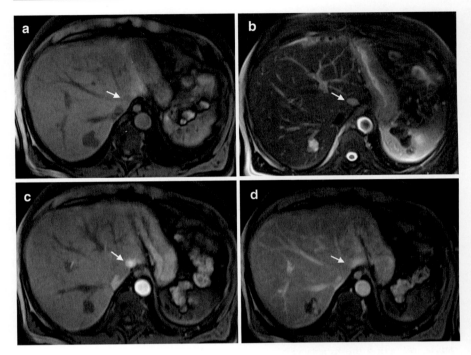

Fig. 2.3 Metastatic liver lesion in a 64-year-old male with history of primary pancreatic neuroen-docrine tumor with incidental hemangioma in the right hepatic lobe. MRI shows T1 hypointense (arrow) (**a**) and T2 faint hyperintense (arrow) (**b**) lesion in the caudate lobe correspond with hyper-vascular lesion in the arterial phase (arrow) (**c**), fading to liver background parenchyma in the portal venous phase (arrow)

Fig. 2.4 Metastatic hepatic neuroendocrine tumor in a 59-year-old male. Multiple metastatic lesions with significant high signal intensity on DWI sequence (b = 800 s/mm²) (arrows). Corresponding ADC map was not shown

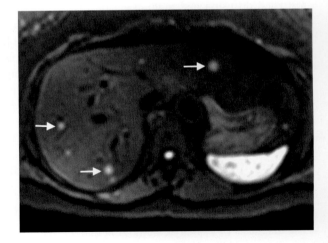

carcinoids do not present with a specific clinical carcinoid syndrome, and imaging may be performed to investigate nonspecific symptom such as vague abdominal discomfort or diarrhea.

CT scan is the principal diagnostic imaging tool for localizing and staging carcinoid tumors. Ultrasound is not a primary imaging modality in localizing the tumor and is predominantly used for guiding biopsy or sometimes for detection of liver metastases. Imaging is also helpful in the diagnosis of synchronized primary tumors, such as gastrointestinal and genitourinary adenocarcinoma, which are frequently described in association with carcinoid neuroendocrine tumors [29, 30].

Foregut Carcinoids, Bronchial Carcinoid

The majority of bronchial carcinoid tumors (80% of cases) are located in the central/middle third of the bronchial tree [2]. These tumors typically present as a mass within the bronchial lumen, usually with an extrabronchial component [31]. A peripherally located tumor (20% of cases) appears as a solitary round or ovoid pulmonary nodule with a smooth or lobulated border (Fig. 2.5). Punctuate or diffuse calcification is rather common as opposed to cavitation and hilar adenopathy [32].

Imaging features of primary bronchial carcinoid are similar regardless of the grade of the tumor [31]. Contrast-enhanced CT usually demonstrates intense homogeneous enhancement, although this is not seen in all cases. Marked enhancement may mimic pulmonary vascular structures and may create diagnostic difficulty as it may be overlooked, or interpreted as a normal vessel [31]. If the tumor is functioning and producing ACTH, then bilateral adrenal hyperplasia may also be seen [33].

Among patients with ectopic ACTH secretion of uncertain etiology, bronchial carcinoids are the most common source. When a pulmonary lesion is suspected but not visualized on CT, MR imaging may play an important role in the diagnosis. Bronchial carcinoids have high signal on T2-weighted images, allowing distinction

Fig. 2.5 Pathologically proven carcinoid tumor in a 42-year-old female. Axial unenhanced CT of the chest demonstrates a large lobulated mass in the left lower lobe (arrow)

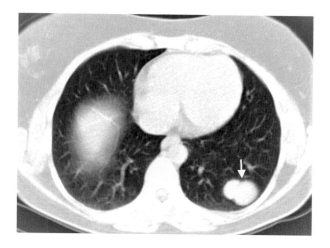

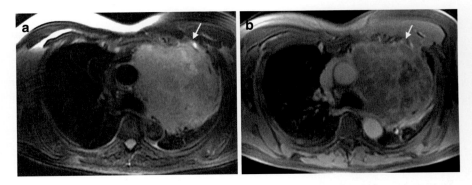

Fig. 2.6 Invasive thymic carcinoid in a 71-year-old female. Axial T2 MRI sequence demonstrates the lesion in the anterior mediastinum with heterogeneous T2 high signal (arrow) (**a**) and partially enhancing on post-contrast sequence with invasion to the left chest wall (**b**)

between a small mass and the pulmonary vascular structure. In some cases, imaging with somatostatin receptor scintigraphy may help in the detection of a small peripheral bronchial lesion [2].

Thymic Carcinoids

These tumors are usually aggressive, and the majority of these lesions present as a partially calcified anterior mediastinal mass that may cause SVC obstruction [33, 34]. There is usually evidence of extension into the pleura, pericardium, great vessels, regional lymph node. Distant metastasis such as bone or liver involvement is also visualized [35, 36] (Fig. 2.6).

Gastric Carcinoids

Gastric carcinoids are divided into three types. With type I, the tumors are multicentric and smaller than <1 cm lesion and are located predominantly in the fundus and body of the stomach. The diagnosis is usually made endoscopically, not on imaging. The disease is almost always benign. Type II tumors are associated with the Zollinger-Ellison syndrome (ZES) and multiple endocrine neoplasia type 1 (MEN 1). CT imaging demonstrates multiple masses within gastric wall, which is diffusely thickened secondary to ZES. Metastasis to regional lymph nodes is common; however, the prognosis is good. Type III tumors are usually solitary and large and may ulcerate. Local invasion and metastases are common [37].

Midgut Carcinoids

The primary tumor may not be seen as it is usually small and invisible against the small bowel or the colon. There may be either single or multiple primary sites. The most frequent imaging findings are secondary features including liver metastasis or tumor-associated desmoplastic fibrosis (Fig. 2.7), which causes tethering of mesentery or may cause small bowel obstruction or intussusception. Bone and lung metastases also can occur. The incidence of metastases from midgut carcinoids increases with tumor size; in tumors >2 cm, metastases occur in approximately 70% of cases [38]. Primary tumors in the small bowel remain one of the most difficult challenges yet to be overcome on imaging [39, 40].

MRI has better sensitivity in detection of primary midgut carcinoids. The best sequence for demonstrating the primary tumor is the post-gadolinium T1-weighted fat-suppressed image. The primary tumor enhances moderately/intensely following gadolinium with a nodular lesion arising from the bowel wall or regional uniform bowel wall thickening [41] (Fig. 2.8).

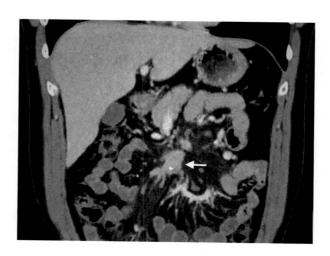

Fig. 2.7 Mesenteric carcinoid tumor in a 46-year-old male. Coronal CT of the abdomen in the portal venous phase shows a 2.8 × 2.2 cm lobulated mesenteric mass with coarse calcification and speculated margins surrounded by fat stranding (arrow)

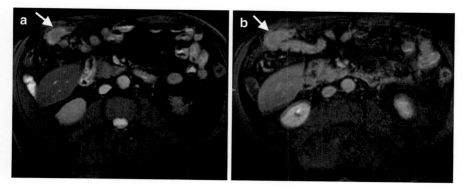

Fig. 2.8 Terminal ileum carcinoid tumor in a 67-year-old male. MRI shows terminal ileum biopsy-proven carcinoid tumor which is hyperintense in T2WI (arrow (**a**) and enhances in arterial phase (**b**)

Hindgut Carcinoids

Hindgut carcinoid lesions are usually diagnosed at endoscopy, although barium studies may demonstrate an extrinsic filling defect. At endoscopy, these lesions appear as solitary submucosal lesions and are typically between 1 cm and 2 cm in diameter in the rectum [42, 43]. Both CT and MRI can be used to stage lymph node disease and distant metastases as part of the preoperative planning; up to 30% of patients have metastatic disease at presentation [43, 44].

Metastases from pancreatic and carcinoid neuroendocrine tumors, particularly from small bowel origin, are common. In a large autopsy series, 29% of patients with a carcinoid tumor were found to have metastatic disease, the majority of which (61%) arise from small bowel carcinoids [45]. The most common sites of metastasis were lymph nodes, followed by the liver [45].

Imaging of Metastases

Liver Metastases

A significant number of patients with midgut carcinoid tumors present with liver metastasis at the time of initial diagnosis, depending on the site of the primary tumor [29]. Forty percent of ileal and up to 80% of cecal lesions have liver metastases at initial diagnosis [29]. The extent of liver metastases is an important prognostic factor for pancreatic NETs. On the other hand, the 5-year survival of patients with no liver metastases is not significantly different from patients with few (less than 5) liver metastases from carcinoid tumors [46]. However, there is a significant decrease in 5-year survival among patients with extensive liver metastases (more than 5) [47]. In addition MRI with quantitative and semi-quantitative visual methods is accurate for assessment of hepatic tumor burden and prediction of overall survival in treated metastatic liver neuroendocrine tumor with TACE [48]. The imaging appearances of metastatic disease in both pancreatic and carcinoid neuroendocrine tumors are similar.

Ultrasound

On transabdominal ultrasound, liver metastases usually demonstrate a hyperechoic lesion. The sensitivity of ultrasound to detect liver metastasis is approximately 60%, although the sensitivity is reduced among patients with a fatty, hyperechoic liver [49, 50].

CT/MRI

Neuroendocrine liver metastases (NELM) are usually hypervascular lesions and may be difficult to identify using single portal venous phase CT exam as the lesions may be isointense to the liver (Fig. 2.3). However, variations are large, and sometimes the NET metastases are hypovascular, which are best delineated on the venous contrast enhancement phase [3]. A combination of arterial and portal venous phase imaging improves the sensitivity of detection of the tumor [51].

On MRI, 75% of NELM appear as low signal intensity on T1-weighted and high signal intensity on T2-weighted images, with a similar appearance on CT images during post-contrast images [41]. Visualization and measurement of neuroendocrine hepatic metastases on DWI alone are comparable with post-contrast images, which allows for the possibility of eliminating post-contrast images [27]. Also, significantly lower mean ADC values are valuable predictors for Grade 2/Grade 3 tumors [28].

Mesenteric Masses and Peritoneal Disease

Secondary mesenteric masses are seen in approximately 50–75% of cases of midgut carcinoid [39, 41]. Masses typically appear as a soft tissue density with peripheral radiating strands. Calcification is seen within 40–70% of mesenteric masses and may be small stippled or bulky calcifications [52, 39] (Fig. 2.7). Masses usually arise within the fat or nodal tissue of the small bowel mesentery, although the exact nidus of metastatic lesion in the mesentery is not certain [52]. Diffuse mesenteric/peritoneal disease with peritoneal studding or ascites is not common and has been reported in 20–30% of cases with GI carcinoid. These tumors may cause bowel obstruction [39, 53]. Peritoneal disease is less common in pancreatic NETs (~11%) [53].

Other Sites of Metastases

Metastases to regional lymph nodes are the most frequent metastatic site at autopsy [45]. Retroperitoneal or mesenteric lymph node enlargement is seen in only 20–30% of patients with a midgut carcinoid [39]. Retroperitoneal fibrosis associated with lymph node involvement may result in ureteral obstruction. In thymic NETs, mediastinal lymph node metastases are present in 60% of patients at the time of surgery [54].

Lung metastases are usually asymptomatic and diagnosis can be made on CT [55]. Bone metastases are more commonly associated with foregut and hindgut carcinoids than midgut carcinoid tumors. The metastases are frequently sclerotic and may be indicative of poor prognosis [33].

Role of Nuclear Medicine Functional Imaging

Somatostatin Receptor-Based Imaging

Somatostatin nuclear imaging techniques play a crucial role in the diagnosis and staging of NETs. Furthermore, somatostatin receptor scintigraphy (SRS) with radiolabeled somatostatin analogs is the only method to select patients for peptide receptor radionuclide therapy (PRRT). In addition, nuclear imaging can play an important role in posttreatment follow-up and evaluation of response to therapy [56].

One of the main characteristics of NETs is overexpression of somatostatin receptors (SSTRs) on the cell surface. Thus, somatostatin analogs labeled with different radionuclides were developed to image patients with NETs. Most radiolabeled somatostatin analogs including ^{99m}TC/^{111}In-DTPA-octreotide and ^{68}Ga-DOTA-TOC/^{68}Ga-DOTATATE are currently available for imaging and have good affinity for the somatostatin receptor subtype 2, which is the most frequent receptor expressed by NETs [3, 56].

In SSTR-positive NETs, unlabeled somatostatin analogs (e.g., octreotide or lanreotide) can be used for therapy. These treatments can reduce hormonal secession in functional NETs, resulting in relief of symptoms, as well as lengthen the time to tumor progression [57].

Somatostatin Receptor-SPECT

^{111}In-Labeled Somatostatin Analogs

The most commonly used SRS radiotracer agent is ^{111}In-pentetreotide [3]. The SNM guidelines [58] recommend an administered activity of 222 MBq and 10 µg of pentetreotide. The relatively long half-life of indium (2.8 days) allows the possibility of imaging at 24 h and an optional 48 h imaging after injection. SPECT/CT of at least the upper abdomen is mandatory for optimal imaging. Normal tissues, such as thyroid, spleen, and the pituitary gland, express SSTR. The tracer also has hepatobiliary and renal excretion, so accumulation of radioactivity is seen in these organs as well [59]. The overall sensitivity and specificity of ^{111}In-DTPA-octreotide for the detection of NETs range from 57% to 93% [60]. The results vary considerably due to variations in the size and locations of the tumors.

Furthermore, imaging of NETs with ^{111}In-DTPA-octreotide is used to select patients for PRRT, which is performed with somatostatin analogs labeled with a β-emitting radionuclide such as Yttrium-90 or Lutetium-177. The level of accumulation in the tumor on the pretherapeutic SRS is an important prognostic factor for the prediction of tumor regression [61].

99mTc-Labeled Somatostatin Analogs

As an alternative to ^{111}In-DTPA-octreotide, somatostatin analogs can be labeled with 99mTechnetium (^{99m}Tc). Currently, the most commonly used ^{99m}Tc-labeled somatostatin analogs are ^{99m}Tc-depreotide and ^{99m}Tc-EDDA/HYNIC-Tyr3-octreotide (^{99m}Tc-EDDA/ HYNIC-TOC) [56]. The main advantage of ^{99m}Tc-labeled somatostatin analogs is the wide availability of ^{99m}Tc and lower radiation burden [61]. However, the disadvantages of ^{99m}Tc are the short half-life of 6 h and higher rate of false-positive results due to nonspecific abdominal tracer accumulation [62]. The recommended imaging protocol is acquisitions 2 and 4 h after injection, complemented with SPECT/CT of the upper abdomen. ^{111}In- and ^{99m}Tc-labeled somatostatin receptor analogs have relatively similar sensitivity in detection of NETs due to nonspecific abdominal tracer accumulation [62].

Somatostatin Receptor PET/CT

Imaging with a positron-emitting radionuclide-labeled compound allows a better image quality compared to imaging with a gamma camera including SPECT. For PET imaging, somatostatin analogs are labeled with the positron emitter Gallium-68 (^{68}Ga) [56]. The most commonly used somatostatin analogs labeled with ^{68}Ga are ^{68}Ga-DOTATOC, ^{68}Ga-DOTANOC, and ^{68}Ga-DOTATATE [56]. The different ^{68}Ga-SSAs perform similarly with regard to sensitivity and specificity [63]. In order to obtain the best imaging quality, an administered activity of at least 100 MBq and less than 50 μg of ^{68}Ga-DOTA-conjugated peptides is recommended. Image acquisition should be done at 60 min after injection [64]. Prior studies demonstrate pooled sensitivity of 93% and specificity of 91% for detection of NETs [63] (Fig. 2.9).

Comparison Between ^{68}Ga-SSA and Non-PET SRS

Several studies have compared ^{68}Ga-SSA to SRS, including ^{111}In-DTPA-octreotide, ^{111}In-DOTATOC, and ^{99m}Tc-EDDA/HYNIC-TOC [65–57]. Overall, ^{68}Ga-PET imaging has many advantages over non-PET SRS including better spatial resolution and higher detection rate of the lesions, less radiation, and shorter study time [66]. A disadvantage of ^{68}Ga-SSA is the higher false-positive results especially in the pancreatic head [56], which can be explained by the higher density of SSTRs in this area of the pancreas [68]. The other disadvantage is that it is not widely available.

Alternative PET Radiotracers

[18]F-fluorodeoxyglucose (^{18}F-FDG) is a glucose analog that accumulates in tumor cells, undergoes phosphorylation by hexokinase, and is trapped intracellularly. ^{18}F-FDG has a limited role in the imaging of NETs [56]. Poorly differentiated tumors (Grade 3) with a high proliferative activity have an increased glucose metabolism [69]. The majority of the more differentiated tumors (Grade 1/Grade 2) have

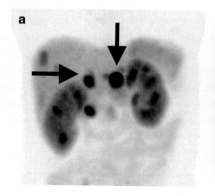
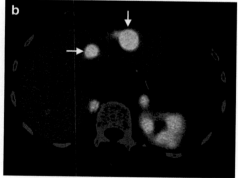

Fig. 2.9 Metastatic neuroendocrine tumor to the liver in a 63-year-old male. Images 67 minutes after injection of 4.3 mCi radiotracer demonstrate multiple ^{68}Ga-Dotatate-avid lesions in the right hepatic lobe in whole-body PET scan (**a**) and fused CT and radionuclide scans (**b**) (arrows)

a normal or slightly increased glucose metabolism [56]. In addition, the increased glucose metabolism, expressed as standardized uptake value (SUV), can provide predictive information in terms of overall survival and progression-free survival (PFS) [70]. ^{18}F-DOPA, a substrate of the catecholamine synthesis pathway, and ^{11}C-5-HTP, a serotonin precursor, are also utilized for research purposes [71, 72].

Imaging Survetillance

Given the slow-growing nature of well-differentiated NETs, surveillance strategies must balance the intensity and duration of imaging surveillance. Indeed, resected well-differentiated gastroenteropancreatic NETs may recur beyond 5 years from surgery. General guidelines have been put forth by the National Comprehensive Cancer Network as well as other organizations and societies. For resected Grade 1 NETs, we typically recommend contrast-enhanced abdominopelvic CT (or chest CT for lung carcinoids) every 6 months for the first 1–2 years and then annually for a total of 10 years following surgery. More frequent surveillance could be considered for more aggressive tumors (e.g., Grade 2 or lymph node-positive disease). Imaging surveillance is generally not recommended for resected low-grade appendiceal NETs <2 cm, rectal NETs <1 cm, or small type I gastric carcinoids.

For patients with metastatic well-differentiated tumors, cross-sectional imaging every 6 months is reasonable, more frequently for those with higher-grade tumors or who are on active systemic therapy. Following liver-directed therapy (e.g., transarterial embolization, ablation), post-procedural contrast-enhanced CT or MRI is recommended to evaluate its effectiveness. Functional imaging is not used for surveillance but performed selectively when the results may influence treatment decision-making (e.g., candidacy for PRRT, assessment of metastatic disease, etc.).

Conclusions

In summary, NETs are a heterogeneous group of tumors that represent a wide spectrum of disease. Imaging plays an essential role in the diagnosis, staging, treatment selection, and follow-up of patients with NETs. Advances in traditional morphological (e.g., CT, MR) and functional imaging have expanded the opportunities for accurate staging, prognostication, and treatment planning. Ongoing developments in somatostatin receptor-based functional imaging should not only improve the early and accurate diagnosis of NETs but also enable new opportunities for theranostics.

References

1. Trouillas J, Vasiljevic A, Jouanneau E, Raverot G. Classification of pituitary neuroendocrine tumors (PitNets). 2019.
2. Reznek RH. CT/MRI of neuroendocrine tumours. Cancer Imaging. 2006;6(Spec No A):S163.
3. Bodei L, Sundin A, Kidd M, Prasad V, Modlin IM. The status of neuroendocrine tumor imaging: from darkness to light? Neuroendocrinology. 2015;101(1):1–17.

4. Modlin IM, Oberg K, Chung DC, Jensen RT, de Herder WW, Thakker RV, et al. Gastroenteropancreatic neuroendocrine tumours. Lancet Oncol. 2008;9(1):61–72.
5. Modlin IM, Latich I, Zikusoka M, Kidd M, Eick G, Chan AK. Gastrointestinal carcinoids: the evolution of diagnostic strategies. J Clin Gastroenterol. 2006;40(7):572–82.
6. Van Heerden JA, Grant CS, Czako PF, Charboneau JW. Occult functioning insulinomas: which localizing studies are indicated? Surgery. 1992;112(6):1010–5.
7. Grant CS. Surgical aspects of hyperinsulinemic hypoglycemia. Endocrinol Metab Clin N Am. 1999;28(3):533–54.
8. Oshikawa O, Tanaka S, Ioka T, Nakaizumi A, Hamada Y, Mitani T. Dynamic sonography of pancreatic tumors: comparison with dynamic CT. Am J Roentgenol. 2002;178(5):1133–7.
9. Ueno N, Tomiyama T, Tano S, Wada S, Aizawa T, Kimura K. Utility of endoscopic ultrasonography with color Doppler function for the diagnosis of islet cell tumor. Am J Gastroenterol. 1996;91(4):772–6.
10. Rösch T, Lightdale CJ, Botet JF, Boyce GA, Sivak MV Jr, Yasuda K, et al. Localization of pancreatic endocrine tumors by endoscopic ultrasonography. N Engl J Med. 1992;326(26):1721–6.
11. Sheth S, Hruban RK, Fishman EK. Helical CT of islet cell tumors of the pancreas: typical and atypical manifestations. Am J Roentgenol. 2002;179(3):725–30.
12. Stafford-Johnson DB, Francis IR, Eckhauser FE, Knol JA, Chang AE. Dual-phase helical CT of nonfunctioning islet cell tumors. J Comput Assist Tomogr. 1998;22(2):335–9.
13. Van Hoe L, Gryspeerdt S, Marchal G, Baert A, Mertens L. Helical CT for the preoperative localization of islet cell tumors of the pancreas: value of arterial and parenchymal phase images. AJR Am J Roentgenol. 1995;165(6):1437–9.
14. Chung M, Choi BI, Han JK, Chung JW, Han M, Bae S. Functioning islet cell tumor of the pancreas: localization with dynamic spiral CT. Acta Radiol. 1997;38(1):135–8.
15. Ichikawa T, Peterson MS, Federle MP, Baron RL, Haradome H, Kawamori Y, et al. Islet cell tumor of the pancreas: biphasic CT versus MR imaging in tumor detection. Radiology. 2000;216(1):163–71.
16. Ahrendt SA, Komorowski RA, Demeure MJ, Wilson SD, Pitt HA. Cystic pancreatic neuroendocrine tumors: is preoperative diagnosis possible? J Gastrointest Surg. 2002;6(1):66–74.
17. Norton JA, Jensen RT. Resolved and unresolved controversies in the surgical management of patients with Zollinger-Ellison syndrome. Ann Surg. 2004;240(5):757.
18. Buetow P, Parrino T, Buck J, Pantongrag-Brown L, Ros P, Dachman A, et al. Islet cell tumors of the pancreas: pathologic-imaging correlation among size, necrosis and cysts, calcification, malignant behavior, and functional status. AJR Am J Roentgenol. 1995;165(5):1175–9.
19. Stark D, Moss A, Goldberg H, Deveney C. CT of pancreatic islet cell tumors. Radiology. 1984;150(2):491–4.
20. Wank S, Doppman J, Miller D, Collen M, Maton P, Vinayek R, et al. Prospective study of the ability of computed axial tomography to localize gastrinomas in patients with Zollinger-Ellison syndrome. Gastroenterology. 1987;92(4):905–12.
21. Maton P, Miller D, Doppman J, Collen M, Norton J, Vinayek R, et al. Role of selective angiography in the management of patients with Zollinger-Ellison syndrome. Gastroenterology. 1987;92(4):913–8.
22. Doppman J, Shawker T, Miller D. Localization of islet cell tumors. Gastroenterol Clin N Am. 1989;18(4):793–804.
23. Kumbasar B, Kamel IR, Tekes A, Eng J, Fishman EK, Wahl RL. Imaging of neuroendocrine tumors: accuracy of helical CT versus SRS. Abdom Imaging. 2004;29(6):696–702.
24. Owen N, Sohaib S, Peppercorn P, Monson J, Grossman A, Besser G, et al. MRI of pancreatic neuroendocrine tumours. Br J Radiol. 2001;74(886):968–73.
25. Semelka RC, Custodio CM, Balci NC, Woosley JT. Neuroendocrine tumors of the pancreas: spectrum of appearances on MRI. J Magn Reson Imaging. 2000;11(2):141–8.
26. Thoeni RF, Mueller-Lisse UG, Chan R, Do NK, Shyn PB. Detection of small, functional islet cell tumors in the pancreas: selection of MR imaging sequences for optimal sensitivity. Radiology. 2000;214(2):483–90.
27. Schmid-Tannwald C, Schmid-Tannwald CM, Morelli JN, Neumann R, Haug AR, Jansen N, et al. Comparison of abdominal MRI with diffusion-weighted imaging to 68 Ga-DOTATATE

PET/CT in detection of neuroendocrine tumors of the pancreas. Eur J Nucl Med Mol Imaging. 2013;40(6):897–907.

28. Liapi E, Geschwind J-F, Vossen JA, Buijs M, Georgiades CS, Bluemke DA, et al. Functional MRI evaluation of tumor response in patients with neuroendocrine hepatic metastasis treated with transcatheter arterial chemoembolization. Am J Roentgenol. 2008;190(1):67–73.

29. Modlin IM, Lye KD, Kidd M. A 5-decade analysis of 13,715 carcinoid tumors. Cancer. 2003;97(4):934–59.

30. Habal N, Sims C, Bilchik AJ. Gastrointestinal carcinoid tumors and second primary malignancies. J Surg Oncol. 2000;75(4):310–6.

31. Jeung M-Y, Gasser B, Gangi A, Charneau D, Ducroq X, Kessler R, et al. Bronchial carcinoid tumors of the thorax: spectrum of radiologic findings. Radiographics. 2002;22(2):351–65.

32. Nessi R, Basso PR, Basso SR, Bosco M, Blanc M, Uslenghi C. Bronchial carcinoid tumors: radiologic observations in 49 cases. J Thorac Imaging. 1991;6(2):47–53.

33. Wollensak G, Herbst EW, Beck A, Schaefer H-E. Primary thymic carcinoid with Cushing's syndrome. Virchows Archiv A Pathol Anat Histopathol. 1992;420(2):191–5.

34. Brown L, Aughenbaugh G, Wick M, Baker B, Salassa R. Roentgenologic diagnosis of primary corticotropin-producing carcinoid tumors of the mediastinum. Radiology. 1982;142(1):143–8.

35. Wang D-Y, Chang D-B, Kuo S-H, Yang P-C, Lee Y-C, Hsu H, et al. Carcinoid tumours of the thymus. Thorax. 1994;49(4):357–60.

36. Brown LR, Aughenbaugh GL. Masses of the anterior mediastinum: CT and MR imaging. AJR Am J Roentgenol. 1991;157(6):1171–80.

37. Binstock AJ, Johnson CD, Stephens DH, Lloyd RV, Fletcher JG. Carcinoid tumors of the stomach: a clinical and radiographic study. Am J Roentgenol. 2001;176(4):947–51.

38. Pinchot SN, Holen K, Sippel RS, Chen H. Carcinoid tumors. Oncologist. 2008; 13(12): 1255–69.

39. Woodard PK, Feldman JM, Paine SS, Baker ME. Midgut carcinoid tumors: CT findings and biochemical profiles. J Comput Assist Tomogr. 1995;19(3):400–5.

40. Sugimoto E, Lörelius L-E, Eriksson B, Öberg K. Midgut carcinoid tumours: CT appearance. Acta Radiol. 1995;36(4–6):367–71.

41. Bader TR, Semelka RC, Chiu VC, Armao DM, Woosley JT. MRI of carcinoid tumors: spectrum of appearances in the gastrointestinal tract and liver. J Magn Reson Imaging. 2001;14(3):261–9.

42. Winburn GB. Multiple rectal carcinoids: a case report. Am Surg. 1998;64(12):1200.

43. Maeda K, Maruta M, Utsumi T, Sato H, Masumori K, Matsumoto M. Minimally invasive surgery for carcinoid tumors in the rectum. Biomed Pharmacother. 2002;56:222s–6s.

44. Danikas D, Theodorou SJ, Matthews WE, Rienzo AA. Unusually aggressive rectal carcinoid metastasizing to larynx, pancreas, adrenal glands, and brain. Am Surg. 2000;66(12):1179.

45. Berge T, Linell F. Carcinoid tumours: frequency in a defined population during a 12-year-period. Acta Pathol Microbiol Scand A Pathol. 1976;84(4):322–30.

46. Yu F, Venzon DJ, Serrano J, Goebel SU, Doppman JL, Gibril F, et al. Prospective study of the clinical course, prognostic factors, causes of death, and survival in patients with long-standing Zollinger-Ellison syndrome. J Clin Oncol. 1999;17(2):615.

47. Janson ET, Holmberg L, Stridsberg M, Eriksson B, Theodorsson E, Wilander E. Carcinoid tumors: analysis of prognostic factors and survival in 301 patients from a referral center. Ann Oncol. 1997;8(7):685–90.

48. Luo Y, Ameli S, Pandey A, Khoshpouri P, Ghasabeh MA, Pandey P, et al. Semi-quantitative visual assessment of hepatic tumor burden can reliably predict survival in neuroendocrine liver metastases treated with transarterial chemoembolization. Eur Radiol. 2019;29(11):5804–12.

49. King C, Reznek R, Dacie J, Wass J. Imaging islet cell tumours. Clin Radiol. 1994;49(5):295–303.

50. London J, Shawker T, Doppman J, Frucht H, Vinayek R, Stark H, et al. Zollinger-Ellison syndrome: prospective assessment of abdominal US in the localization of gastrinomas. Radiology. 1991;178(3):763–7.

51. Paulson EK, McDermott VG, Keogan MT, DeLong DM, Frederick MG, Nelson RC. Carcinoid metastases to the liver: role of triple-phase helical CT. Radiology. 1998;206(1):143–50.

52. Pantongrag-Brown L, Buetow PC, Carr NJ, Lichtenstein JE, Buck JL. Calcification and fibrosis in mesenteric carcinoid tumor: CT findings and pathologic correlation. AJR Am J Roentgenol. 1995;164(2):387–91.
53. Vasseur B, Cadiot G, Zins M, Fléjou JF, Belghiti J, Marmuse JF, et al. Peritoneal carcinomatosis in patients with digestive endocrine tumors. Cancer. 1996;78(8):1686–92.
54. Fukai I, Masaoka A, Fujii Y, Yamakawa Y, Yokoyama T, Murase T, et al. Thymic neuroendocrine tumor (thymic carcinoid): a clinicopathologic study in 15 patients. Ann Thorac Surg. 1999;67(1):208–11.
55. Khan JH, McElhinney DB, Rahman SB, George TI, Clark OH, Merrick SH. Pulmonary metastases of endocrine origin: the role of surgery. Chest. 1998;114(2):526–34.
56. Brabander T, Kwekkeboom DJ, Feelders RA, Brouwers AH, Teunissen JJ. Nuclear medicine imaging of neuroendocrine tumors. In: Neuroendocrine tumors a multidisciplinary approach, vol. 44. New York: Karger Publishers; 2015. p. 73–87.
57. Rinke A, Muller H, Schade-Brittinger C, Klose K-J, Barth P, Wied M, et al. Placebo-controlled, double-blind, prospective, randomized study on the effect of octreotide LAR in the control of tumor growth in patients with metastatic neuroendocrine midgut tumors: a report from the PROMID study group. J Clin Oncol. 2009;27(28):4656–63.
58. Balon HR, Brown TL, Goldsmith SJ, Silberstein EB, Krenning EP, Lang O, et al. The SNM practice guideline for somatostatin receptor scintigraphy 2.0. J Nucl Med Technol. 2011;39(4):317–24.
59. Kwekkeboom DJ, Kam BL, Van Essen M, Teunissen JJ, van Eijck CH, Valkema R, et al. Somatostatin receptor-based imaging and therapy of gastroenteropancreatic neuroendocrine tumors. Endocr Relat Cancer. 2010;17(1):R53–73.
60. Modlin IM, Kidd M, Latich I, Zikusoka MN, Shapiro MD. Current status of gastrointestinal carcinoids. Gastroenterology. 2005;128(6):1717–51.
61. Kwekkeboom DJ, de Herder WW, Kam BL, van Eijck CH, van Essen M, Kooij PP, et al. Treatment with the radiolabeled somatostatin analog [177Lu-DOTA0, Tyr3] octreotate: toxicity, efficacy, and survival. J Clin Oncol. 2008;26(13):2124–30.
62. Gabriel M, Decristoforo C, Donnemiller E, Ulmer H, Rychlinski CW, Mather SJ, et al. An intrapatient comparison of 99mTc-EDDA/HYNIC-TOC with 111In-DTPA-octreotide for diagnosis of somatostatin receptor-expressing tumors. J Nucl Med. 2003;44(5):708–16.
63. Geijer H, Breimer LH. Somatostatin receptor PET/CT in neuroendocrine tumours: update on systematic review and meta-analysis. Eur J Nucl Med Mol Imaging. 2013;40(11):1770–80.
64. Virgolini I, Ambrosini V, Bomanji JB, Baum RP, Fanti S, Gabriel M, et al. Procedure guidelines for pet/ct tumour imaging with 68 Ga-dota-conjugated peptides: 68 Ga-dota-toc, 68 Ga-dota-noc, 68 Ga-dota-tate. Eur J Nucl Med Mol Imaging. 2010;37(10):2004–10.
65. Gabriel M, Decristoforo C, Kendler D, Dobrozemsky G, Heute D, Uprimny C, et al. 68Ga-DOTA-Tyr3-octreotide PET in neuroendocrine tumors: comparison with somatostatin receptor scintigraphy and CT. J Nucl Med. 2007;48(4):508–18.
66. Buchmann I, Henze M, Engelbrecht S, Eisenhut M, Runz A, Schäfer M, et al. Comparison of 68 Ga-DOTATOC PET and 111 in-DTPAOC (Octreoscan) SPECT in patients with neuroendocrine tumours. Eur J Nucl Med Mol Imaging. 2007;34(10):1617–26.
67. Krausz Y, Freedman N, Rubinstein R, Lavie E, Orevi M, Tshori S, et al. 68 Ga-DOTA-NOC PET/CT imaging of neuroendocrine tumors: comparison with 111 in-DTPA-Octreotide (OctreoScan®). Mol Imaging Biol. 2011;13(3):583–93.
68. Wang X, Zielinski MC, Misawa R, Wen P, Wang T-Y, Wang C-Z, et al. Quantitative analysis of pancreatic polypeptide cell distribution in the human pancreas. PLoS One. 2013;8(1):e55501.
69. Adams S, Baum R, Rink T, Schumm-Dräger P-M, Usadel K-H, Hör G. Limited value of fluorine-18 fluorodeoxyglucose positron emission tomography for the imaging of neuroendocrine tumours. Eur J Nucl Med. 1998;25(1):79–83.
70. Binderup T, Knigge U, Loft A, Federspiel B, Kjaer A. 18F-fluorodeoxyglucose positron emission tomography predicts survival of patients with neuroendocrine tumors. Clin Cancer Res. 2010;16(3):978–85.

71. Jager PL, Chirakal R, Marriott CJ, Brouwers AH, Koopmans KP, Gulenchyn KY. 6-L-18F-fluorodihydroxyphenylalanine PET in neuroendocrine tumors: basic aspects and emerging clinical applications. J Nucl Med. 2008;49(4):573–86.
72. Orlefors H, Sundin A, Garske U, Juhlin C, Oberg K, Skogseid B, et al. Whole-body 11C-5-hydroxytryptophan positron emission tomography as a universal imaging technique for neuroendocrine tumors: comparison with somatostatin receptor scintigraphy and computed tomography. J Clin Endocrinol Metabol. 2005;90(6):3392–400.

Pathology of Neuroendocrine Neoplasms in the Digestive System

Zhaohai Yang

Introduction

The digestive system is the largest diffuse neuroendocrine system, where the neuroendocrine and exocrine cells have shared origin, topographical distribution, and functional interplay. Neuroendocrine neoplasms (NENs) can arise from various organs such as the esophagus, stomach, small intestine, colon, rectum, appendix, and pancreas. Some of them are functional as defined by associated clinically evident hormonal syndromes due to inappropriate secretion of excess hormonal peptides, while others are nonfunctional. NENs of the digestive system show common morphological features; however, the behavior of the tumors can be unpredictable. Now there is a uniform classification and grading scheme that separates NENs into two major types: well-differentiated neuroendocrine tumor (WDNET) and poorly differentiated neuroendocrine carcinoma (PDNEC). The former often grows slowly, and the patients can live for many years even after liver metastasis, while the latter has a much precipitous clinical course and worse outcome. NENs of certain organs also display some unique clinico-pathological features, which will be covered in this chapter as well.

Neuroendocrine Cells

Neuroendocrine cells are present in almost every organ in the digestive system. In the luminal gastrointestinal (GI) tract, those cells are often dispersed in the epithelial layer. Although the percentage of the neuroendocrine cells is small (1% or less

Z. Yang (✉)

Department of Pathology and Laboratory Medicine, University of Pennsylvania Perelman School of Medicine, Hospital the University of Pennsylvania, Philadelphia, PA, USA
e-mail: Zhaohai.yang@pennmedicine.upenn.edu

© Springer Nature Switzerland AG 2021
J. M. Cloyd, T. M. Pawlik (eds.), *Neuroendocrine Tumors*,
https://doi.org/10.1007/978-3-030-62241-1_3

of total epithelial cells), due to its large volume, the digestive system constitutes the largest diffuse neuroendocrine system [1].

There are multiple types of neuroendocrine cells even in the same GI organ. Those cells are intimately associated with the exocrine epithelial cells, and both are derived from pluripotent stem cells of the endoderm. Different types of neuroendocrine cells often contain different neurosecretory granules with various peptides. The topographical distribution between the neuroendocrine and exocrine cells and the delicate balance among different neuroendocrine cells allow tight regulation of secretory, kinetic, and proliferative functions at both the local and systemic levels [1]. At least some of them also function as sensory or effector cells of the central nervous system and thus are part of the brain-gut axis.

At least five different types of neuroendocrine cells are identified in the gastric fundus/body and antrum, respectively. In the gastric fundus/body, the neuroendocrine cells are typically located at the periphery of deep oxyntic glands. The most prevalent type of cell is the enterochromaffin-like (ECL) cell that secretes histamine. However, in the antrum the neuroendocrine cells are mostly located in the neck region with gastrin-secreting G cells being the most abundant. Somatostatin-secreting D cells are present in both the body and antrum, which inhibit both ECL and G cells (Table 3.1) [1]. The neuroendocrine cells in the stomach play a central role in the negative feedback mechanism of gastric acid secretion: central nervous stimulus, food ingestion, and elevated pH in the antrum allow G cells to secrete gastrin, which directly stimulates parietal cells to secrete hydrochloric acid and also stimulates ECL cells to secrete histamine. Histamine in turn stimulates parietal cells to secrete hydrochloric acid as well. This process is inhibited by somatostatin secreted by D cells when the pH is lowered [2].

Table 3.1 Major types of neuroendocrine cells in the digestive system

Organ	Cells	Peptides
Stomach (fundus and body)	ECL cell	Histamine
	D cell	Somatostatin
Stomach (antrum)	G cell	Gastrin
	D cell	Somatostatin
Duodenum	G cell	Gastrin
	D cell	Somatostatin
	EC cell	Serotonin
Jejunum/ileum/colon	EC cell	Serotonin
	D cell	Somatostatin
Rectum	L cell	Glucagon-like peptide, pancreatic peptide/peptide YY
Pancreas	B/β cell	Insulin
	A/α cell	Glucagon
	D/δ cell	Somatostatin
	PP cell	Pancreatic polypeptide

ECL enterochromaffin-like, *EC* enterochromaffin, *PP* pancreatic polypeptide

There are at least 15 different types of neuroendocrine cells in the intestine, and many of them are scattered in the basolateral crypts, with basally located fine secretory granules facing the stroma and capillary, consistent with their endocrine/paracrine function [1, 3]. G cells are concentrated in the duodenum, L cells are more abundant in the distal colon/rectum, while serotonin-secreting EC (enterochromaffin) cells and D cells are present throughout the entire intestine (Table 3.1).

In the pancreas, the neuroendocrine cells form distinct clusters with delicate capillary network (islets of Langerhans), which are surrounded by the exocrine pancreas (acini). The cells are relatively uniform, with round or ovoid nuclei and salt-and-pepper chromatin [1]. Insulin-secreting B or β cells are most abundant (~70%) and distributed throughout the entire islet, glucagon-secreting A or α cells (~10%) are predominantly at the periphery of the islet, and D or δ cells are few in number (~5%) and scattered in the islet (Fig. 3.1). Pancreatic

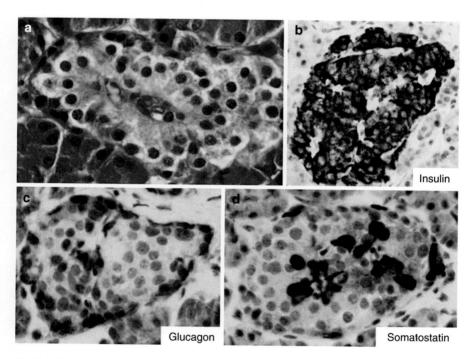

Fig. 3.1 Pancreatic islets of Langerhans. **a**, the islet of Langerhans consists of a tightnest of uniform neuroendocrine cells with rich capillary. It is surrounded by exocrine acini. **b**, immunohistochemistry for insulin shows that the majority of neuroendocrine cells are B/β cells diffusely distributed in the islet. **c**, immunohistochemistry for glucagon shows that a smaller number of cells are A/α cells which are mostly located at the periphery of the islet. **d**, immunohistochemistry for somatostatin shows few D/δ cells scattered in the islet

polypeptide-secreting PP cells account for the remaining 15% of pancreatic neuro-endocrine cells (Table 3.1) [4, 5].

Common Features and Markers of Neuroendocrine Tumors

The neuroendocrine tumors (NETs) in the digestive system are thought to arise from neuroendocrine cells. They share some common features. The tumor typically has an organoid pattern, forming ribbons, trabeculae, acini, glands, or solid nests, with rich vasculature. The cells are similar to their normal counterpart, relatively uniform in size and shape, with moderate clear, eosinophilic or amphophilic cyto-plasm, sometimes with visible secretory granules. The nuclei are round or ovoid, with salt-and-pepper chromatin (Fig. 3.2) [6]. The behavior of the tumor can be unpredictable and appears unrelated to the morphology; however, most tumors (WDNETs; see below) grow slowly and present with protracted clinical course.

A pathologic diagnosis of NET generally requires the demonstration of epithelial origin (based on morphology and sometimes coupled with expression of

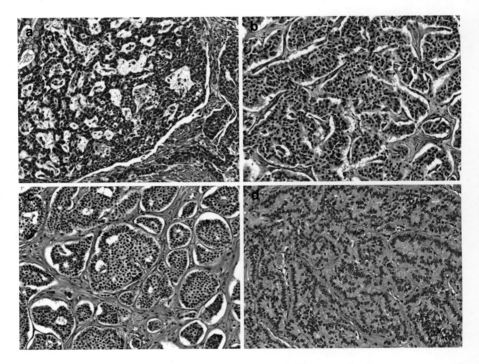

Fig. 3.2 Representative morphologic patterns of luminal GI neuroendocrine tumors. **a**, type I ECL cell NET of the stomach, with anastomosing cords and trabeculae. **b**, functional gastrin-producing NET (gastrinoma) of the duodenum, with gyriform or irregular trabecular patterns. **c**, EC cell NET of the small intestine (the prototype midgut carcinoid), with regular solid nest or cribriform growth. Note the peripheral palisading and delicate fibrous stroma between the tumor nests. **d**, L cell NET of the rectum, with uniform tumor cells and thin delicate trabecular growth

cytokeratin) and confirmation of neuroendocrine differentiation. The general neuro-endocrine markers include chromogranin A, synaptophysin, protein gene product 9.5 (PGP 9.5), CD56 (neural cell adhesion molecule, NCAM), and neuron-specific enolase (NSE). Chromogranin A and synaptophysin are considered the most

Table 3.2 Common neuroendocrine markers

Marker	Chromogranin A [9, 10]	Synaptophysin [11, 12]	CD56 (NCAM) [8]	INSM1 [14, 15]
Protein	Granin family of acidic secretory proteins	Synaptic vesicle glycoprotein	Glycoprotein of Ig superfamily	Zinc-finger transcription factor
Location	Secretory vesicles of neurons and endocrine cells	Secretory vesicle membrane	Surface of neurons, glia, and skeletal muscle	Nuclear
Function	Induces and promotes the generation of secretory granules	Regulates endocytosis, ensures vesicle availability during and after sustained neuronal activity	Cell-cell adhesion, neurite outgrowth, synaptic plasticity, and learning and memory	Controls expression of neuroendocrine phenotype
Staining	Granular cytoplasmic	Cytoplasmic	Membranous	Nuclear
Sensitivity/ specificity in GI NETs [16]	88%/87%	99%/86%	93%/86%	83%/96%
Expression in other tumors	Desmoplastic small round cell tumor, middle ear adenoma, parathyroid cyst, pituitary adenoma; fetal-type tumors	Adrenocortical adenoma and carcinoma, fetal-type lung adenocarcinoma, desmoplastic small round cell tumor, glomus tumor, myxoid chondrosarcoma	Various myeloid and lymphoid neoplasms, alveolar rhabdomyosarcoma, meningiomas, intrahepatic cholangiocarcinoma, solid pseudopapillary neoplasm	Extraskeletal myxoid chondrosarcoma, etc.
Comment	More positive in the upper GI and pancreas, less so in the rectum and ovary (chromogranin B typically positive). Also useful as a serum marker			

NCAM neural cell adhesion molecule, *INSM1* insulinoma-associated protein 1, *Ig* immunoglobulin specific neuroendocrine markers, while CD56 is less useful in the digestive organs (Table 3.2) [1, 7, 8]. Chromogranin A belongs to the granin family of acidic neuro-endocrine secretory proteins and is expressed in the secretory vesicles of neurons and neuroendocrine cells [9, 10]. Synaptophysin is a transmembrane synaptic vesicle glycoprotein [11, 12]. Chromogranin A is slightly more specific than synaptophysin, while the latter appears more widely expressed especially in the lower GI tract where chromogranin B is predominantly expressed (Table 3.2). In addition, chromogranin A is also a valuable serum marker whose serum level correlates with tumor burden [13].

More recently, a new neuroendocrine marker, insulinoma-associated protein 1 (INSM1), has gained recognition. INSM1 is a zinc-finger transcription factor predominantly expressed in the nucleus of developing neuroendocrine tissues and nervous system and involved in early embryonic neurogenesis [14, 15]. INSM1 is slightly less sensitive but more specific than chromogranin A and synaptophysin for NETs of the digestive system (Table 3.2) [16]. It was also reported to be a sensitive and specific marker for small cell carcinoma of the lung, where its expression may be associated with a worse prognosis [17].

Somatostatin receptors (SSTRs) are a family of five transmembrane G protein-coupled receptors that mediate inhibitory effects in mammals. SSTR2 is widely distributed in human tissues [18] and thus not useful as a specific neuroendocrine marker. SSTR2 expression can be detected by immunohistochemical staining, octreotide scan, or (68)Ga-DOTA-NOC PET/CT scan. Immunohistochemical expression of SSTR2A in NETs was associated with clinical efficacy to somatostatin analogs [19] and also correlated with (68)Ga-DOTA-NOC PET/CT scans [20]. However, octreotide and PET/CT scans often provide additional imaging and staging information and thus unlikely to be replaced by in vitro SSTR2A staining, except under special situation such as during COVID-19 pandemic when in-person clinical encounter is discouraged or when the cost of the scan is too prohibitive.

Terminology, Classification, and Grading of Neuroendocrine Neoplasms

The old term "carcinoid" (carcinoma-like) was proposed in 1907 due to the perception of it being a benign tumor [21], and this term is still in use for luminal GI tract in some literatures today. For pancreatic tumor it was previously called islet cell tumor. Now it is well recognized that all neuroendocrine tumors have malignant potential, and a more generic term, "neuroendocrine tumor," which was initially proposed by Capella in 1995 [7], has been endorsed by the World Health Organization (WHO) since 2010 [22].

Earlier classifications of NETs were based on embryonic origin and/or morphologic patterns (Fig. 3.2) [23, 24]. With the exception of midgut NET which often demonstrates characteristic solid or cribriform tumor nests with peripheral palisading set in delicate fibrous stroma, those criteria are difficult to apply to NETs at other sites and have no prognostic value, and thus have lost favor. The modern classification started from 1995, when Capella et al. incorporated prognostic factors such as tumor size, angioinvasion, and functional status in their proposal [7]. Over the years, multiple parameters have been reported to show prognostic significance, including tumor size, depth of invasion, lymphovascular invasion, functional status, proliferation rate, necrosis, local invasion, and metastasis, some of which were included in the WHO classifications of GI and pancreatic tumor in 2000 and 2004, respectively [25, 26].

To provide a simplified and uniform approach for the grading (the degree of inherent tumor aggressiveness) of all NENs in the digestive system and also separate from the newly proposed staging criteria (the extent of tumor involvement), the European Neuroendocrine Tumour Society (ENETS) chose to use proliferation rate alone, as assessed by mitotic count and/or Ki-67 labeling index, to stratify NENs into three progressive grades [27, 28]. The WHO adopted this classification in 2010, with minor modifications: low grade (Grade 1, G1) and intermediate grade (Grade 2, G2) tumors were considered well-differentiated NETs, while high grade (Grade 3, G3) was termed poorly differentiated neuroendocrine carcinoma (PDNEC), conceptually similar to small cell carcinoma or large cell neuroendocrine carcinoma (LCNEC) of the lung (Table 3.3) [22]. The WHO recommends to use the mitotically active area (hot spot) for grading purpose. When there is discrepancy between mitotic grade and Ki-67 grade, the higher grade (typically the Ki-67 grade) dictates the final grade. The prognostic significance of this grading scheme was validated in multiple studies, in both pancreatic NENs [29] and metastatic NENs of various GI origins [30].

The high-grade PDNEC in the 2010 WHO classification had been the subject of debate, and accumulative evidence suggested that it was a heterogeneous group. In the NORDIC NEC study which included 305 patients with WHO G3/NEC (primary sites: pancreas 23%, colon 20%, unknown 32%), patients whose tumor had a Ki-67 index of <55% were less responsive to platinum-based chemotherapy but showed longer survival, compared to patients with Ki-67 index of >55% [31]. A multicenter European study of 204 patients with gastroenteropancreatic (GEP) G3 tumors (37 NET and 167 NEC) showed that the average Ki-67 index in NEC was much higher than that of NET (80% vs 30%) and platinum-based chemotherapy was effective in NEC but not in NET, supporting the separation of NET from NEC in the WHO G3

Table 3.3 WHO classification of neuroendocrine neoplasms in the digestive system

Terminology	Mitotic rate	Ki-67 index	WHO 2010 grade [22]	WHO 2019 grade [35]
WDNET	< 2/2 mm^2	< 3%	G1/low	G1/low
	2–20/2 mm^2	3–20%	G2/intermediate	G2/intermediate
	> 20/2 mm^2	> 20%		G3/high
PDNEC	> 20/2 mm^2	> 20%	G3/high	High
Mixed			Poorly differentiated	Well or poorly differentiated

WDNET well-differentiated neuroendocrine tumor, *PDNEC* poorly differentiated neuroendocrine carcinoma category [32]. In a study conducted at Memorial Sloan-Kettering Cancer Center (MSKCC), three groups of pancreatic NENs were included: grade-concordant (WHO G2 by both mitotic rate and Ki-67 index), grade-discordant (WHO G2 by mitotic rate and G3 by Ki-67 index), and PDNEC (WHO G3 by both mitotic rate and Ki-67 index). The average mitotic rates (per 2 mm^2)/Ki-67 indices were 3.5/8.1%, 7.6/40%, and 42/69% for the three groups, respectively. The disease-specific survival in the grade-discordant group was slightly worse than that of the grade-concordant group, but without statistical significance. However, the PDNEC group showed significantly worse survival than the grade-discordant group ($p < 0.002$) [33].

All above studies supported the notion that the 2010 WHO G3 NEC group consisted of two different categories: one with lower mitotic rate and Ki-67 index (typically 20–55%) which is less responsive to platinum-based chemotherapy but survives longer, and another with higher mitotic rate and Ki-67 index (typically >55%) which is more responsive to platinum-based chemotherapy but with shorter survival. This led to the revised WHO classification of pancreatic NENs in 2017, in which a G3 NET category was introduced and separated from bona fide PDNEC (Fig. 3.3c), though the proliferation rate criterion was the same for both categories [34]. This modified classification was subsequently expanded to all NENs in the entire digestive system and reflected in the most recent 2019 WHO classification of

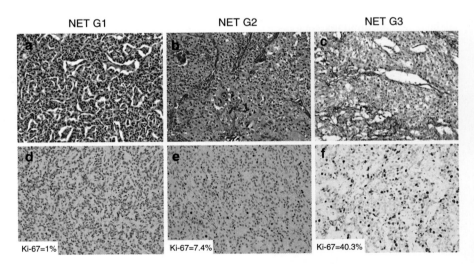

Fig. 3.3 Representative pancreatic neuroendocrine tumors of different grades. **a** and **d**, Grade 1 nonfunctional NET of the pancreas with anastomosing trabecular growth, in a patient with multiple endocrine neoplasia type 1. **b** and **e**, Grade 2 nonfunctional NET of the pancreas with solid nest/broad trabeculae, in a patient with von Hippel-Lindau syndrome. Note the atypical nuclei and abundant eosinophilic cytoplasm. **c** and **f**, Grade 3 NET of the pancreas with solid nest/broad trabeculae. Note the evident mitosis and high Ki-67 index. All examples show organoid growth pattern and rich vasculature

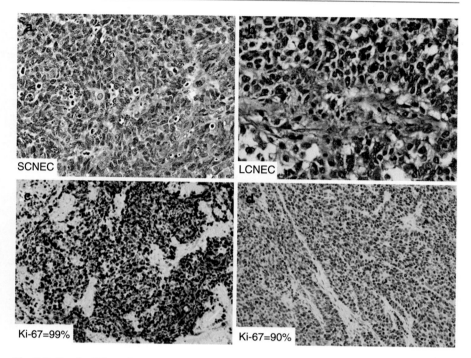

Fig. 3.4 Poorly differentiated neuroendocrine carcinoma. **a** and **c**, small cell neuroendocrine carcinoma of the ampulla. Note the compact growth with nuclear molding, minimal cytoplasm, delicate fine chromatin, and prominent mitotic and apoptotic activities. **b** and **d**, large cell neuroendocrine carcinoma of the gallbladder. Note the solid growth more abundant cytoplasm, and large nuclei with vesicular chromatin and some prominent nucleoli. There is extensive tumor necrosis elsewhere in this tumor. The Ki-67 index in both tumors is well above 55%

digestive system tumors, where PDNEC was no longer graded but considered high grade by definition (Table 3.3) [35].

As mentioned earlier, conceptually PDNEC consists of small cell carcinoma and LCNEC, similar to its counterparts in the lung. Small cell carcinoma typically shows small- to medium-sized nuclei with scant cytoplasm, high nuclear/cytoplasmic ratio, and finely dispersed chromatin with indiscernible nucleoli. Nuclear molding is frequent. LCNEC often consists of medium-sized to large tumor cells with moderate to abundant cytoplasm and large nuclei with vesicular chromatin and prominent nucleoli. Both small cell carcinoma and LCNEC often grow in solid nests or sheets, and necrosis is common (Fig. 3.4). Admittedly the distinction between the two subcategories can be difficult at times, and combined small cell carcinoma and LCNEC is also recognized at least in the lung [36]. These tumors often present at advanced stage with dismal survival.

In the 2010 WHO classification, mixed adenoneuroendocrine carcinoma was a high-grade carcinoma with both adenocarcinoma and PDNEC component, each accounting for at least 30% of the tumor [22]. Occasionally PDNEC can be associated with a precursor glandular component such as tubulovillous adenoma; however, this is not considered mixed adenoneuroendocrine carcinoma. To accommodate rare examples of mixed NET and adenocarcinoma, the mixed category was further expanded and renamed mixed neuroendocrine-non-neuroendocrine neoplasm in the 2019 WHO classification, which can be either well-differentiated or poorly differentiated (Table 3.3). Mixed squamous cell carcinoma-neuroendocrine carcinoma, typically occurring in the esophagus or anus, was also included in this category [35]. Of note, goblet cell carcinoid of the appendix has been renamed goblet cell adenocarcinoma in the new WHO classification and no longer considered a neuroendocrine neoplasm [37].

Issues and Approaches in Histologic Grading of Neuroendocrine Neoplasms

As alluded earlier, intratumoral heterogeneity, manifested as different tumor grade in different areas of the same tumor, is common in NETs. Couvelard et al. studied 29 metastatic pancreatic NETs and found that 12 of them (41%) showed both G1 and G2 areas and 4 (14%) had areas spanning from G1 to G3 [38]. Yang et al. studied 45 metastatic NETs to the liver and showed that 21 (47%) tumors had both G1 and G2 areas when graded by Ki-67 index and most homogeneous cases were G1. In addition, when the final grade was defined by the highest rather than mean Ki-67 index, there was a better separation between G1 and G2 tumors in terms of patient survival, supporting the WHO recommendation that the final grade should be determined by the hot spot [39].

The cutoff of mitotic rate between NET G1 and G2 is set at only 2 mitoses/2 mm^2; thus, accurate count of mitotic rate is critical for accurate grading of NETs. Both the WHO and College of American Pathologists (CAP) recommend to count 40–50 high power fields (40x objective) and average to 2 mm^2 [22, 40]. Although for the old microscopes, 2 mm^2 is generally equivalent to 10 high power fields (HPFs), modern microscopes may have different field diameters; thus, the required numbers of HPFs to achieve 2 mm^2 are different. The CAP cancer protocol includes a detailed table listing the field diameter, area, and number of HPFs equivalent to 2 mm^2 for most microscopes. For example, for an eyepiece with a field diameter of 0.55 mm, the area is 0.238 mm^2, and 8 HPFs are equivalent to 2 mm^2 [40].

The mitotic rate can vary from one area to another in the same tumor, and finding the hot spot based on routine H&E staining is difficult, if not impossible [1, 6]. In addition, differentiating a true mitotic figure from karyorrhexis, apoptosis, darkly stained nuclei, or nuclei with irregular nuclear membrane is also challenging. Phosphohistone H3 (PHH3), which accumulates during M phase of cell cycle, is a sensitive and specific marker for mitosis. Using immunostaining for PHH3, more mitotic figures were identified in pancreatic NETs, and with a modified cutoff of 4 mitoses/2 mm^2, the histologic grade determined by PHH3 was significantly associated with patient survival. PHH3 immunostaining makes it much easier to find the mitotic hot spot; the tumor grade can thus be determined by counting just one low or intermediate power hot spot field rather than 40–50 HPFs. PHH3 also improved interobserver agreement and reduced the time spent on counting mitosis to about 1 min [41].

Ki-67 is a DNA-binding protein that is expressed in G, S, and M phases of cell cycle and thus is widely used as a proliferation marker in various tumor types [42]. Multiple studies have confirmed its prognostic significance in NETs, using various cutoffs anywhere between 2% and 5% [1, 6]. The ENETS and WHO chose to use 2% (3% when using decimal) as the cutoff between G1 and G2 NETs. In 2017 WHO acknowledged that there were different opinions about the optimal cutoff and it was possible that 5% may be better, but decided to keep 3% for consistency [34]. The fundamental issue is that Ki-67 is a continuous variable, and using any number between 2% and 8% as the cutoff will likely achieve statistically significant difference between G1 and G2 tumors; thus, the optimal cutoff point may be influenced by the patient cohort, methods of assessment, and outcome measurement, and the same cutoff may not apply to every situation [41].

The Ki-67 index is expressed as a percentage of positively stained nuclei over total tumor nuclei. The WHO recommends to count at least 500–2000 cells in the hot spot, which can be laborious. Various methods have been used to assess Ki-67 labeling index [43]. The WHO further recommends to photograph the hot spot and manually count on printed color copy [34]. With improvement and wide availability of imaging software in the era of digital pathology [43], counting Ki-67 may become an easy task with just a few clicks or completely undertaken by artificial intelligence.

Mitotic rate and Ki-67 index generally correlate with each other; however, since mitosis only occurs in M phase while Ki-67 is expressed in G, S, and M phases of cell cycle, discrepancy does occur. When there is discordance between tumor grades determined by mitotic rate and Ki-67 index, it is recommended that the higher grade define the final grade. McCall et al. studied 297 pancreatic NETs, and 36% showed discordant grades with the majority being G2 by Ki-67 index and G1 by mitotic rate. Those tumors were similar to G2 tumors by mitotic rate while different from concordant G1 tumors, in terms of frequencies of lymphovascular and perineural invasion, infiltrative growth, lymph node and distant metastasis, and prognosis [44]. Nowadays it is generally expected that both mitotic rate and Ki-67 index be included in the pathology report and the final grade be determined by the higher grade [40]. In small liver biopsies where there are often less than 40 HPFs, Ki-67 is especially important and may be the only means to grade the tumor. Some authorities advocate the sole use of Ki-67 index, since in most cases the grade determined by Ki-67 index is either equivalent to or higher than the grade by mitotic rate and thus would define the final grade. Nevertheless, mitotic rate determined on routine H&E staining obviates any delay due to performance of immunohistochemistry and may add additional value in certain cases such as differentiation between NET G3 and NEC (see below).

Pathologic Staging of NENs

The American Joint Commission on Cancer (AJCC)/Union for International Cancer Control (UICC) cancer staging is based on tumor, node, and metastasis (TNM). TNM staging systems for GI NETs were first proposed by ENETS in 2006 and 2007 at the same time when the aforementioned uniform histologic grading was introduced, which included separate schemes for stomach, foregut small bowel, midgut small bowel, colon/rectum, appendix, and pancreas. The T group was based on tumor size and depth of invasion for luminal GI NETs and size for pancreatic NETs, respectively, and the same scheme applied to all three grades of tumors including what is now considered PDNEC [27, 28]. The 2010 AJCC seventh edition adopted the ENETS schemes with the following modifications: (1) the new NET staging only applied to WDNETs (G1 and G2), while adenocarcinoma staging schemes were used for PDNEC; (2) the same staging scheme applied to the foregut and midgut small bowel; and (3) in the pancreas, the adenocarcinoma staging scheme applied to all pancreatic NENs including WDNETs and PDNECs [45]. This modification was also endorsed by WHO in 2010 [22]. Multiple studies confirmed the prognostic value of the new staging system [46, 47].

In light of the differences between ENETS and AJCC staging schemes, an international study conducted on 1072 pancreatic NENs showed that the ENETS TNM staging system allocated patients into 4 statistically significantly different and equally populated risk groups better than the UICC/AJCC/WHO 2010 TNM staging system, with tighter 95% confidence intervals for each stage, suggesting that the ENETS TNM staging system was superior to the UICC/AJCC/WHO 2010 TNM staging system [48]. In the most recent UICC/AJCC 2017 eighth edition staging system, a separate pancreatic NET staging scheme was adopted, much similar to the ENETS system. Recognizing the unique features of duodenal NETs, a separate staging for duodenal NETs was also introduced by AJCC [49]. The new AJCC jejunal/ileal NET staging system included an N2 category, when there are either more than 12 positive lymph nodes or large mesenteric tumor deposit of more than 2 cm (presumably matted lymph nodes) [49]. However, the prognostic significance of a large mesenteric tumor deposit has been questioned [50].

NENs of Major Digestive Organs

The incidence of NETs has been steadily increasing since 1985, partially due to increased awareness and improved detection. In 2007, the incidence of GEP NET reached 3.65 per 100,000 populations, with a mean age of 63 at diagnosis [51]. Despite the common features as described previously, NETs from different GI organs show differences in incidence, aggressiveness, morphological features, and molecular changes. In terms of overall incidence, the most common site is the small intestine, followed by the rectum. For localized disease, rectum NET is most common, followed by small intestine and stomach; for regional disease, small intestinal NET stands out, followed by colon at a distance; and for metastatic disease, the three most common primary sites are the small intestine, pancreas, and colon. The overall 5-year survival was 68.1%, with the best survival seen in rectal NETs, followed by appendix, small intestine, stomach, colon, and pancreatic NET being the worst [51].

Esophagus

NENs in the esophagus are exceedingly rare, with more than 90% being PDNEC, some of which are associated with squamous cell carcinoma or Barrett dysplasia/adenocarcinoma. Small cell carcinoma may show similar morphology to basaloid squamous cell carcinoma, and immunohistochemistry is often needed to confirm the diagnosis [52]. Pure PDNEC showed slightly worse prognosis than mixed PDNEC; however, when stratified by stage, the survival difference appeared not statistically significant [53].

Stomach

Most gastric NETs arise from ECL cells in the oxyntic mucosa, in which well-characterized precursor lesions with a hyperplasia-dysplasia-neoplasia sequence have been described [54]. Two common predisposing conditions are autoimmune atrophic gastritis (AAG) and Zollinger-Ellison syndrome (ZES). The former is caused by autoimmune destruction of oxyntic glands in the gastric fundus and body, which through the previously described feedback mechanism results in hypergastrinemia [55]. The latter is caused by a gastrinoma (see below), mostly in the duodenum, which constitutively produces gastrin [56]. In addition to stimulating ECL cells to secrete histamine with resultant stimulation of acid secretion by parietal cells, gastrin also stimulates ECL cells to proliferate, which morphologically manifests as simple hyperplasia, linear hyperplasia, and/or micronodular hyperplasia. Some of them go on to develop neuroendocrine dysplasia. Neoplasia (NET) is diagnosed when the cells show infiltrative growth, or solid growth of over 0.5 mm [54].

Accordingly, three types of gastric ECL cell NETs have been described: the most common type is type I NET which arises from AAG and accounts for 80–90% of the cases (Fig. 3.2a). Type II NET arises from ZES and accounts for 5–7%. Both types I and II are associated with hypergastrinemia and can be multiple, and most are Grade 1 tumors. Type III NET accounts for 10–15% and arises from normal gastric mucosa without hypergastrinemia or abnormal acid secretion. Most type III NETs are Grade 2. The prognosis and survival are also different, with type I showing the lowest stage and best prognosis, type II with varied stages and intermediate prognosis, and type III more frequently presenting at higher stage (including stage IV) and worse prognosis, which is usually managed with surgical resection [57]. With the wide use of proton pump inhibitors (PPI), ECL cell NET can rarely develop in those patients, and the pathogenesis and clinical features appear similar to type I NET [58].

Gastric PDNEC is rare, and most are LCNECs. The clinical presentation is often nonspecific, with systemic and/or local symptoms related to tumor growth and metastasis. The tumor typically shows solid, tubular, or scirrhous patterns. The prognosis is much worse than adenocarcinoma, with a median survival of about 20 months and 5-year survival of less than 30%. The survival of mixed adenoneuroendocrine carcinoma appears to be in between [59].

Duodenum (Including Ampulla of Vater)

Despite its short length, duodenum is the common site for some interesting NENs. Most tumors occur in the first or second portion of the duodenum, in particular the ampulla. In fact, PDNEC of the small intestine almost exclusively occurs in the ampullary region (Fig. 3.4a). Most duodenal NETs are small (< 2 cm) polypoid lesions. The patient is often asymptomatic with incidental finding of NET at endoscopy. When symptomatic, nonfunctional NETs often present with mass effect which when involving the ampulla can cause obstructive jaundice. Functional NETs, by definition, present with systemic symptom due to abnormal hormonal secretion [60].

The most common functional duodenal NET is gastrinoma which causes ZES with intractable peptic ulcer disease, as mentioned earlier. Duodenal gastrin-producing NET accounts for 60–75% of sporadic and all multiple endocrine neoplasia type 1 (MEN1)-associated duodenal NETs, and about 50% of sporadic tumors are functional. The average size of sporadic tumor is about 0.8 cm, while those associated with MEN1 can be multiple and tiny (may <1 mm). Despite the small size, it can metastasize to the lymph node, and when the primary tumor is difficult to find, it may be mistaken as pancreatic or primary lymph node NET. Morphologically duodenal gastrinoma shows broad gyriform or trabeculae and is often Grade 2 (Fig. 3.2b). Functional tumor has a worse prognosis, likely due to associated ZES [22].

Duodenal somatostatin-producing NET is typically located in the peri-ampullary region and presents during the fourth to fifth decades of life. It is often nonfunctional, with an average size of 1.8 cm. Microscopically the tumors frequently show tubuloglandular growth, some of them also have psammomatous calcifications. About two thirds of the tumors are Grade 2. This tumor may be associated with MEN1 or neurofibromatosis type 1 (NF1). There is significant risk of lymph node metastasis especially when the tumor involves muscularis propria, larger than 2 cm, or Grade 2 [22].

Gangliocytic paraganglioma is a peculiar tumor which almost exclusively occurs in the peri-ampullary region. It is often polypoid, with a mean size of 1.7 cm. This tumor shows triphasic growth containing neuroendocrine cells, ganglion cells, and spindly Schwannian cells, though the proportion of each component varies depending on the individual tumor. Gangliocytic paraganglioma may be associated with NF1. It is usually benign, though larger tumor (> 2 cm) may have lymph node metastasis from the epithelial component [22].

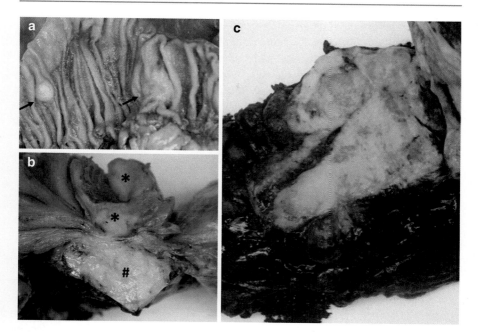

Fig. 3.5 Gross images of neuroendocrine tumors. **a** & **b**, small intestinal NET. Two yellow tumor nodules are noted from the mucosal side (arrow). The cross section shows deep invasion through the full thickness of intestinal wall (*), forming a large mesenteric mass (#). **c**, a large pancreatic NET, which is well-circumscribed with multinodular growth and red-white-yellow cut surface

Jejunum and Ileum

Jejunoileal NET predominantly occurs in the distal ileum, with rare cases involving the Meckel diverticulum. Smaller lesions often present as golden yellow mucosal nodules, and about a third of the cases show multiple nodules (Fig. 3.5a). Deep infiltration into the muscle and serosa is common, which can cause stricture, serosal adhesion, and small bowel obstruction. Metastasis to the mesenteric lymph nodes can cause desmoplastic reaction and mesenteric retraction. Some tumors form a large mesenteric mass, which presumably represents matted lymph nodes (Fig. 3.5b). When the fibrosis encases the mesenteric artery, ischemia ensues. Most jejunoileal NETs are serotonin-producing EC cell NETs and show the prototypic morphology of classic midgut carcinoid (Fig. 3.2c); most are Grade 1, though both G2 and G3 tumors do occur. About 10% of patients show carcinoid syndrome, which occurs only after liver metastasis. The overall 5-year survival is about 60.5% [22, 60].

Appendix

Appendiceal NET accounts for 50–77% of appendiceal tumors, most are incidental findings observed in 0.3–0.9% of appendectomy specimens The patient is typically young to middle aged, though children are not uncommon. Grossly the tumor often shows a well-circumscribed lesion in the distal tip of the appendix, with a firm, gray-white or yellow cut surface. Most appendiceal NETs are EC cell tumor morphologically similar to the ileal NET. A rare variant shows tubular morphology which should not be mistaken as adenocarcinoma. Deep invasion is common in appendiceal NET, but metastasis is rare. The size of the tumor is the most important indicator of metastatic potential. Most patients have a tumor of less than 2 cm, with excellent prognosis [22, 61].

Colon and Rectum

Most colonic NETs are serotonin-producing EC cell NETs. They are typically larger with an average size of 4.9 cm and otherwise similar to their counterpart in the small intestine. Rectal NET is much more common. It is readily detectable as a solitary submucosal polypoid rectal nodule, generally <2 cm. About half of the patients are asymptomatic, and the other half show local symptoms. Most tumors are Grade 1 L cell NET, with uniform tumor cells forming delicate trabeculae (Fig. 3.2d). They typically express synaptophysin, chromogranin B, and peptide YY. The prognosis is favorable, with a 5-year survival of 88.3%. High-risk factors include larger size (> 2 cm), deeper invasion into muscularis propria, lymphovascular invasion, atypical morphology, and higher grade (G2 or G3) [22, 62].

Pancreas

Pancreatic NET is relatively uncommon, which accounts for less than 5% of pancreatic tumors. Unlike the stomach, no confirmed precursor lesion is identified in the pancreas except for tumors associated with a familial syndrome. Pancreatic NET is typically solitary and well-circumscribed, with tan red to yellow cut surface (Fig. 3.5c). The microscopic growth patterns are variable, including trabecular, acinar, glandular, and solid (Fig. 3.3). Rare variants with oncocytic, pleomorphic, or clear cell morphology have been described. Most pancreatic NETs can be readily diagnosed on cytology specimen obtained by fine needle aspiration (FNA), obviating more invasive procedures such as standard core needle biopsy or surgical biopsy. Differentiation between WDNET from PDNEC is generally achievable on cytology specimen; however, grading of WDNET based on Ki-67 index is unreliable due to the scant and disrupted nature of cytology specimen [63].

Over half of the pancreatic NETs are nonfunctional; those tumors may secrete one or more peptides but do not produce clinically evident hormonal syndrome. The TNM stage is mostly based on the size of the tumor: tumors smaller than 2 cm are often indolent, while tumors larger than 3 cm tend to have a higher risk of metastasis. When the tumor is small (< 5 mm), it is considered neuroendocrine microadenoma which is often nonfunctional and clinically benign [63]. Serotonin-producing pancreatic NET may abut the main duct and show prominent stromal fibrosis,

Table 3.4 Pathologic features of nonfunctional and common functional NETs in the pancreas [63]

	Clinical features	Frequency	Location	Size	Growth pattern	Grade	Metastasis rate	Five-year survival
Nonfunctional	Symptoms due to tumor growth or metastasis	> 60%	Head>tail	2–5 cm	Variable	G1, G2, G3	55–75%	65–86%
Insulinoma	Hypoglycemia	4–20%	Head = tail	1–2 cm	Trabecular or solid, may have amyloid	G1, G2, G3	10%	96% (<2 cm); 75% (>2 cm) [97]
Glucagonoma	Necrolytic migratory erythema, diabetes, weight loss; may also have angular stomatitis, cheilitis, or atrophic glossitis	1–2%	Tail>head	3–7 cm	Trabecular	G1, G2, G3	49% [98]	70%
Gastrinoma	ZES, peptic ulcer disease	4–8%	Head = tail	3.8 cm	Trabecular or glandular	G1, G2, G3	40%	73% [65]
VIPoma	WDHA syndrome (watery diarrhea, hypokalemia, achlorhydria)	0.6–1.5%	Tail>head	4.5–5.3 cm	Variable	G1, G2	50–80%	68% [99]
Somatostatinoma	Diabetes, cholelithiasis, steatorrhea	<1%	Head>tail	5–6 cm	Trabecular, solid, or acinar, rarely psammomatous calcification	Mostly G2	19%	75% [66]

VIP vasoactive intestinal peptide, *ZES* Zollinger-Ellison syndrome causing pancreatic duct obstruction and dilatation and clinically mimicking intra-ductal papillary mucinous neoplasm [64].

Common functional pancreatic NETs include insulinoma, glucagonoma, VIPoma (vasoactive intestinal peptide), gastrinoma, and somatostatinoma [63], and their main pathologic features are listed in Table 3.4. Insulinoma is the most common functional pancreatic NET; it confers the best prognosis likely owing to its smaller size, and enucleation is often considered adequate treatment. Compared to their extrapancreatic counterparts (mostly in the duodenum), pancreatic gastrinoma and somatostatinoma tend to be larger, and metastatic pancreatic gastrinoma preferen-tially involves the liver rather than lymph node [65, 66].

PDNEC in the pancreas is very rare, accounting for <1% of pancreatic tumors. The tumor resembles the PDNEC in the lung, often forming solid nests and sheets with prominent tumor necrosis. Mitosis is frequent (typically >20/2 mm^2), and Ki-67 index tends to be well above 50%. A study of 44 cases of pancreatic PDNEC showed that 88% of tumors had lymph node or liver metastasis and 77% of patients died of disease. The median survival was 11 months, with a 2-year survival of 22.5% and 5-year survival of 16.1%. There was no significant survival difference between small cell carcinoma and LCNEC [67]. Common mixed neuroendocrine-non-neuroendocrine neoplasms in the pancreas include mixed ductal-neuroendocrine carcinoma and mixed acinar-neuroendocrine carcinoma; the former appears to behave slightly better than PDNEC, while the latter behaves similarly to acinar cell carcinoma [63].

Metastatic NENs

Up to 40% of NETs of the digestive system present with distant metastasis, mostly to the liver [68]. The most common primary sites of metastatic GI NET include the small intestine, pancreas, and colon [51], and the most common metastatic non-GI neuroendocrine tumor is lung carcinoid. In about 11% of metastatic NETs, no pri-mary site is identified despite extensive clinico-radiological workup, thus consid-ered tumor of unknown primary [69]. Those tumors pose special challenges to oncologists and surgeons, as knowledge of primary site is crucial for local therapy as well as optimal prognosis.

Multiple efforts have been devoted to characterize site-specific markers, mostly for the pancreas, midgut (small intestine and colon), and lung. Tissue-specific tran-scription factors, due to their nuclear expression, ease of interpretation, and high specificity, have been the favored markers in most studies. Thyroid transcription factor 1 (TTF1) is expressed in lung carcinoids with moderate sensitivity (35–95%) and high specificity, and caudal type homeobox 2 transcription factor (CDX2) is expressed in 52–100% midgut NET (mostly serotonin-producing EC cell NET) but much less in pancreas and almost nil in the lung, making them the preferred markers for lung and midgut NETs, respectively. Their value in differentiating between lung and midgut NETs has been validated in multiple studies [70–73]. Several markers have been reported for pancreatic NET, including PDX1 (pancreatic duodenal homeobox 1), ISL1 (insulin gene enhancer protein ISL1), PAX8, and NKX6-1. ISL1 appears to be the preferred marker, with a sensitivity of 88.9% for pancreatic NET and 100% for duodenal NET [74]. As such, multiple panels with either three or four markers have been proposed, mostly based on the expression profile in primary tumors. Yang et al. focused exclusively on metastatic NETs to the liver and demonstrated that a three-marker panel composed of TTF1, CDX2, and ISL1 showed an overall accuracy of 82% in predicting the site of origin, which reduced the percentage of NET of unknown primary from 12% to 5% [75]. It should be noted that TTF1 is also expressed in medullary thyroid carcinoma, which can be distinguished from lung carcinoid by relevant clinical history and inclusion of additional thyroid-specific markers such as PAX8 and calcitonin. Rectal NETs may show similar immunoprofile to pancreatic NETs, likely reflecting their similarities in hormonal profile [75, 76]. Since rectum is easily accessible by endoscopy, this generally does not cause any clinical confusion. More recently special AT-rich sequence binding protein-2 (SATB2) was shown to be a sensitive marker for lower GI tumors including rectal NET, which may aid in the differentiation from pancreatic NET [77].

The utility of CDX2, TTF1, and ISL1 was also studied in PDNEC. GI PDNECs appeared to preferentially express CDX2, while lung PDNECs showed higher expression of TTF1 and ISL1. Whether this finding reflects some degree of tissue specificity or merely the difference between LCNEC and small cell carcinoma (most GI PDNECs in the cohort were LCNEC) was unclear, and these three markers seemed to have little value in pinpointing to a specific primary site within the digestive system [78]. Nevertheless, bona fide metastatic PDNECs are generally treated with systemic chemotherapy, and for clinical management, the knowledge of the exact primary site is less important [79].

Familial Syndromes Associated with NENs of the Digestive System

About 10% of NETs in the digestive system are associated with a familial syndrome. The elucidation of their germline mutations provides the first insight into the molecular basis of NENs (Table 3.5) [80, 81].

Multiple endocrine neoplasia type 1 (MEN1) is an autosomal dominant syndrome characterized by germline *MEN1* mutation. The patients develop multiple endocrine tumors involving multiple organs such as the parathyroid, anterior pituitary, duodenum, and pancreas, etc. The frequency of pancreatic NET is 30–75%, including multiple neuroendocrine microadenomas, nonfunctional NETs (Fig. 3.3a), and functional NET (mostly insulinoma). About 50–80% of patients also have multiple duodenal gastrinomas (Fig. 3.2b), leading to ZES and type II gastric ECL cell NET. *MEN1* codes for menin, which functions as a tumor suppressor and scaffold protein; interacts with many protein partners that are implicated in histone modifications, chromatin remodeling, and telomere maintenance; and regulates cell growth and proliferation [80, 81].

Table 3.5 Familial syndromes associated with neuroendocrine tumors of the digestive system [80, 81]

	Chromosome	Protein function	Pancreatic NET	Luminal GI NET	Other tumors
MEN1	11q13	Menin: Histone modifications, chromatin remodeling, and telomere maintenance	30–75%: Functional (10–30% insulinoma, rare glucagonoma, VIPoma), nonfunctional, microadenomas	50–80%: Duodenal gastrinoma, type II gastric NET	Parathyroid, pituitary, thymic/ bronchial carcinoid, adrenal cortical tumor, cutaneous lipoma, and angiofibroma
VHL	3p25.3	pVHL: Target HIF1α protein for degradation	11–17%: Nonfunctional clear cell type, half multiple; microadenoma	Rare: Clear cell NET in duodenum, gallbladder, bile duct	RCC, HB, pancreatic serous cystadenoma and cysts (91%), pheochromocytoma/ paraganglioma, endolymphatic sac tumor
NF1	17q11.2	Neurofibromin: Inactivate Ras-GTP, interact with cytoskeleton	10%: Somatostatin or insulin-producing NET	Peri-ampullary somatostatin-producing NET, gangliocytic paraganglioma	Neurofibroma, MPNST, pheochromocytoma, glioma, GIST
TSC	*TSC1:* 9q34 *TSC2:* 16p13.3	TSC1/Hamartin TSC2/Tuberlin (mTOR pathway)	1.8–9%: Insulin-producing or nonfunctional NET	ND	Astrocytic hamartomas, cardiac rhabdomyoma, PEComas, bone cyst
MEN4	*CDKN1B:* 12p13	P27: Cell cycle inhibitor	Pancreatic NET	Intestinal, gastric NET	Similar to MEN1
GCHN	*GCGR:* 17q25	Glucagon receptor	Glucagon cell hyperplasia and neoplasia	ND	ND
Familial insulinomatosis [100]		MAFA: Glucose-stimulated insulin secretion	Multifocal trabecular insulin-producing NET		

MEN multiple endocrine neoplasia, *VHL* Von Hippel-Lindau syndrome, *NF* neurofibromatosis, *TSC* tuberous sclerosis complex, *GCHN* glucagon cell hyperplasia and neoplasia, *HIF* hypoxia-inducible factor, *mTOR* mammalian target of rapamycin, *RCC* renal cell carcinoma, *HB* hemangioblastoma, *MPNST* malignant peripheral nerve sheath tumor, *GIST* gastrointestinal stromal tumor, *PEComa* perivascular epithelioid cell tumor, *ND* no data, *MAFA* V-Maf avian musculoaponeurotic fibrosarcoma oncogene homolog A

Multiple endocrine neoplasia type 4 (MEN4) is a similar tumoral syndrome but caused by germline *CDKN1B* mutation. *CDKN1B* encodes p27, which is a cyclin-dependent kinase inhibitor whose loss of function promotes cell cycle progression and cell growth. MEN4 patients may develop pancreatic, gastric, and small intestine NETs [80, 81].

Von Hippel-Lindau syndrome (VHL) is an autosomal dominant syndrome caused by *VHL* germline mutation. Patients may have renal cell carcinoma, hemangioblastoma, pheochromocytoma, and paraganglioma. About 11–17% of patients develop pancreatic nonfunctional NET, whose characteristic morphology includes rich vasculature, nuclear atypia, and clear or eosinophilic cytoplasm (Fig. 3.3b). Serous cystic lesion is also common in the pancreas, and clear cell NETs have been rarely observed in other GI organs. pVHL is part of the E3 ubiquitin ligase complex that targets hypoxia-inducible factor (HIF) 1α for ubiquitiration and degradation. Mutation of *VHL* gene leads to disruption of pVHL function, subsequent stabilization of HIF1α and its heterodimerization with HIF1β, and activation of downstream genes [80, 81].

Tuberous sclerosis (TSC) is caused by mutations in *TSC1* or *TSC2* gene. *TSC1* and *TSC2* encode hamartin and tuberin, respectively. They form a dimer to regulate phosphatidylinositol 3-kinase (PI3K) and mammalian target of rapamycin (mTOR) signaling pathway, which further regulates cell growth. TSC is characterized by benign hamartomas, and pancreatic NET is rarely associated with TSC [81].

Neurofibromatosis type 1 (NF1) is an autosomal dominant syndrome characterized by multiple neurofibromas, café-au-lait spots, axillary or groin freckles, and bone dysplasia. In addition to gastrointestinal stromal tumor (GIST), about 30% of duodenal somatostatin-producing NETs as well as some gangliocytic paragangliomas are associated with NF1, though functional tumor is essentially unheard of. Germline mutation of *NF1* gene leads to inactivation of neurofibromin, an inhibitor of RAS activity, and resultant upregulation of RAS/MAPK pathway signaling [80, 81]. Neurofibromin also inhibits the mTOR pathway [81].

Molecular Pathology of Neuroendocrine Neoplasms

The molecular pathology of neuroendocrine neoplasms is better characterized in the pancreas. Expanding the knowledge of gene mutations learned from familial cases, exomic sequencing of non-familial pancreatic NETs identified the following gene mutations: *MEN1* (44%), histone H3.3 binding proteins *DAXX* (death-domain-associated protein) or *ATRX* (a thalassemia/mental retardation syndrome X-linked) (43%, mutually exclusive), as well as genes in the mTOR pathway (14%). The above mutant spectrum of pancreatic NET is very different from ductal adenocarcinoma which predominantly shows mutations in *TP53* and *KRAS*, and to a lesser degree, *TGFBR1*, *SMAD3*, and *SMAD4* [82]. More recently in a coordinated effort by the International Cancer Genome Consortium (ICGC), whole-genome sequencing of 98 primary pancreatic NETs found that clinically sporadic tumors contained various germline mutations in 17% of patients, and somatic mutations were commonly clustered in 4 main pathways: chromatin remodeling (~11%, e.g., *MEN1*, *SETD2*, *ARID1A*, and *MLL3*), DNA damage repair (~11%, e.g., *MUTYH*, *CHEK2*, and *BRCA2*), activation of mTOR signaling (~12%, e.g., *PTEN*, *TSC2*, *TSC1*, and *DEPDC5*), and telomere maintenance (~32%, e.g., *DAXX* or *ATRX*), with *MEN1* (~41%) playing a broad role and affecting all 4 pathways [83, 84]. In addition, DAXX/ATRX loss was associated with a worse prognosis in G2 tumors [85].

Small intestinal NET is the most common malignancy in the small intestine and most common metastatic NET from the luminal GI tract. Loss of heterozygosity (LOH) at chromosome 18 is the most common genetic alteration, identified in 11 of 18 tumors [86]. A whole exome study of 48 small intestinal NETs found similarly low mutation rate as pancreatic NETs. The commonly mutated genes were implicated in PI3K/Akt/mTOR signaling (e.g., mutually exclusive amplification of *AKT1* or *AKT2*), TGF-β pathway (alterations in *SMAD* genes), and *SRC* oncogene. Notably, there was little overlap with genes commonly mutated in adenocarcinoma (e.g., *KRAS*, *NRAS*, *TP53*, *PTEN*, *APC*, *CTNNB1*, *EGFR*) and pancreatic NETs (e.g., *ATRX*, *DAXX*, *PTEN*, *TSC1*, *TSC2*) [87]. A separate study focusing on *APC* gene identified a mutation in 23% of ileal NET cases. The *APC* mutational profiles were different from those reported in colorectal or other carcinomas, suggesting a different mechanism [88]. Using exome and genome sequence analysis, Francis et al. found that in small intestinal NETs statistically significant alterations existed in only a single gene *CDKN1B* at a frequency of 8%, which results in heterozygous inactivation [89]. Karpathakis et al. performed integrated molecular analysis of 97 small intestinal NETs. Epigenetic mutations were common with a recurrence rate of up to 85%, and the most commonly affected genes included *CDX1*, *CELSR3*, *FBP1*, and *GIPR*. Based on copy-number alterations, epigenetic profile, and *CDKN1B* status, the authors proposed to classify small intestinal NETs into three prognostically different groups that showed significantly different progression-free survival after surgical resection [90].

Differentiation Between WDNET G3 and PDNEC

Although WHO introduced the NET G3 category, the threshold of proliferation rate is the same as that of PDNEC (Table 3.3) [34, 35]. In light of different prognosis and treatment response, it is especially important to differentiate those two types of high-grade neuroendocrine neoplasms [31–33]. The mitotic rate of PDNECs is often higher than 20/2 mm^2 and Ki-67 index typically >55%, and NET G3 usually shows a lower mitotic rate of <20/2 mm^2 and Ki-67 is between 20% and 55%. However, there is wide variability and sufficient overlap in proliferation rates that makes them less reliable criteria. As mentioned previously, WDNETs often show organoid growth with rich capillary. There is considerable intratumoral heterogeneity [38, 39], as well as intertumoral heterogeneity with grade progression in a third of the tumors upon metastasis [91]. PDNECs are more uniform with solid nests or sheets of tumor cells and prominent necrosis; and a subset are mixed with a component of adenocarcinoma or squamous cell carcinoma. Thus a metachronous or synchronous lower-grade NET or significant intratumoral heterogeneity favors NET G3; and a history or component of adenocarcinoma or squamous cell carcinoma in the same location favors PDNECs.

Advances in the molecular pathology of pancreatic neuroendocrine neoplasms have provided invaluable tools in this important distinction. The vast majority of PDNECs harbor mutations in *TP53* and *Rb1*, and some also have *SMAD4* mutation, very similar to pancreatic adenocarcinoma; while pancreatic NETs including NET G3 typically show mutations in *MEN1* and *DAXX/ATRX* in about half of the cases and changes in mTOR pathway in a smaller percentage [82, 92, 93]. Using an algorithmic approach, Tang et al. studied 33 high-grade pancreatic NENs and found that morphology was helpful in differentiating NET G3 from PDNEC in 11 cases (33%), a history of or coexistent tumor component was helpful in 23 cases (70%), immunohistochemical expression of affected proteins (DAXX, ATRX, p53, Rb1, SMAD4) was helpful in 20 cases (61%), and a combination of the above features successfully separated all but one case (3%) into either NET G3 or NEC category [94]. However, rarely *TP53* mutation may be present in a small percentage (<5%) of WDNETs [83, 95].

Molecular changes in WDNETs of luminal GI organs are less consistent. *CDKN1B* mutation occurs in only 8% of small intestinal NETs and there is no correlation with p27 protein expression [96]; currently there is no readily available protein marker for luminal GI WDNETs. For PDNECs, the genetic changes especially *TP53* and *Rb1* mutations appear to be common even in non-pancreatic tumors, thus immunohistochemical staining for p53 and Rb1 may help with the distinction [83, 95].

Summary

The behavior of NETs had been elusive, and the terminology and classification had been ever changing for a century after the initial description of carcinoid tumor. It was largely settled with the WHO classification in 2010 and subsequent fine-tuning in 2017 and 2019, though some issues and controversies will likely continue. Despite recent advancement in the diagnosis and management, many patients with NETs will eventually succumb to disease. More recent efforts focus on the molecular basis of NENs especially for the pancreatic and small intestinal tumors, with the hope of finding targetable molecules for personalized therapy. This is just the beginning of the molecular era in NENs, and much remains to be learned in the coming years.

References

1. Yang Z, Tang LH, Klimstra DS. Gastroenteropancreatic neuroendocrine neoplasms: historical context and current issues. Semin Diagn Pathol. 2013;30(3):186–96.
2. Itoh Z, Takeuchi S, Aizawa I, Honda R. The negative feedback mechanism of gastric acid secretion: significance of acid in the gastric juice in man and dog. Surgery. 1975;77(5):648–60.

3. Sjolund K, Sanden G, Hakanson R, Sundler F. Endocrine cells in human intestine: an immunocytochemical study. Gastroenterology. 1983;85(5):1120–30.
4. Grube D, Bohn R. The microanatomy of human islets of Langerhans, with special reference to somatostatin (D-) cells. Arch Histol Jpn. 1983;46(3):327–53.
5. Stefan Y, Grasso S, Perrelet A, Orci L. A quantitative immunofluorescent study of the endocrine cell populations in the developing human pancreas. Diabetes. 1983;32(4):293–301.
6. Klimstra DS, Yang Z. Pathology, classification, and grading of neuroendocrine tumors arising in the digestive system. In: Goldberg RM, Savarese DF, editors. UpToDate. Waltham: UpToDate; 2020.
7. Capella C, Heitz PU, Hofler H, Solcia E, Kloppel G. Revised classification of neuroendocrine tumours of the lung, pancreas and gut. Virchows Arch. 1995;425(6):547–60.
8. Pernick N. CD56. 2020. http://www.pathologyoutlines.com/topic/cdmarkerscd56.html
9. Levine MA, Dempsey MA, Helman LJ, Ahn TG. Expression of chromogranin-A messenger ribonucleic acid in parathyroid tissue from patients with primary hyperparathyroidism. J Clin Endocrinol Metab. 1990;70(6):1668–73.
10. Pernick N. Chromogranin. 2020. http://www.pathologyoutlines.com/topic/stainschromogranin.html
11. Calhoun ME, Jucker M, Martin LJ, Thinakaran G, Price DL, Mouton PR. Comparative evaluation of synaptophysin-based methods for quantification of synapses. J Neurocytol. 1996;25(12):821–8.
12. Pernick N. Synaptophysin. 2020. http://www.pathologyoutlines.com/topic/stainssynaptophysin.html
13. Eriksson B, Oberg K, Stridsberg M. Tumor markers in neuroendocrine tumors. Digestion. 2000;62(Suppl 1):33–8.
14. Lan MS, Breslin MB. Structure, expression, and biological function of INSM1 transcription factor in neuroendocrine differentiation. FASEB J. 2009;23(7):2024–33.
15. Rooper LM. INSM1. July 31, 2019 ed: Pathologyoutlines.com website.; 2019.
16. McHugh KE, Mukhopadhyay S, Doxtader EE, Lanigan C, Allende DS. INSM1 is a highly specific marker of neuroendocrine differentiation in primary neoplasms of the gastrointestinal tract, appendix, and pancreas. Am J Clin Pathol. 2020;153(6):811–20.
17. Sakakibara R, Kobayashi M, Takahashi N, et al. Insulinoma-associated protein 1 (INSM1) is a better marker for the diagnosis and prognosis estimation of small cell lung carcinoma than neuroendocrine phenotype markers such as Chromogranin A, Synaptophysin, and CD56. Am J Surg Pathol. 2020;
18. Ballian N, Brunicardi FC, Wang XP. Somatostatin and its receptors in the development of the endocrine pancreas. Pancreas. 2006;33(1):1–12.
19. Kasajima A, Papotti M, Ito W, et al. High interlaboratory and interobserver agreement of somatostatin receptor immunohistochemical determination and correlation with response to somatostatin analogs. Hum Pathol. 2018;72:144–52.
20. Kaemmerer D, Peter L, Lupp A, et al. Molecular imaging with (6)(8)Ga-SSTR PET/CT and correlation to immunohistochemistry of somatostatin receptors in neuroendocrine tumours. Eur J Nucl Med Mol Imaging. 2011;38(9):1659–68.
21. Kloppel G. Oberndorfer and his successors: from carcinoid to neuroendocrine carcinoma. Endocr Pathol. 2007;18(3):141–4.
22. Bosman F, Carneiro F, Hruban R, Theise N, editors. WHO classification of tumours of the digestive system. Lyon: IARC Press; 2010.
23. Williams ED, Sandler M. The classification of carcinoid tum ours. Lancet. 1963;1(7275):238–9.
24. Soga J, Tazawa K. Pathologic analysis of carcinoids. Histologic reevaluation of 62 cases. Cancer. 1971;28(4):990–8.
25. Hamilton SR, Aaltonen LA, editors. World Health Organization classification of tumours: pathology and genetics of tumours of the digestive system. Lyon: IARC Press; 2000.
26. Heitz PU, Komminoth P, Perren A, et al. Pancreatic endocrine tumours: introduction. In: DeLellis RA, Lloyd RV, Heitz PU, Eng C, editors. Pathology and genetics of tumours of endocrine organs. Lyon: IARC Press; 2004. p. 177–82.

27. Rindi G, Kloppel G, Alhman H, et al. TNM staging of foregut (neuro)endocrine tumors: a consensus proposal including a grading system. Virchows Arch 2006;449(4):395–401.
28. Rindi G, Kloppel G, Couvelard A, et al. TNM staging of midgut and hindgut (neuro) endocrine tumors: a consensus proposal including a grading system. Virchows Arch. 2007;451(4):757–62.
29. Strosberg JR, Cheema A, Weber J, Han G, Coppola D, Kvols LK. Prognostic validity of a novel American joint committee on cancer staging classification for pancreatic neuroendocrine tumors. J Clin Oncol. 2011;29(22):3044–9.
30. Strosberg J, Nasir A, Coppola D, Wick M, Kvols L. Correlation between grade and prognosis in metastatic gastroenteropancreatic neuroendocrine tumors. Hum Pathol. 2009;40(9):1262–8.
31. Sorbye H, Welin S, Langer SW, et al. Predictive and prognostic factors for treatment and survival in 305 patients with advanced gastrointestinal neuroendocrine carcinoma (WHO G3): the NORDIC NEC study. Ann Oncol. 2013;24(1):152–60.
32. Heetfeld M, Chougnet CN, Olsen IH, et al. Characteristics and treatment of patients with G3 gastroenteropancreatic neuroendocrine neoplasms. Endocr Relat Cancer. 2015;22(4):657–64.
33. Basturk O, Yang Z, Tang LH, et al. The high-grade (WHO G3) pancreatic neuroendocrine tumor category is morphologically and biologically heterogenous and includes both well differentiated and poorly differentiated neoplasms. Am J Surg Pathol. 2015;39(5):683–90.
34. Neoplasms of the neuroendocrine pancreas. In: Lloyd RV, Osamura RY, Kloppel G, Rosai J, editors. WHO classification of tumours of endocrine organs. 4th ed. Lyon: IARC; 2017. p. 209–239.
35. Klimstra DS, Kloeppel G, La Rosa S, Rindi G. Classification of neuroendocrine neoplasms of the digestive system. In: WHO Classification of Tumours Editorial Board, editor. Digestive system tumours, 1 vol. 5th ed. Lyon: IARC; 2019. p. 16–19.
36. Tumours of the lung. In: Travis WD, Brambilla E, Burke AP, Marx A, Nicholson AG, editors. WHO classification of tumours of the lung, pleura, thymus and heart. 4th ed. Lyon: IARC; 2015. p. 1–151.
37. Misdraji J, Carr NJ, Pai RK. Appendiceal goblet cell adenocarcinoma. In: WHO Classification of Tumours Editorial Board, editor. Digestive system tumours. Lyon: IARC; 2019. p. 149–51.
38. Couvelard A, Deschamps L, Ravaud P, et al. Heterogeneity of tumor prognostic markers: a reproducibility study applied to liver metastases of pancreatic endocrine tumors. Mod Pathol. 2009;22(2):273–81.
39. Yang Z, Tang LH, Klimstra DS. Effect of tumor heterogeneity on the assessment of Ki67 labeling index in well-differentiated neuroendocrine tumors metastatic to the liver: implications for prognostic stratification. Am J Surg Pathol. 2011;35(6):853–60.
40. Shi C, Adsay V, Bergsland EK et al. Protocol for the examination of specimens from patients with tumors of the endocrine pancreas 2020. https://documents.cap.org/protocols/cp-endocrine-pancreas-endocrine-20-4002.pdf
41. Voss SM, Riley MP, Lokhandwala PM, Wang M, Yang Z. Mitotic count by phosphohistone H3 immunohistochemical staining predicts survival and improves interobserver reproducibility in well-differentiated neuroendocrine tumors of the pancreas. Am J Surg Pathol. 2015;39(1):13–24.
42. Menon SS, Guruvayoorappan C, Sakthivel KM, Rasmi RR. Ki-67 protein as a tumour proliferation marker. Clin Chim Acta. 2019;491:39–45.
43. Tang LH, Gonen M, Hedvat C, Modlin IM, Klimstra DS. Objective quantification of the Ki67 proliferative index in neuroendocrine tumors of the gastroenteropancreatic system: a comparison of digital image analysis with manual methods. Am J Surg Pathol. 2012;36(12):1761–70.
44. McCall CM, Shi C, Cornish TC, et al. Grading of well-differentiated pancreatic neuroendocrine tumors is improved by the inclusion of both Ki67 proliferative index and mitotic rate. Am J Surg Pathol. 2013;37(11):1671–7.
45. Edge SB, Byrd DR, Compton CC, Fritz AG, Greene FL, Trotti A, editors. AJCC cancer staging manual. 7th ed. New York: Springer; 2010.

46. Pape UF, Jann H, Muller-Nordhorn J, et al. Prognostic relevance of a novel TNM classification system for upper gastroenteropancreatic neuroendocrine tumors. Cancer. 2008;113(2):256–65.
47. Ekeblad S, Skogseid B, Dunder K, Oberg K, Eriksson B. Prognostic factors and survival in 324 patients with pancreatic endocrine tumor treated at a single institution. Clin Cancer Res. 2008;14(23):7798–803.
48. Rindi G, Falconi M, Klersy C, et al. TNM staging of neoplasms of the endocrine pancreas: results from a large international cohort study. J Natl Cancer Inst. 2012;104(10): 764–77.
49. Amin MB, Edge SB, Greene FL, editors. AJCC cancer staging manual. 8th ed. New York: Springer; 2017.
50. Gonzalez RS, Cates JMM, Shi C. Number, not size, of mesenteric tumor deposits affects prognosis of small intestinal well-differentiated neuroendocrine tumors. Mod Pathol. 2018;31(10):1560–6.
51. Lawrence B, Gustafsson BI, Chan A, Svejda B, Kidd M, Modlin IM. The epidemiology of gastroenteropancreatic neuroendocrine tumors. Endocrinol Metab Clin N Am. 2011;40(1):1–18. vii
52. Scoazec JY, Rindi G. Oesophageal neuroendocrine neoplasms. In: WHO Classification of Tumours Editorial Board, editor. Digestive system tumours, 1 vol. 5th ed. Lyon: IARC; 2019. p. 56–58.
53. Maru DM, Khurana H, Rashid A, et al. Retrospective study of clinicopathologic features and prognosis of high-grade neuroendocrine carcinoma of the esophagus. Am J Surg Pathol. 2008;32(9):1404–11.
54. Solcia E, Fiocca R, Villani L, Luinetti O, Capella C. Hyperplastic, dysplastic, and neoplastic enterochromaffin-like-cell proliferations of the gastric mucosa. Classification and histogenesis. Am J Surg Pathol. 1995;19(Suppl 1):S1–7.
55. Torbenson M, Abraham SC, Boitnott J, Yardley JH, Wu TT. Autoimmune gastritis: distinct histological and immunohistochemical findings before complete loss of oxyntic glands. Mod Pathol. 2002;15(2):102–9.
56. De Angelis C, Cortegoso Valdivia P, Venezia L, Bruno M, Pellicano R. Diagnosis and management of Zollinger-Ellison syndrome in 2018. Minerva Endocrinol. 2018;43(2):212–20.
57. La Rosa S, Rindi G, Solcia E, Tang LH. Gastric neuroendocrine neoplasms. In: WHO Classification of Tumours Editorial Board, editor. Digestive system tumours, 1 vol. 5th ed. Lyon: IARC; 2019. p. 104–109.
58. Trinh V Q-H, Shi C, Ma C. Gastric neuroendocrine tumours from long-term proton pump inhibitor users are indolent tumours with good prognosis. Histopathology. 2020 Jul 23. https://doi.org/10.1111/his.14220. Online ahead of print. PMID: 32702178. https://doi.org/10.1111/his.14220.
59. Jiang SX, Mikami T, Umezawa A, Saegusa M, Kameya T, Okayasu I. Gastric large cell neuroendocrine carcinomas: a distinct clinicopathologic entity. Am J Surg Pathol. 2006;30(8):945–53.
60. Perren A, Basturk O, Bellizzi AM, Scoazec JY, Sipos B. Small intestinal and ampullary neuroendocrine neoplasms. In: WHO Classification of Tumours Editorial Board, editor. Digestive system tumours, 1 vol. 5th ed. Lyon: IARC; 2019. p. 131–134.
61. Couvelard A, Perren A, Sipos B. Appendiceal neuroendocrine neoplasms. In: WHO Classification of Tumours Editorial Board, editor. Digestive system tumours, 1 vol. Lyon: IARC; 2019. p. 152–155.
62. Rindi G, Komminoth P, Scoazec JY, Shia J. Colorectal neuroendocrine neoplasms. In: WHO Classification of Tumours Editorial Board, editor. Digestive system tumours, 1 vol. 5th ed. Lyon: IARC; 2019. p. 188–191.
63. Gill AJ, Klimstra DS, Lam AK, Washington MK. Tumours of the pancreas. In: WHO Classification of Tumours Editorial Board, editor. Digestive system tumours, 1 vol. Lyon: IARC; 2019. p. 295–372.

64. McCall CM, Shi C, Klein AP, et al. Serotonin expression in pancreatic neuroendocrine tumors correlates with a trabecular histologic pattern and large duct involvement. Hum Pathol. 2012;43(8):1169–76.
65. Soga J, Yakuwa Y. The gastrinoma/Zollinger-Ellison syndrome: statistical evaluation of a Japanese series of 359 cases. J Hepato-Biliary-Pancreat Surg. 1998;5(1):77–85.
66. Soga J, Yakuwa Y. Somatostatinoma/inhibitory syndrome: a statistical evaluation of 173 reported cases as compared to other pancreatic endocrinomas. J Exp Clin Cancer Res. 1999;18(1):13–22.
67. Basturk O, Tang L, Hruban RH, et al. Poorly differentiated neuroendocrine carcinomas of the pancreas: a clinicopathologic analysis of 44 cases. Am J Surg Pathol. 2014;
68. Ramage JK, Davies AH, Ardill J, et al. Guidelines for the management of gastroenteropancreatic neuroendocrine (including carcinoid) tumours. Gut. 2005;54(Suppl 4):iv1–16.
69. Catena L, Bichisao E, Milione M, et al. Neuroendocrine tumors of unknown primary site: gold dust or misdiagnosed neoplasms? Tumori. 2011;97(5):564–7.
70. Folpe AL, Gown AM, Lamps LW, et al. Thyroid transcription factor-1: immunohistochemical evaluation in pulmonary neuroendocrine tumors. Mod Pathol. 1999;12(1):5–8.
71. Lin X, Saad RS, Luckasevic TM, Silverman JF, Liu Y. Diagnostic value of CDX-2 and TTF-1 expressions in separating metastatic neuroendocrine neoplasms of unknown origin. Appl Immunohistochem Mol Morphol. 2007;15(4):407–14.
72. Oliveira AM, Tazelaar HD, Myers JL, Erickson LA, Lloyd RV. Thyroid transcription factor-1 distinguishes metastatic pulmonary from well-differentiated neuroendocrine tumors of other sites. Am J Surg Pathol. 2001;25(6):815–9.
73. Saqi A, Alexis D, Remotti F, Bhagat G. Usefulness of CDX2 and TTF-1 in differentiating gastrointestinal from pulmonary carcinoids. Am J Clin Pathol. 2005;123(3):394–404.
74. Hermann G, Konukiewitz B, Schmitt A, Perren A, Kloppel G. Hormonally defined pancreatic and duodenal neuroendocrine tumors differ in their transcription factor signatures: expression of ISL1, PDX1, NGN3, and CDX2. Virchows Arch. 2011;459(2):147–54.
75. Yang Z, Klimstra DS, Hruban RH, Tang LH. Immunohistochemical characterization of the origins of metastatic well-differentiated neuroendocrine tumors to the liver. Am J Surg Pathol. 2017;41(7):915–22.
76. Koo J, Zhou X, Moschiano E, De Peralta-Venturina M, Mertens RB, Dhall D. The immunohistochemical expression of islet 1 and PAX8 by rectal neuroendocrine tumors should be taken into account in the differential diagnosis of metastatic neuroendocrine tumors of unknown primary origin. Endocr Pathol. 2013;24(4):184–90.
77. Li Z, Yuan J, Wei L, et al. SATB2 is a sensitive marker for lower gastrointestinal well-differentiated neuroendocrine tumors. Int J Clin Exp Pathol. 2015;8(6):7072–82.
78. Lee H, Fu Z, Koo BH, et al. The expression of TTF1, CDX2 and ISL1 in 74 poorly differentiated neuroendocrine carcinomas. Ann Diagn Pathol. 2018;37:30–4.
79. NCCN Guideline Panel. Neuroendocrine and adrenal tumors: National Comprehensive Cancer Network; 2019.
80. Inherited tumour syndromes. In: Lloyd RV, Osamura RY, Kloeppel G, Rosai J, eds. *WHO classification of tumours of endocrine organs.* 4th ed. Lyon, France: IARC; 2017:242–283.
81. Pipinikas CP, Berner AM, Sposito T, Thirlwell C. The evolving (epi)genetic landscape of pancreatic neuroendocrine tumours. Endocr Relat Cancer. 2019;26(9):R519–44.
82. Jiao Y, Shi C, Edil BH, et al. DAXX/ATRX, MEN1, and mTOR pathway genes are frequently altered in pancreatic neuroendocrine tumors. Science. 2011;331(6021):1199–203.
83. Scarpa A, Chang DK, Nones K, et al. Whole-genome landscape of pancreatic neuroendocrine tumours. Nature. 2017;543(7643):65–71.
84. Mafficini A, Scarpa A. Genomic landscape of pancreatic neuroendocrine tumours: the international cancer genome consortium. J Endocrinol. 2018;236(3):R161–7.
85. Singhi AD, Liu TC, Roncaioli JL, et al. Alternative lengthening of telomeres and loss of DAXX/ATRX expression predicts metastatic disease and poor survival in patients with pancreatic neuroendocrine tumors. Clin Cancer Res. 2017;23(2):600–9.

86. Kulke MH, Freed E, Chiang DY, et al. High-resolution analysis of genetic alterations in small bowel carcinoid tumors reveals areas of recurrent amplification and loss. Genes Chromosomes Cancer. 2008;47(7):591–603.
87. Banck MS, Kanwar R, Kulkarni AA, et al. The genomic landscape of small intestine neuroendocrine tumors. J Clin Invest. 2013;123(6):2502–8.
88. Bottarelli L, Azzoni C, Pizzi S, et al. Adenomatous polyposis coli gene involvement in ileal enterochromaffin cell neuroendocrine neoplasms. Hum Pathol. 2013;44(12):2736–42.
89. Francis JM, Kiezun A, Ramos AH, et al. Somatic mutation of CDKN1B in small intestine neuroendocrine tumors. Nat Genet. 2013;45(12):1483–6.
90. Karpathakis A, Dibra H, Pipinikas C, et al. Prognostic impact of novel molecular subtypes of small intestinal neuroendocrine tumor. Clin Cancer Res. 2016;22(1):250–8.
91. Dumars C, Foubert F, Touchefeu Y, et al. Can PPH3 be helpful to assess the discordant grade in primary and metastatic enteropancreatic neuroendocrine tumors? Endocrine. 2016;53(2):395–401.
92. Tang LH, Untch BR, Reidy DL, et al. Well-differentiated neuroendocrine tumors with a morphologically apparent high-grade component: a pathway distinct from poorly differentiated neuroendocrine carcinomas. Clin Cancer Res. 2016;22(4):1011–7.
93. Yachida S, Vakiani E, White CM, et al. Small cell and large cell neuroendocrine carcinomas of the pancreas are genetically similar and distinct from well-differentiated pancreatic neuroendocrine tumors. Am J Surg Pathol. 2012;36(2):173–84.
94. Tang LH, Basturk O, Sue JJ, Klimstra DS. A practical approach to the classification of WHO grade 3 (G3) well-differentiated neuroendocrine tumor (WD-NET) and poorly differentiated neuroendocrine carcinoma (PD-NEC) of the pancreas. Am J Surg Pathol. 2016;40(9):1192–202.
95. Coriat R, Walter T, Terris B, Couvelard A, Ruszniewski P. Gastroenteropancreatic well-differentiated grade 3 neuroendocrine tumors: review and position statement. Oncologist. 2016;21(10):1191–9.
96. Crona J, Gustavsson T, Norlen O, et al. Somatic mutations and genetic heterogeneity at the CDKN1B locus in small intestinal neuroendocrine tumors. Ann Surg Oncol. 2015;22(Suppl 3):S1428–35.
97. Wang L, Yang M, Zhang Y, Xu S, Tian BL. Prognostic validation of the WHO 2010 grading system in pancreatic insulinoma patients. Neoplasma. 2015;62(3):484–90.
98. Song X, Zheng S, Yang G, et al. Glucagonoma and the glucagonoma syndrome. Oncol Lett. 2018;15(3):2749–55.
99. Soga J, Yakuwa Y. Vipoma/diarrheogenic syndrome: a statistical evaluation of 241 reported cases. J Exp Clin Cancer Res. 1998;17(4):389–400.
100. Iacovazzo D, Flanagan SE, Walker E, et al. MAFA missense mutation causes familial insulinomatosis and diabetes mellitus. Proc Natl Acad Sci U S A. 2018;115(5):1027–32.

Perioperative Management

4

J. Bart Rose and Rui Zheng-Pywell

Introduction

Neuroendocrine neoplasms (NENs) are a diverse class of tumors that may secrete bioactive substances requiring careful consideration in the perioperative setting. While they most often occur sporadically, patients may be predisposed due to familial cancer syndromes such as MEN1, MEN2A, MEN2B, neurofibromatosis I, von Hippel-Lindau, or tuberous sclerosis. A genetic work-up ought to be pursued with a family history suggestive of one of these syndromes (e.g., hyperparathyroidism, pituitary adenoma, or paragangliomas) and/or physical findings on exam (e.g., skin angiomas, lipomas, macules, or Lisch nodules). The majority of NENs do not secrete bioactive substances and are referred to as nonfunctioning. These nonfunctional NENs are either generally discovered incidentally on axial imaging or present with symptoms related to mass effect. Functional NENs can present with a litany of signs and symptoms related to the bioactive substance secreted. The following sections will discuss the perioperative management of both of these NEN subtypes.

Nonfunctional Neuroendocrine Neoplasms

Nonfunctional NENs are tumors that do no induce substance-related symptoms. While some are truly non-secretory, others may secrete bioactive substances at asymptomatic levels [1]. Patients often remain asymptomatic until there is significant tumor burden, after which symptoms attributed to tumor mass effect (e.g.,

J. B. Rose (✉)
Division of Surgical Oncology, University of Alabama Birmingham, Birmingham, AL, USA
e-mail: jbrose@uabmc.edu

R. Zheng-Pywell
Department of General Surgery, University of Alabama Birmingham, Birmingham, AL, USA
e-mail: rzheng@uabmc.edu

© Springer Nature Switzerland AG 2021
J. M. Cloyd, T. M. Pawlik (eds.), *Neuroendocrine Tumors*,
https://doi.org/10.1007/978-3-030-62241-1_4

abdominal pain, anorexia, weight loss, nausea, intra-abdominal bleeding, or jaundice) become apparent. Preoperative biochemical work-up is recommended to evaluate serum chromogranin A (CgA) levels [2]. If a nonfunctional GI or pancreatic tumor is suspected, urinary 5-hydroxyindoleacetic acid (5-HIAA) or pancreatic polypeptide levels can be measured, respectively [3, 4].

Perioperative Somatostatin Analog Use

Somatostatin is a cyclic peptide that essentially functions as the "brakes of the GI system" in that it inhibits hypothalamic hormones, gastrin, insulin, glucagon, pancreatic amylase, cholecystokinin, vasoactive intestinal peptide, and secretin production. The effect of somatostatin is dependent on the receptors expressed by the target tissues. Most somatostatin analogs (SSAs) target somatostatin receptor 2 (SSTR2). SSAs have been shown to be effective agents both in addressing secretory symptoms and in inhibiting tumor proliferation [5–7].

The first SSA developed was the eight-amino-acid-long synthetic peptide called octreotide. It has a stronger affinity for SSTR2 than SSTR5, and it does not cause rebound hormone hypersecretion [8, 9]. Subsequently, the long-acting SSAs lanreotide and pasireotide were developed and FDA approved for treatment of secretory syndromes [9]. Current recommendations for SSA therapy involve starting with short-acting octreotide before transitioning to lanreotide or long-acting repeatable octreotide [10].

Gastrin-Secreting Neoplasms (Gastrinomas)

This subset of functional tumors secrete gastrin, a peptide that stimulates the parietal cells to increase acid secretion. The overexpression of gastrin is responsible for Zollinger-Ellison syndrome, a constellation of symptoms characterized by peptic ulcer disease, acid hypersecretion, and a culprit lesion. Sporadic gastrinomas (i.e., those unrelated to hereditary mutations) are found 85% of the time within the so-called gastrinoma triangle, a region bounded by the cystic duct, the junction between the second and third portions of the duodenum, and the pancreatic neck (see Fig. 4.1) [11]. There are multiple secondary causes to increased acid secretion including but not limited to gastric outlet obstruction and a retained gastric antrum.

Symptoms of this condition include abdominal pain and diarrhea. Preoperative management includes prevention of acid secretion to allow for symptom relief. Perioperatively, patients will need biochemical determination looking at fasting serum gastrin levels (off PPI for 1–2 weeks as tolerated). Should serum gastrin levels be >1000 pg/ml, then they likely have a gastrinoma [13]. However, if the serum gastrin level is indeterminate and the diagnosis is suspect, gastric pH sampling can be performed as well as a secretin stimulation test. A gastric pH >2 would exclude a diagnosis of gastrinoma [14]. To perform a secretin stimulation test, intravenous secretin is administered, and serum gastrin levels are collected at 5 min intervals for

Fig. 4.1 The gastrinoma triangle is demarcated by the dotted lines as the region where most sporadic gastrinomas originate [12]

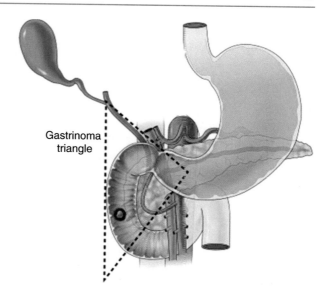

Gastrinoma triangle

30 min. Patients with gastrinomas have a paradoxical rise in serum gastrin >200 pg/ml over basal level after secretin stimulation [13]. In young patients, patients with a positive family history of endocrinopathies, or patients with personal or family history of neuroendocrine tumors, genetic testing ought to be considered [2, 15].

Patients should be started on proton pump inhibitor (PPI) therapy after diagnosis due to the high risk of gastrointestinal perforation and hemorrhage. Goal titration is to aim for acid secretion of ≤10 mEq/hr, or lower should the patient have had previous reflux or acid-reducing surgery. Gastric pH > 4 is the therapeutic target to protect the gastric mucosa [14]. High doses of PPI are often prescribed (i.e., pantoprazole starting at 60–80 mg daily) and titrated according to response. The PPI should be continued for up to 3 months postoperatively given the persistent risk of perforation and hemorrhage in the postoperative period [15].

Special consideration should be given for patients with MEN1-associated gastrinomas. In general, genetic testing is indicated among patients with gastrinomas given this strong association with MEN1. A thorough history, physical examination, and biochemical work-up should be conducted to rule out co-existing hyperparathyroidism and/or hyperpituitarism. Patients with MEN1-associated hypergastrinemia and concomitant hyperparathyroidism should usually undergo parathyroidectomy first because achieving normocalcemia may decrease serum gastrin levels and improve perioperative safety of the pancreatectomy.

Vasoactive Intestinal Peptide-Secreting Neoplasms (VIPomas)

Vasoactive intestinal peptide (VIP) is a small peptide that acts on the gastrointestinal tract to relax smooth muscle and increase luminal water secretion. Overproduction results in a secretory diarrhea syndrome known as either watery diarrhea, hypokalemia, and achlorhydria syndrome, Verner-Morrison syndrome, or pancreatic cholera syndrome. Fasting VIP levels range from 0 to 190 pg/mL, while those with VIPomas generally have elevated levels [16].

Patients tend to experience secretory diarrhea leading to hypokalemia, hypomagnesemia, hypophosphatemia, achlorhydria, metabolic acidosis, and dehydration. Abnormal electrolyte levels associated with depleted levels of magnesium and phosphorus are often present. SSAs are often used concurrently with intravenous (IV) hydration and electrolyte repletion preoperatively to decrease symptoms and correct acid-base balance prior to resection [16, 17].

Glucagon-Secreting Neoplasms (Glucagonomas)

Glucagon is a catabolic hormone that increases serum glucose and fatty acid levels. Overproducing tumors are rare and associated with the constellation of diabetes, dermatitis (i.e., necrolytic migrating erythema), deep vein thrombosis (DVT), depression, and severe weight loss [17, 18]. A normal fasting glucagon level ranges between 70 pg/mL and 160 pg/mL, while a level > 500 pg/mL is diagnostic of a glucagonoma [19].

Patients presenting with cachexia secondary to glucagon-induced vitamin deficiencies and decreased fat and protein stores require nutritional optimization. These patients should be started on supplemental enteral nutrition with excess of basic caloric needs [18]. Additionally, IV amino acids and antibiotics can be initiated to treat symptoms of dermatitis. Prophylactic high-dose anticoagulation (i.e., heparin) is recommended to decrease risk of DVTs and pulmonary embolisms, which are a significant cause of patient morbidity and mortality [18]. Hyperglucagonemia does not appear to affect postoperative glucose homeostasis, and pancreatic alpha-cell responsiveness can be expected to be restored [20].

Somatostatin-Secreting Neoplasms (Somatostatinomas)

Somatostatinomas are typically found in the head of the pancreas and often associated with neurofibromatosis type 1 (von Recklinghausen's disease) and intra-adrenal paragangliomas (pheochromocytomas). Patients tend to present with steatorrhea, diabetes, malabsorption, and cholelithiasis. Fasting somatostatin levels ought to be checked, and a level > 160 pg/mL is suggestive of the disease. Correction of malnutrition and hyperglycemia should be addressed preoperatively. Pancreatic enzyme replacement may help with steatorrhea. Preoperative evaluation for gallstones should be performed, and a prophylactic cholecystectomy should be considered during resection.

Insulin-Secreting Neoplasms (Insulinomas)

Insulinomas are typically benign, and overproduction of insulin results in severe hypoglycemia. Symptoms vary between patients who may complain of fatigue, weakness, fearfulness, hunger, tremor, diaphoresis, and tachycardia. Classically, insulinomas are suspected of causing a patient's hypoglycemia when they meet the criteria of Whipple's triad: neuroglycopenic symptoms, low plasma glucose levels when symptomatic, and relief of symptoms with administration of glucose. However, there are many conditions that may cause similar findings, including exogenous insulin use, autoimmune hypoglycemia, and noninsulinoma pancreatogenous hypoglycemia syndrome. To discern between these etiologies, measurements of plasma glucose, insulin, C peptide, proinsulin, and beta-hydroxybutyrate levels should be obtained during an episode of spontaneous hypoglycemia [21]. Diagnosis of insulinoma can be made with a serum glucose level ≤ 40 mg/dL (≤ 2.2 mmol), concomitant elevated insulin levels >6 µU/mL (≥ 36 pmol/L), elevated C-peptide levels ≥ 200 mol/L, elevated proinsulin levels ≥ 5 pmol/l, low beta-hydroxybutyrate levels ≤ 2.7 mmol/L, and no metabolites of sulfonylureal antiglycemic agents in plasma or urine. The gold standard to evaluate for hypoglycemia is a 72-h monitored fast, though 48-h monitored fast may be adequate per consensus guidelines [10].

Perioperative treatment for both initial and refractory hypoglycemia includes diazoxide (3 mg/kg either BID or TID) and intramuscular (IM) glucagon or intravenous (IV) glucose as needed [2]. Concurrent hypokalemia will require potassium repletion. Side effects of diazoxide include edema and hirsutism. Intraoperatively and postoperatively, glucose infusions are held to assist with glucose monitoring [17]. Perioperative use of somatostatin receptor analogs (SSAs) can be considered. While SSA may help prevent hypoglycemia in patients that express somatostatin receptor 2, SSAs may worsen hypoglycemia in others [10].

Carcinoid Syndrome-Associated Neoplasms

Carcinoid syndrome is predominantly associated with overproduction of serotonin. However carcinoid tumors may secrete other substances such as 5-HTP, tachykinins (substance P and neurokinin A), bradykinin, prostaglandins, and rarely histamine. These tumors are mostly found in the gastrointestinal tract (small intestines, rectum, appendix, colon, and stomach in decreasing incidence) and the bronchopulmonary system [22, 23]. They are rarely found in the pancreas, comprising only approximately 1% of NENs in this organ [24, 25]. Associated findings include cutaneous flushing (typically change in color of the face, neck, or upper chest skin with concomitant sensation of burning), diarrhea, intestinal obstructive symptoms from desmoplastic fibrotic reactions, and dyspnea from bronchospasms. A sudden systemic release of these substances can occur during surgery triggering a life-threatening carcinoid crisis manifested by blood pressure lability, hyperthermia, and bronchospasm. While previously thought to be related to intraoperative release of serotonin, this has not been shown in a prospective study. Rather pre-incision serotonin levels greater than 1064 ng/mL seem to be predictive of the distributed shock associated with carcinoid crisis [26]. Given the poor outcomes associated with carcinoid crisis, several prophylactic steps may be necessary in the perioperative period [22].

It is crucial to determine if the patient has evidence of carcinoid heart disease (CHD) if these tumors are suspected, and a thorough cardiac physical exam focusing on the presence of a murmur, typically diastolic, and jugular venous distention should be performed. For patients with metastatic disease, concerning physical findings of CHD, or serotonin or 5-HIAA levels 5X the upper limit of normal, echocardiography should be considered to evaluate for carcinoid heart disease [3]. N-terminal prohormone brain natriuretic peptide (NT-proBNP) is a good screening tool for CHD. A cutoff of 260 pg/mL helps detect CHD with a sensitivity and specificity of 92% and 91%, respectively. Prognostically, it can be correlated with CgA to predict overall mortality. Five-year survival was 16% in those with elevated CgA and NT-proBNP levels, 44% in those with normal NT-proBNP levels but elevated CgA, and finally 81% in patients with normal levels of both NT-proBNP and CgA [27]. Should CHD be diagnosed, the patient should be evaluated by a cardiologist prior to surgical intervention. If CHD is severe, the patient may require valve replacement prior to tumor resection.

Patients may be dehydrated from chronic diarrhea and require resuscitation, electrolyte repletion, and replacement of nutrient deficiencies. Patients may have underlying tryptophan deficiencies due to conversion to serotonin, leading to hypoproteinemia and niacin deficiencies. They may also have deficiencies of other fat-soluble vitamins due to SA use [17, 22].

Preoperative measurements of serum chromogranin A and the serotonin metabolite 5-hydroxyindoleacetic acid (5-HIAA), either plasma or 24-hr urine, can help determine probability of triggering a carcinoid crisis [2, 17, 21, 22]. Given the risk of carcinoid crisis that may occur with any midgut NEN, especially metastatic of those with carcinoid syndrome, patients are often treated prophylactically with SSAs preoperatively [17]. For symptom management, no agents are found to significantly impact flushing. The mechanism is multifactorial and suspected to be more related to histamine rather than serotonin [22, 28]. SSAs are typically first-line treatment for diarrheal symptoms. If SSAs fail to improve diarrhea, then the peripheral tryptophan hydroxylase (TPH) inhibitor telotristat should be started regardless of 5-HIAA level [22, 28]. TPH is the rate-limiting enzyme in serotonin synthesis. Consideration should also be given to the possibility of a mass effect of the tumor on the pancreas leading to ductal obstruction and pancreatic insufficiency, in which case pancreatic enzyme therapy may be an appropriate adjunct therapy.

Many considerations are taken for anesthetic use for patients with carcinoid syndrome to minimize risk of carcinoid crisis. Sympathetically stimulating drugs and drugs that increase histamine release ought to be avoided, such as morphine and depolarizing neuromuscular blockers. Hypotension related to a carcinoid crisis is often refractory to volume, and administration of catecholamines or calcium may make the condition worse [17, 29]. Intraoperative subcutaneous or continuous intravenous administration of octreotide has been used successfully to reverse a carcinoid crisis. Postoperatively, patients should be slowly weaned from SSAs. Avoid postoperative hypovolemia and uncontrolled pain to prevent sympathetic stimulation [17].

Catecholamine-Secreting Neoplasms (Sympathetic Paragangliomas)

Paragangliomas are NENs arising from the paravertebral axis (termed extra-adrenal) or the adrenal medulla (termed intra-adrenal or pheochromocytoma) and are further subcategorized as either parasympathetic or sympathetic. While those arising from parasympathetic origins are generally non-secretory, those arising from sympathetic tissues can secrete catecholamines [30]. The majority of sympathetic paragangliomas are intra-adrenal or extra-adrenal arising from the organ of Zuckerkandl at the level of the inferior mesenteric artery origin or aortic bifurcation. Patients may present with hypertension (baseline or paroxysmal), palpitations, diaphoresis, and end-organ damage as a result of prolonged hypertension.

Perioperative optimization of blood pressure and intravascular volume is important due to hemodynamic instability. Therapy is targeted to inhibit the alpha-mediated effects of vasoconstriction and beta-1-mediated effects of inotropy and tachycardia from the extra catecholamine release. Preoperative alpha-blockade is achieved with either a selective (e.g., doxazosin) or non-selective (e.g., phenoxybenzamine) agent [31]. Unlike selective alpha-1 blockers, phenoxybenzamine crosses the blood-brain barrier to act on both the peripheral and central alpha-1 and alpha-2 receptors resulting in side effects such as orthostatic hypotension, tachycardia, dizziness, headaches, and drowsiness. When dosing phenoxybenzamine, it is often titrated until orthostatic hypotension develops. Due to its non-selective nature, selective blockers may be preferred [31, 32]. Calcium channel blockers can serve as adjuncts to alpha-antagonists to assist with hypertension control. No differences in intraoperative hemodynamic stability were observed comparing preoperative alpha-blockade with calcium blocker use [33]. Cardioselective beta-antagonists may be added on after the initiation of alpha-blockade to assist with side effects from strict alpha-blockade, such as rebound tachycardia [31]. Therapy is recommended for 5–15 days prior to surgical intervention [32]. Given the vasodilatory effects of alpha-antagonism, patients should be fluid-resuscitated vigorously preoperatively.

Patients may experience hypotension in the postoperative period due to catecholamine withdrawal. Typically, patients are treated with fluid resuscitation and vasopressors. Monitoring in an intensive care unit may be necessary. Severe hypoglycemia can occur from rebound hyperinsulinemia in the postoperative period, and close glucose monitoring is recommended [17].

Parathyroid Hormone-Related Peptide-Secreting Neoplasms

A parathyroid hormone receptor agonist called parathyroid hormone-related peptide can be produced by NENs causing a paraneoplastic hypercalcemia via the activation of osteoblasts and increased bone reabsorption. Symptoms related to hypercalcemia include fatigue, altered mental status, lethargy, dehydration, nephrolithiasis, polyuria, nausea, vomiting, and bone pain [34]. Perioperative treatment involves symptom control and hydration. Hypophosphatemia needs to be corrected to prevent worsening hypercalcemia. Intravenous bisphosphonates (pamidronate or zoledronic acid), denosumab, and calcitonin may be started to treat malignant hypercalcemia. All oral calcium agents ought to be stopped [35]. Definitive treatment requires removal of underlying secretory tumor if localized.

Ectopic Adrenocorticotropic Hormone-Secreting Neoplasms

Ectopic release of adrenocorticotropic hormone (ACTH) can be secreted by some NENs, resulting in overproduction of cortisol by the adrenal glands (Cushing's syndrome). Patients tend to present with a spectrum of findings including weight gain with centripetal fat, hypertension, striae, proximal muscle weakness, depression, fatigue, facial plethora, hirsutism, and menstrual irregularities [34, 36]. To confirm the diagnosis, the source of ACTH release needs to be isolated to either the pituitary gland (Cushing's disease) or a secretory tumor. Preliminary testing can be any of the following: 24-h urine free cortisol, overnight 1-mg dexamethasone suppression test, or late night salivary cortisol testing. If endogenous cortisol hypersecretion is confirmed, then an 8-mg high-dose dexamethasone suppression to determine source of ACTH, pituitary axis (central) versus ectopic, can follow [36].

Perioperative management focuses on addressing the comorbidities accompanying hypercortisolemia. Oral agents and insulin may be necessary for glycemic control. Patients often have concurrent dyslipidemia; thus, those with confirmed diagnosis will require screening and treatment. Blood pressure should be optimized and electrolyte disturbances corrected. These patients are at increased risk of DVTs; thus, perioperative deep vein thrombosis prophylaxis is essential. Finally, given the psychiatric symptoms from excess cortisol, appropriate mental health care and psychiatry referral may be necessary [6, 7, 37].

Conclusion

Neuroendocrine neoplasms are a diverse class of tumors that are associated with multiple syndromes due to tumor secretion of bioactive substances. While surgical excision is the curative treatment for NENs, many steps are necessary in the perioperative period to minimize patient morbidity and mortality (summarized in Table 4.1). Given that perioperative management differs significantly among

Table 4.1 Recommended perioperative management of specific neuroendocrine tumors

Tumor	Bioactive substance(s)	Biochemical evaluation	Perioperative testing	Perioperative management
Nonfunctional	Minimal to none	Chromogranin A 5-HIAA		
Gastrinoma	Gastrin	Chromogranin A Fasting gastrin (off PPI for 2 weeks if safe)	Gastric pH Secretin stimulation test[a] Gastric pH sampling[a]	Proton pump inhibitors Genetic testing[b]
VIPoma	VIP	Chromogranin A Fasting VIP	Biochemical profile	Hydration Electrolyte and acid-base correction Somatostatin analog
Glucagonoma	Glucagon	Chromogranin A Fasting glucagon	Nutrition evaluation	DVT prophylaxis Antibiotics[c] Caloric support[a] Correction of vitamin and amino acid deficiencies[a]
Somatostatinoma	Somatostatin	Chromogranin A Fasting somatostatin	Right upper quadrant ultrasound	
Insulinoma	Insulin	Chromogranin A Glucose Insulin Proinsulin C peptide Beta-hydroxybutyrate	72-hour monitored fast	Diazoxide Dextrose infusions Glucagon Potassium repletion Somatostatin analog[d] Genetic testing[b]
Carcinoid	Serotonin[e] 5-HTP Prostaglandins Tachykinins Bradykinin Histamine	Chromogranin A 5-HIAA	Echocardiography NT-proBNP[f] TGF FGF	Somatostatin analog Anti-diarrheal agents Telotristat

(continued)

Table 4.1 (continued)

Tumor	Bioactive substance(s)	Biochemical evaluation	Perioperative testing	Perioperative management
Catecholamine-secreting	Norepinephrine Epinephrine	Chromogranin A Metanephrines and normetanephrines[g]		Alpha-blockade Genetic testing Beta-blocker[h] Hydration[h]
PTHrP	PTHrP	Calcium PTHrP	Biochemical profile	Bisphosphonates Calcitonin Stop calcium supplements
Ectopic ACTH	ACTH[i]	24-hour urine cortisol[j] Low-dose dexamethasone suppression test[j] Late night salivary cortisol testing[j] High-dose dexamethasone suppression test	Biochemical profile	Antihypertensives[a] Antiglycemics[a] Electrolyte correction Psychiatric interventions[a]

VIP vasoactive intestinal peptide, *PTHrP* parathyroid hormone-related peptide, *ACTH* adrenocorticotropic hormone, *MTC* medullary thyroid carcinoma, *5-HIAA* 5-hydroxyindoleacetic acid, *Ab* antibody, *DVT* deep vein thrombosis, *5-HTP* 5-hydroxytryptophan, *BNP* brain natriuretic peptide, *TGF* transforming growth factor, *FGF* fibroblast growth factor

[a] As needed

[b] Consider genetic testing, specifically for MEN1 (multiple endocrine neoplasia), in young patients or those with positive personal or family history of NENs or endocrinopathies

[c] May be necessary in treating infections associated with necrolytic migrating erythema

[d] Depending on somatostatin receptor status, somatostatin analogs may help with hypoglycemia. However they may also worsen hypoglycemia in other patients

[e] Most common secreted substance though the others listed may also be present

[f] For assessment of severity of CHD (carcinoid heart disease)

[g] Multiple consensus groups note that either urine or plasma levels are acceptable

[h] May be started after adequate alpha-blockade from the effects of vasodilation

[i] Should ACTH results conflict with clinical diagnosis, consider repeating ACTH levels with alternate ACTH test [38]

[j] Any of these three tests can be a preliminary test for separating exogenous cortisol from endogenous cortisol

various NENs, biochemical work-up is crucial for accurate diagnosis and preoperative management. In addition, utilizing appropriate perioperative therapies (i.e., SSAs) is crucial to patient care and improve overall morbidity and mortality.

References

1. Cloyd JM, Poultsides GA. Non-functional neuroendocrine tumors of the pancreas: advances in diagnosis and management. World J Gastroenterol. 2015;21(32):9512–25.
2. Kunz PL, Reidy-Lagunes D, Anthony LB, Bertino EM, Brendtro K, Chan JA, et al. Consensus guidelines for the management and treatment of neuroendocrine tumors. Pancreas. 2013;42(4):557–77.
3. Howe JR, Merchant NB, Conrad C, Keutgen XM, Hallet J, Drebin JA, et al. The North American neuroendocrine tumor society consensus paper on the surgical management of pancreatic neuroendocrine tumors. Pancreas. 2020;49(1):1–33.
4. Network NCC. Neuroendocrine and adrenal tumors (version 1.2019) 2019. Available from: https://www.nccn.org/professionals/physician_gls/pdf/neuroendocrine_blocks.pdf
5. Stueven AK, Kayser A, Wetz C, Amthauer H, Wree A, Tacke F, et al. Somatostatin analogues in the treatment of neuroendocrine tumors: past, present and future. Int J Mol Sci. 2019;20(12)
6. Rinke A, Wittenberg M, Schade-Brittinger C, Aminossadati B, Ronicke E, Gress TM, et al. Placebo-controlled, double-blind, prospective, randomized study on the effect of Octreotide LAR in the control of tumor growth in patients with metastatic neuroendocrine midgut tumors (PROMID): results of long-term survival. Neuroendocrinology. 2017;104(1):26–32.
7. Caplin ME, Pavel M, Ruszniewski P. Lanreotide in metastatic enteropancreatic neuroendocrine tumors. N Engl J Med. 2014;371(16):1556–7.
8. Saltz L, Trochanowski B, Buckley M, Heffernan B, Niedzwiecki D, Tao Y, et al. Octreotide as an antineoplastic agent in the treatment of functional and nonfunctional neuroendocrine tumors. Cancer. 1993;72(1):244–8.
9. Wolin EM. The expanding role of somatostatin analogs in the management of neuroendocrine tumors. Gastrointest Cancer Res. 2012;5(5):161–8.
10. Jensen RT, Cadiot G, Brandi ML, de Herder WW, Kaltsas G, Komminoth P, et al. ENETS consensus guidelines for the management of patients with digestive neuroendocrine neoplasms: functional pancreatic endocrine tumor syndromes. Neuroendocrinology. 2012;95(2):98–119.
11. Passaro E Jr, Howard TJ, Sawicki MP, Watt PC, Stabile BE. The origin of sporadic gastrinomas within the gastrinoma triangle: a theory. Arch Surg. 1998;133(1):13–6; discussion 7.
12. Metz DC. Diagnosis of the Zollinger–Ellison syndrome. Clin Gastroenterol Hepatol. 2012;10(2):126–30.
13. McGuigan JE, Wolfe MM. Secretin injection test in the diagnosis of gastrinoma. Gastroenterology. 1980;79(6):1324–31.
14. Banasch M, Schmitz F. Diagnosis and treatment of gastrinoma in the era of proton pump inhibitors. Wien Klin Wochenschr. 2007;119(19–20):573–8.
15. Norton JA, Foster DS, Ito T, Jensen RT. Gastrinomas: medical or surgical treatment. Endocrinol Metab Clin N Am. 2018;47(3):577–601.
16. Vinik A. Vasoactive intestinal peptide tumor (VIPoma). In: Feingold KR, Anawalt B, Boyce A, Chrousos G, Dungan K, Grossman A, et al., editors. Endotext. South Dartmouth: MDText. com, Inc. Copyright © 2000–2020, MDText.com, Inc.; 2000.
17. Kaltsas G, Caplin M, Davies P, Ferone D, Garcia-Carbonero R, Grozinsky-Glasberg S, et al. ENETS consensus guidelines for the standards of care in neuroendocrine tumors: pre- and perioperative therapy in patients with neuroendocrine tumors. Neuroendocrinology. 2017;105(3):245–54.

18. Jin XF, Spampatti MP, Spitzweg C, Auernhammer CJ. Supportive therapy in gastroentero-pancreatic neuroendocrine tumors: often forgotten but important. Rev Endocr Metab Disord. 2018;19(2):145–58.
19. John AM, Schwartz RA. Glucagonoma syndrome: a review and update on treatment. J Eur Acad Dermatol Venereol. 2016;30(12):2016–22.
20. Holst JJ, Helland S, Ingemannson S, Pedersen NB, von Schenck H. Functional studies in patients with the glucagonoma syndrome. Diabetologia. 1979;17(3):151–6.
21. Kanakis G, Kaltsas G. Biochemical markers for gastroenteropancreatic neuroendocrine tumours (GEP-NETs). Best Pract Res Clin Gastroenterol. 2012;26(6):791–802.
22. Ito T, Lee L, Jensen RT. Carcinoid-syndrome: recent advances, current status and controversies. Curr Opin Endocrinol Diabetes Obes. 2018;25(1):22–35.
23. Pinchot SN, Holen K, Sippel RS, Chen H. Carcinoid tumors. Oncologist. 2008;13(12):1255–69.
24. Modlin IM, Lye KD, Kidd M. A 5-decade analysis of 13,715 carcinoid tumors. Cancer. 2003;97(4):934–59.
25. Soga J. Carcinoids of the pancreas: an analysis of 156 cases. Cancer. 2005;104(6):1180–7.
26. Condron ME, Jameson NE, Limbach KE, Bingham AE, Sera VA, Anderson RB, et al. A prospective study of the pathophysiology of carcinoid crisis. Surgery. 2019;165(1):158–65.
27. Hayes AR, Davar J, Caplin ME. Carcinoid heart disease: a review. Endocrinol Metab Clin N Am. 2018;47(3):671–82.
28. Kulke MH, Hörsch D, Caplin ME, Anthony LB, Bergsland E, Öberg K, et al. Telotristat ethyl, a tryptophan hydroxylase inhibitor for the treatment of carcinoid syndrome. J Clin Oncol. 2017;35(1):14–23.
29. Vaughan DJ, Brunner MD. Anesthesia for patients with carcinoid syndrome. Int Anesthesiol Clin. 1997;35(4):129–42.
30. Else T, Greenberg S, Fishbein L. Hereditary paraganglioma-pheochromocytoma syndromes. In: Adam MP, Ardinger HH, Pagon RA, Wallace SE, Bean LJH, Stephens K, et al., editors. GeneReviews(®). Seattle: University of Washington, Seattle. Copyright © 1993–2020, University of Washington, Seattle. GeneReviews is a registered trademark of the University of Washington, Seattle. All rights reserved.; 1993.
31. Davison AS, Jones DM, Ruthven S, Helliwell T, Shore SL. Clinical evaluation and treatment of phaeochromocytoma. Ann Clin Biochem. 2018;55(1):34–48.
32. Ramachandran R, Rewari V. Current perioperative management of pheochromocytomas. Indian J Urol. 2017;33(1):19–25.
33. Brunaud L, Boutami M, Nguyen-Thi PL, Finnerty B, Germain A, Weryha G, et al. Both preoperative alpha and calcium channel blockade impact intraoperative hemodynamic stability similarly in the management of pheochromocytoma. Surgery. 2014;156(6):1410–7; discussion 7–8.
34. Guilmette J, Nosé V. Paraneoplastic syndromes and other systemic disorders associated with neuroendocrine neoplasms. Semin Diagn Pathol. 2019;36(4):229–39.
35. Zagzag J, Hu MI, Fisher SB, Perrier ND. Hypercalcemia and cancer: differential diagnosis and treatment. CA Cancer J Clin. 2018;68(5):377–86.
36. Nieman LK, Biller BM, Findling JW, Newell-Price J, Savage MO, Stewart PM, et al. The diagnosis of cushing's syndrome: an endocrine society clinical practice guideline. J Clin Endocrinol Metab. 2008;93(5):1526–40.
37. Schreiner F, Anand G, Beuschlein F. Perioperative management of endocrine active adrenal tumors. Exp Clin Endocrinol Diabetes. 2019;127(2–03):137–46.
38. Greene LW, Geer EB, Page-Wilson G, Findling JW, Raff H. Assay-specific spurious ACTH results lead to misdiagnosis, unnecessary testing, and surgical misadventure-a case series. J Endocr Soc. 2019;3(4):763–72.

Neoadjuvant and Adjuvant Treatment Strategies for Well-Differentiated Neuroendocrine Tumors

5

Satya Das, Heloisa Soares, and Arvind Dasari

Incidence and Recurrence Patterns of Locoregional NETs

The incidence of neuroendocrine tumors (NETs) has increased globally over the last several decades, with most of this increase occurring in well-differentiated NETs [1–4]. Well-differentiated NETs presenting with locoregional involvement have increased disproportionately compared to NETs presenting with metastatic spread. Poorly differentiated neuroendocrine carcinomas have a much more aggressive biology and propensity for metastatic involvement at diagnosis and will not be discussed in this chapter. In a population-based study of the United States Surveillance, Epidemiology, and End Results (SEER) program, age-adjusted incidence rate of NETs increased 6.4-fold from 1973 (1.09 cases per 100,000) to 2012 (6.98 cases per 100,000). Among stage groups, the incidence increased the most in localized NETs by 15-fold, from 0.21 cases per 100,000 in 1973 to 3.15 cases per 100,000 in 2012 [1]. In a Canadian population-based study evaluating epidemiological trends from 1994 to 2009, the incidence of NETs increased from 2.48 to 5.86 cases per 100,000 per year representing a 2.36-fold increase [4]. The proportion of patients presenting

S. Das
Vanderbilt University Medical Center, Department of Medicine, Division of Hematology and Oncology, Nashville, TN, USA
e-mail: satya.das@vumc.org

H. Soares
Huntsman Cancer Institute at University of Utah, Division of Oncology, Salt Lake City, UT, USA
e-mail: Heloisa.Soares@hci.utah.edu

A. Dasari (✉)
The University of Texas MD Anderson Cancer Center, Department of Gastrointestinal Medical Oncology, Division of Cancer Medicine, Houston, TX, USA
e-mail: ADasari@mdanderson.org

© Springer Nature Switzerland AG 2021
J. M. Cloyd, T. M. Pawlik (eds.), *Neuroendocrine Tumors*,
https://doi.org/10.1007/978-3-030-62241-1_5

with metastatic disease at the time of diagnosis however, decreased from 29% to 13% over the same time period. Given these trends, more NETs are being resected or being considered for surgical resection. In many other solid tumors, neoadjuvant and/or adjuvant therapies are staples of standard treatment in the management of locoregional disease with a goal of eradicating micrometastatic disease and thus improving disease-free survival (DFS) and overall survival (OS) [5–8]. The value of these approaches for patients with locoregional NETs remains to be determined.

Perhaps the value of perioperative therapy in NET patients can only be contextualized in the context of understanding the recurrence risk for these tumors. In a large 936 cohort study of patients with resected gastroenteropancreatic (GEP) NETs, the cumulative risk of recurrence was 23.3%, 33.5%, 48.5%, and 58.3% at 3, 5, 10, and 15 years, respectively [9]. In a retrospective analysis of 129 midgut NET patients with resected disease, the cumulative risk of recurrence at 1, 5, and 10 years was 15%, 50%, and 85%, respectively [10]. Concerning lung NETs, in a cohort study of 337 patients, recurrence patterns of atypical and typical NETs were assessed [11]. Of patients with atypical lung NETs, 26% experienced recurrence; among patients with typical lung NETs, 6% experienced recurrence. In another analysis, among 142 resected lung NET patients, the 5- and 10-year DFS rates for atypical and typical NETs were 72% & 32% and 92% & 85%, respectively [12]. In most other solid tumors (e.g., gastrointestinal cancers such as colorectal cancers), the risk of recurrence is highest in the first 2–3 years after surgery (80% of all recurrences in the case of colorectal adenocarcinomas occur in the first 3 years) and is minimal after the 5-year mark when typically surveillance for recurrence is stopped. In contrast, as the above studies show, in NETs, irrespective of primary site of origin, only about a third of the recurrences occur within the first 5 years and the risk of recurrence appears to persist for a much longer duration, up to 10–15 years.

Risk Factors for Recurrence

As discussed above, the objective of perioperative therapy is to eradicate micrometastatic disease. Since there are no reliable detection methods for such metastatic spread, identifying NETs with the highest predisposition for recurrence may be the first step to defining the patient population who may benefit from systemic treatment in the perioperative setting.

Pancreatic NETs are clinically and biologically distinct from NETs arising from other sites. Multiple studies have shown worse survival for patients with metastatic pancreatic NETs compared to other NETs. In a population-based study, the hazard ratio for OS for patients with pancreatic NETs compared to those with small intestinal NETs was 1.65 (HR 1.53–1.78) [3]. Similar trends have been reported for resected pancreatic NETs that appear to have an increased recurrence risk compared to other gastrointestinal NETs [13]. In the above mentioned 936 patient cohort study, the corresponding cumulative incidence rates of recurrence for pancreatic NETs were 26.5%, 39.6%, 57%, and 69.4% at 3, 5, 10, and 15 years, respectively [9]. Furthermore, of all the sites, recurrences occurred earliest among patients with pancreatic NETs. Reflecting these trends and worse prognosis for pancreatic NETs, recurrence in these tumors has been best studied of all the NET sites. Data from over 1000 patients with nonfunctioning well-differentiated pancreatic NET were used to develop and validate a Recurrence Risk Score (RRS) generated from several clinicopathologic features. These features included regional lymph node positivity, primary tumor size >2 cm, symptomatic primary tumor (defined as jaundice, pain, and/ or bleeding) and Ki-67 index >3 [14]. Patients were grouped into low (RRS ≤ 2; 54% of all patients); intermediate (RRS 3–5; 44% of all patients), and high risk (RRS 6–10; 0.02% of all patients). After a median follow-up of 41 months, patients with high and intermediate risk scores had a hazard ratio for recurrence of 22.5 and 3.7, relative to low risk score patients, respectively. At 24 months, 33% of high RRS, 14% of intermediate, and only 2% of low RRS recurred. Several other studies have evaluated these and other risk factors including elevated chromogranin levels, perineural invasion, lymphovascular invasion, tumor location, and number of lymph nodes involved [15, 16]. The management of pancreatic NETs <2 cm pose a clinical conundrum with significant debate around the incremental benefit of surgical intervention over observation. In patients with these tumors that do undergo resection, one study suggested that patients with lymph node positive tumors had a 5-year recurrence free survival of 80% compared to 96% in patients with lymph node negative tumors [17]. This study also suggested that location (distal vs proximal) and Ki-67 index (<3% vs ≥ 3%) could be used to categorize such tumors into low, intermediate, and high risk of regional lymph node involvement (3.2% vs 13.8% vs 20.5%, respectively). In another study of 210 patients with resected pancreatic NETs <2 cm, patients with tumors ≤1 cm were disease-free at last follow-up; while 1-, 3- and 5-year DFS rates for patients with tumors sized 1.1–2 cm were 95.1%, 91.0%, and 87.3%, respectively [18]. It should be noted that the data for recurrence risk for smaller pancreatic NETs is confounded by the lack of consensus around the clinical criteria used for selection for surgery and the extent of surgery (enucleation vs resection) that may not always provide information regarding regional lymph node involvement [19].

Pancreatic NETs, in contrast to other NETs, are characterized by a myriad of mutational changes that converge on the following four pathways: DNA damage repair, cell cycle regulation, PI3K/mTOR signaling, and telomere maintenance. *DAXX* and *ATRX* encode nuclear proteins that regulate the deposition of histone variant H3.3 during the assembly of pericentromeric and telomeric chromatin and mutations in these genes are associated with alternative lengthening of telomeres (ALT). Although initial studies suggested better prognosis in metastatic pancreatic NETs with ALT, subsequent studies have suggested that ALT positive tumors are more likely to present with advanced primary tumors with worse outcomes after surgical resection [20]. ALT-positive NETs, may be characterized by higher rates of lymphovascular invasion, perineural invasion, lymph node positivity, and recurrence compared to ALT-negative NETs. In a study of 321 patients with resected pancreatic NETs, the 5-year DFS of patients with ALT-positive and DAXX/ATRX-negative pancreatic NETs was 40% as compared with 96% for patients with ALT-negative tumors. Similar results were noted in another study of patients with resected pancreatic NETs with the 5-year DFS for ALT-positive vs ALT-negative tumors being 38.7% vs 79.2% [21]. A recent study classified nonfunctional pancreatic NETs using epigenomes and transcriptomes into two major subtypes partially resembling islet α- and β cells that could be identified based on expression patterns of transcription factors ARX and PDX1 [22]. In a cohort of 103 patients with pancreatic NETs, recurrences were noted almost exclusively in those with ARX$^+$PDX1$^-$ tumors and, within this subtype, in cases only with ALT-positive disease.

A retrospective study of 129 patients with resected small intestinal NETs, with a median follow-up of 81 months, revealed that 31% of patients developed disease recurrence, with a median DFS time of 138 months. Stage I tumors appeared to have a lower risk of recurrence as compared to stages II, III tumors [10]. Sequencing efforts have shown that small bowel NETs have a lower mutation burden compared to pancreatic NETs. In contrast to these rare mutational events, most small intestinal NETs have segmental losses of chromosome 18. In a study of 97 patients with resected small intestinal NETs, with nearly 10 years of follow-up, those with chromosomal 18 loss of heterozygosity (LOH) tended to have the best DFS (not reached) compared to those with NETs with CpG island methylator phenotype and no copy number variations (CNVs), CNVs (56 months) or those with multiple CNVs (21 months) [23]. Multiple smaller studies have evaluated epigenetic changes and microRNAs as potential prognostic biomarkers for small intestinal NETs but need validation [24].

While several clinicopathologic features and molecular features are associated with more aggressive disease biology, and higher recurrence rates for GEP NETs, these have not consistently been used to select patients being considered for adjuvant or neoadjuvant systemic treatment. Perhaps until this patient selection improves, it will be challenging to draw meaningful conclusions about the role for perioperative therapies for patients with resected NETs.

Neoadjuvant and Adjuvant Therapies for NETs

No randomized studies exist which demonstrate benefit for neoadjuvant or adjuvant therapy in patients with locoregional well differentiated NETs. Still, given the high recurrence rate of these tumors, the aggressive behavior of certain NETs, and the introduction of potent systemic therapies such as capecitabine plus temozolomide and peptide receptor radionuclide therapy (PRRT), several analyses have examined the impact of perioperative therapy on patient outcomes. We will discuss some of these studies by tumor type.

Pancreatic NETs

A 237-patient pragmatic study from China assessed DFS and OS in patients with resected grade 2 pancreatic NETs treated with 6 months of adjuvant octreotide or observation [25]. Of the included patients, 66 received adjuvant octreotide while

171 patients were observed. Patient characteristics were balanced between the two arms with the following exception: octreotide treated patients possessed tumors with more microvascular invasion and peri-pancreatic invasion. Rates of 24-month, 36-month, and 60-month DFS were 95.5%, 93.9%, and 90.9% and 85.4%, 81.3%, and 76% in octreotide and observation arms, respectively OS was also longer for octreotide-treated patients compared to patients who were observed, though this did not meet statistical significance ($p = 0.056$).

A recently presented retrospective analysis explored the possible utility of neoadjuvant capecitabine plus temozolomide in 30 patients with locally advanced or oligometastatic (to liver) pancreatic NETs [26]. In this analysis, patients received a median of four cycles of capecitabine plus temozolomide. Of the included patients, 87% were able to undergo surgery. No difference in partial response rate was observed between tumors of different WHO grade. The median progression-free survival (PFS) for all patients was 28.2 months while 5-year OS was 63%.

In a single-institution retrospective analysis, a group from MD Anderson published their experience with neoadjuvant fluorouracil, doxorubicin, and streptozocin (FAS) chemotherapy in patients with locoregional pancreatic NETs [27]. Between 2000–2012, 29 patients who received FAS were identified. Patients received a median of four treatment cycles of FAS prior to surgery. Only 7% of patients experienced a partial response while 90% of patients maintained stable disease. Similarly, only 21% of patients experienced a reduction of primary tumor vascular abutment. Among included patients, 44.8% were not considered for resection while 48.2% underwent pancreatectomy. Median OS of all patients was 108 months; median OS for resected patients was 112 months, and was 41 months for unresected patients. In contrast to the response rate of this regimen at the primary site, the response rate of FAS at metastatic sites was 39% suggesting differential responses between primary and metastatic pancreatic NET sites [28]. Another retrospective study by the same group evaluated the role of preoperative FAS in patients with pancreatic NETs metastatic to the liver [29]. Of the 67 patients included, 27 received preoperative FAS, whereas 40 did not. Although the patients receiving preoperative therapy had more advanced tumors with higher rates of synchronous disease, lymph node metastases, and larger tumor size, they demonstrated comparable OS (108.2 months vs. 107.0 months) and a trend toward improved DFS (25.1 months vs. 18.0 months $p = 0.16$) as patients who did not. In fact, in the 46 patients who presented with synchronous liver metastases, the median OS (97.3 months vs. 65.0 months, $p = 0.001$) and DFS (24.8 months vs. 12.1 months, $p = 0.003$) were significantly better in the patients who received preoperative FAS compared to OS and DFS in patients who did not receive the therapy. Though the retrospective nature of these studies limits definitive conclusions, these data suggest that the benefit of perioperative cytotoxic chemotherapy in pancreatic NETs may not be primary tumor regression but rather risk recurrence reduction by eliminating micrometastatic disease.

Multiple published case reports have touted the ability of PRRT to convert initially unresectable localized pancreatic NETs into resectable tumors; however, only few larger studies have been reported [30–32]. A Dutch retrospective analysis explored the role for neoadjuvant PRRT in 29 pancreatic NET patients with borderline-resectable or unresectable disease [33]. All patients included in the analysis received PRRT with ^{177}Lu-octreotide up to a maximum cumulative dose of 29.6 gigabecquerel (GBq). Of the included patients, 31% were able to undergo curative resection. Median PFS of all patients was 55 months; median PFS was 69 months in patients who were able to undergo surgical resection, while it was 49 months for the other patients; however this difference was not statistically significant ($p = 0.22$). The median OS in the included patients was greater than 105 months. A retrospective Italian analysis assessed postoperative outcomes in 23 resectable or borderline-resectable pancreatic NETs who were matched by tumor characteristics in a 1:1 fashion with 23 patients who underwent upfront surgical resection [34]. Of the PRRT treated patients, 87% completed five cycles of neoadjuvant therapy with ^{90}Y-DOTATOC while the others received therapy with ^{177}Lu-DOTATATE. Tumor downsizing was observed in the PRRT treated patients; however no differences in R0 resection rates were observed between the groups. No differences in disease-specific survival or PFS were seen in the two groups though patients treated with neoadjuvant therapy demonstrated lower rates of postoperative pancreatic fistulae ($p = 0.11$).

A large retrospective analysis queried the National Cancer Database to identify localized (Stage I–III) pancreatic NETs diagnosed between 2006 and 2014 [35]. Of the 4892 cases identified, 301 patients who underwent perioperative systemic therapy followed by surgery were analyzed. Among these patients, 21% received neoadjuvant therapy, 55% received adjuvant therapy, 2.3% received both, and 22% received perioperative systemic therapy of unclear sequence. Patients were matched in a 1:1 fashion based upon tumor characteristics to patients in the database who underwent surgery alone. The types of systemic therapy that patients received were not specified. In the matched cohort, the treated patients experienced a significantly shorter OS compared to patients who underwent surgery alone ($p = 0.037$) likely reflecting confounding by indication. Multivariable Cox proportional hazards analysis showed the HR for OS in the perioperative systemic therapy cohort was 1.45 ($p = 0.006$). Among patients with grade 1/2 pancreatic NETs, those who received neoadjuvant therapy demonstrated no difference in OS from patients who underwent surgery alone. Patients with grade 1/2 pancreatic NETs who received adjuvant therapy demonstrated a significantly shorter OS than patients who underwent surgery alone.

GI NETs

Data regarding perioperative systemic therapy is even scarcer in patients with small intestinal NETs. Locoregional therapy in the adjuvant setting however, has been explored. A single-institution retrospective analysis examined outcomes in small intestinal NET patients with bulky mesenteric lymphadenopathy (it is unclear how many patients had distant metastatic disease) who underwent cytoreductive surgery between 2003 and 2012 [36]. In this study, 86 patients underwent placement of 5-FU saturated gel strips into their mesenteric resection sites while 103 patients did not (served as matched controls). Mortality rates for patients treated with and without the 5-FU saturated gel strips were no different at 30, 60, and 90 days. Median OS was 236 months versus 148 months for the experimental group and standard treatment groups though this difference was not statistically significant ($p = 0.15$).

A multicenter analysis assessed outcomes between GEP NET patients who received adjuvant therapy after curative intent resection versus observation from 2000 to 2016 [37]. Among the 1662 patients with Stage I–III disease, 91 patients received adjuvant therapy with cytotoxic therapy or somatostatin analogs. Five-year relapse-free survival (RFS) and OS in the patients who received adjuvant therapy was 49% and 83%, respectively. Five-year RFS and OS in the patients who received no adjuvant therapy was 81% and 89%, respectively. Notably, there was imbalance in certain high-risk tumor characteristics (higher Ki-67 index %, mitoses, lymph node positivity, clinical jaundice, hypoalbuminemia) between patients who received adjuvant therapy and those who did not with patients who received adjuvant therapy being enriched for a number of these features [38].

The single ongoing study in this space is the NeoLuPaNET study [NCT 04385992]. This is a single arm phase II study of neoadjuvant PRRT with ^{177}Lu-dotatate in resectable pancreatic NETs with high risk features. Some of the key eligibility criteria for patients includes primary tumor size >4 cm, Ki-67 index >10%, resectable disease with some vascular involvement and lymph node involvement. The primary outcomes of the study are 90-day postoperative mortality and 90-day postoperative morbidity and the secondary outcome of the study is radiographic response. Several other studies were initiated; however, they have been terminated due to slow accrual. The TERAVECT study was a randomized phase III study, which randomized resected small intestinal NET patients with oligometastatic disease to the liver to PRRT to ^{111}In-pentetreotide or observation. The study was terminated as only four patients were enrolled over a 2-year period. Another study (NCT02031536) was designed as a double-blinded randomized phase II trial that allocated patients with resected liver-limited pancreatic NETs to everolimus or placebo. This study accrued only two patients over a 3-year period. Finally, the NEO-LEBE study [NCT01201096] was a single-arm prospective case control study of PRRT prior to liver transplantation in gastrointestinal NETs with liver metastases (< 50% hepatic tumor burden). No updates have been provided for this study since 2010.

Bronchial NETs

A retrospective analysis querying the National Cancer Data Base, assessed outcomes in typical lung NET patients with lymph node involvement who were treated with adjuvant chemotherapy post-lobectomy [39]. Of the 4612 patients identified, 629 had positive lymph node involvement; 37 of these patients received adjuvant chemotherapy. No baseline differences existed between patients who did and did not receive adjuvant chemotherapy. After propensity matching, no significant difference in 5-year survival was observed between the patient groups (69.7% versus

80.9%, $p = 0.096$). The specific chemotherapy regimen that patients received was not specified.

The role for adjuvant chemotherapy in atypical lung NETs was also explored in a retrospective National Cancer Data Base analysis [40]. A total of 581 patients with resected atypical lung NETs were identified of whom 62.5% were found to be node negative while 37.5% had node positive disease. Adjuvant chemotherapy was utilized in 4.1% of patients with node negative disease and 40.8% of patients with node positive disease. Of propensity matched node positive patients, 1 year-survival was no different between patients who did and did not receive chemotherapy ($p = 0.15$). Five-year survival appeared to favor the patients who received chemotherapy; however this difference was not statistically significant (72.5% versus 47.9%, $p = 0.15$). Among propensity-matched patients with node negative disease, no difference in 1-year and 5-year survival was seen between the adjuvant and no treatment arms.

Recommendations from Consensus Guideline Panels

None of the consensus guidelines strongly advocate for perioperative therapy. The North American Neuroendocrine Tumor Society guidelines do not definitively recommend neoadjuvant or adjuvant therapy for well-differentiated NETs citing the lack of data for these approaches at this time [41]. The European Neuroendocrine Tumor Society guidelines also do not support the routine use of adjuvant therapy for resected well-differentiated GEP NETs given the lack of prospective evidence; however, do suggest consideration of neoadjuvant treatment for local pancreatic NETs with high risk features instead of upfront surgery [42]. The National Comprehensive Cancer Network guidelines do not suggest any adjuvant therapy for resected GEP NETs; however, do recommend consideration of cytotoxic chemotherapy for resected atypical lung NETs (category 2B recommendation) [43]. Thus, routine use of perioperative therapy in GI and lung NETs should not be considered standard of care at this time and on occasion, may be considered after multidisciplinary discussion.

Challenges and Future Directions

Several pertinent challenges exist concerning designing perioperative studies for NET patients. Firstly, although the incidence of NETs is rising, they are still relatively rare tumors. Also, a significant proportion of NET patients continue to be diagnosed with unresectable, metastatic disease at diagnosis, precluding consideration of these approaches. Furthermore, given the differences in biology and clinical outcomes, it is likely that trials would need to be done separately for NETs arising from different sites such as pancreas and small intestine. Together, these factors pose limitations on the number of patients who can be enrolled onto trials and thus the study sizes. Study sizes may be reduced by adopting one or both of two approaches: (a) by increasing event rate (recurrences) by limiting study populations to those at the highest risk of recurrence and (b) by evaluating therapies that provide the highest chance of benefit toward reducing the number needed to treat. There has been significant progress made in the systemic therapy of NETs with several therapies showing impressive improvements in progression-free survival of metastatic patients. The NETTER-1 trial evaluating PRRT vs octreotide LAR in small bowel NETs reduced the risk of progression by 79% corresponding to a hazard ratio, HR, of 0.21 and showed a trend toward improvement in OS [44]. The ECOG 2211 study demonstrated an improved PFS in patients treated with capecitabine to temozolomide compared to those treated with temozolomide with a HR of 0.58, and also a trend toward improvement in OS [45]. Impressively, both trials had active control arms and likely would have shown even more significant improvements against placebo, as would be the case in an adjuvant trial. There are rapidly accumulating data as discussed above evaluating histopathological factors and molecular features that may help identify patients at the highest risk of recurrence. Acknowledging the hurdles associated with enrollment, broad consensus must be obtained during the planning stages of potential adjuvant studies and be conducted through the National Cancer Institute's Cooperative groups or international consortiums. These studies should also incorporate interim analyses for futility and/or efficacy or may also consider adaptive designs that can use accumulating data to decide how to modify design aspects without undermining the validity and integrity of the study. Secondly, as discussed above, recurrences in patients with resected NETs may occur up to 10–15 years. Also, the indolent clinical course even after metastatic spread coupled with the recent improvements in systemic therapies has resulted in prolonged OS of up to 10 years at some sites [1]. In this context, the work by multiple groups evaluating outcomes over shorter periods and developing nomograms for recurrence post-resection should be used to identify and validate robust surrogate endpoints for DFS and OS. Thirdly, limited cytoreductive treatment options exist for NET patients outside of capecitabine plus temozolomide and PRRT; whether therapies such as somatostatin analogs and tyrosine kinase inhibitors (everolimus, sunitinib) would have activity in the adjuvant setting is uncertain. Efforts are ongoing toward developing preclinical models for testing adjuvant therapies in multiple solid tumors and similar efforts should be carried out in NETs as well building on available models such as RipTag, and those recapitulating the MEN-1 biological milieu [46]. Although the confluence of these issues hinder perioperative studies in NETs, the plethora of recent advances in systemic therapies and in understanding the biologic underpinnings of NETs coupled with the long-standing tradition of fruitful collaborative efforts among NET researchers will hopefully bear fruit soon.

References

1. Dasari A, Shen C, Halperin D, Zhao B, Zhou Z, Xu Y, et al. Trends in the incidence, prevalence, and survival outcomes in patients with neuroendocrine tumors in the United States. JAMA Oncol. 2017;3(10):1335–42.
2. Chauhan A, Kohn E, Del Rivero J. Neuroendocrine tumors-less well known, often misunderstood, and rapidly growing in incidence. JAMA Oncol. 2020;6(1) 21–2.

3. Yao JC, Hassan M, Phan A, Dagohoy C, Leary C, Mares J, et al. One hundred years after "carcinoid": epidemiology of and prognostic factors for neuroendocrine tumors in 35,825 cases in the United States. J Clin Oncol. 2008;26(18):3063–72.

4. Hallet J, Law C, Cukier M, Saskin R, Liu N, Singh S. Exploring the rising incidence of neuroendocrine tumors: a population-based analysis of epidemiology, metastatic presentation, and outcomes. Cancer. 2015;121(4):589–97.

5. Al-Batran S, Homann N, Pauligk C, Goetze T, Meiler J, Kasper S, et al. Lancet. 2019;393(10184):1948–57.

6. Conroy T, Hammel P, Hebbar M, Abdelghani M, Wei A, Raoul J, et al. FOLFIRINOX or gemcitabine as adjuvant therapy for pancreatic cancer. N Engl J Med. 2018;379(25):2395–406.

7. van Hagen P, Hulshof M, van Lanschot J, Steyerberg E, Henegouwen v WB, et al. Preoperative chemoradiotherapy for esophageal or junctional cancer. N Engl J Med. 2012;366:2074–84.

8. Grothey A, Sobrero A, Shields A, Yoshino T, Paul J, Paul J, et al. Duration of adjuvant chemotherapy for stage III colon cancer. N Engl J Med. 2018;378:1177–88.

9. Singh S, Chan D, Moody L, Liu N, Fischer H, Austin P, et al. Recurrence in resected gastroenteropancreatic neuroendocrine tumors. JAMA Oncol. 2018;4(4):583–5.

10. Cives M, Anaya D, Soares H, Coppola D, Strosberg J. Analysis of postoperative recurrence in stage I–III midgut neuroendocrine tumors. J Natl Cancer Inst. 2018;110(3):282–9.

11. Lou F, Sarkaria I, Pietanza C, Healy D, Rusch V, Huang J, et al. Recurrence of pulmonary carcinoid tumors after resection: implications for postoperative surveillance. Ann Thorac Surg. 2013;96(4):1156–62.

12. Lee P, Osakwe N, Narula N, Port J, Paul S, Stiles B, et al. Predictors of disease-free survival and recurrence in patients with resected bronchial carcinoid tumors. Thorac Cardiovasc Surg. 2016;64(2):159–65.

13. Singh S, Moody L, Chan D, Metz D, Strosberg J, Amis T, et al. Follow-up recommendations for completely resected gastroenteropancreatic neuroendocrine tumors. JAMA Oncol. 2018;4(11):1597–604.

14. Zaidi M, Lopez-Aguilar A, Switchenko J, Lipscomb J, Andreasi V, Partelli S, et al. A novel validated recurrence risk score to guide a pragmatic surveillance strategy after resection of pancreatic neuroendocrine tumors. Ann Surg. 2019;270(3):422–33.

15. Tsutumi K, Ohtsuka T, Fujino M, Nakshima H, Aishima S, Ueda J, et al. Analysis of risk factors for recurrence after curative resection of well-differentiated pancreatic neuroendocrine tumors based on the new grading classification. J Hepatobiliary Pancreatic Sci. 2014;21(6):418–25.

16. Genc CG, Falconi M, Partelli S, Muffatti F, van Eeden S, Doglioni C, et al. Recurrence of pancreatic neuroendocrine tumors and survival predicted by Ki67. Ann Surg Oncol. 2018;25(8):2467–74.

17. Lopez-Aguilar A, Ethun C, Zaidi M, Rocha F, Poultsides G, Dillhoff M, et al. The conundrum of < 2-cm pancreatic neuroendocrine tumors: a preoperative risk score to predict lymph node metastases and guide surgical management. Surgery. 2019;166(1):15–21.

18. Sallinen V, Le Large T, Tieftrunk E, Galeev S, Kovalenko Z, Haugvik S, et al. Prognosis of sporadic resected small (≤2 cm) nonfunctional pancreatic neuroendocrine tumors – a multi-institutional study. HPB (Oxford). 2017;20(3):251–9.

19. Mansour J, Chavin K, Morris-Stiff G, Warner S, Cardona K, et al. Management of asymptomatic, well-differentiated PNETs: results of the Delphi consensus process of the Americas Hepato-Pancreato-Biliary Association. HPB (Oxford). 2019;21(5):515–23.

20. Kim J, Brosnan-Cashman J, An S, Kim S, Song K, Kim M, et al. Alternative lengthening of telomeres in primary pancreatic neuroendocrine tumors is associated with aggressive clinical behavior and poor survival. Clin Cancer Res. 2017;23(6):1598–606.

21. Singhi A, Liu T, Roncaioli J, et al. Alternative lengthening of telomeres and loss of DAXX/ATRX expression predicts metastatic disease and poor survival in patients with pancreatic neuroendocrine tumors. Clin Cancer Res. 2017;23(2):600–9.

22. Cejas P, Drier Y, Dreijerink K, Lodewijk DV, Epstein C, et al. Enhancer signatures stratify and predict outcomes of non-functional pancreatic neuroendocrine tumors. Nat Med. 2019;25(8):1260–5.

23. Karpathakis A, Dibra H, Pipinkas C, Feber A, Morris T, Francis J, et al. Prognostic impact of novel molecular subtypes of small intestinal neuroendocrine tumor. Clin Cancer Res. 2016;22(1):250–8.
24. Stalberg P, Westin G, Thirlwell C. Genetics and epigenetics in small intestinal neuroendocrine tumours. J Intern Med. 2016;280(6):584–94.
25. Shi X, Xu X, Zhang Y, Gao S, Li B, Ma H, et al. Using long-acting somatostatin analogue as adjuvant therapy for post resection grade 2 pancreatic neuroendocrine tumor: interim results from an ongoing multicenter real-world study in China. ENETS. 2019; Abstract #2899
26. Squires M, Worth P, Konda B, Shah M, Dillhoff M, Abdel-Misih S, et al. Neoadjuvant capecitabine/temozolomide for locally advanced or metastatic pancreatic neuroendocrine tumors. Pancreas. 2020;49(3):355–60.
27. Prakash L, Bhosale P, Cloyd J, Kim M, Parker N, Yao J, et al. Role of fluorouracil, doxorubicin, and streptozocin therapy in the preoperative treatment of localized pancreatic neuroendocrine tumors. J Gastrointest Surg. 2017;21(1):155–63.
28. Kouvaraki M, Ajani J, Hoff P, Wolff R, Evans D, Lozano R, et al. Fluorouracil, doxorubicin, and streptozocin in the treatment of patients with locally advanced and metastatic pancreatic endocrine carcinomas. J Clin Oncol. 2004;22(23):4762–71.
29. Lam M, Rogers J, Halperin D, Dagohoy C, Yao J, Dasari A. Outcomes with 5-Fluorouracil, Doxorubicin, and Streptozocin (FAS) and subsequent therapies in patients with well differentiated Pancreatic Neuroendocrine Tumors (PanNETs). Pancreas. 2019;48(3):427–57.
30. Perysinakis I, Aggeli C, Kaltsas G, Zografos G. Neoadjuvant therapy for advanced pancreatic neuroendocrine tumors: an emerging treatment modality? Hormones (Athens). 2016;15(1):15–22.
31. Sabet A, Biersack H-J, Ezziddin S, et al. Advances in peptide receptor radionuclide therapy. Semin Nucl Med. 2016;46(1):40–6.
32. Sowa-Staszczak A, Hubalewska-Dydejczyk A, Tomaszuk M. PRRT as neoadjuvant treatment in NET. Recent Results Cancer Res. 2013;194:479–85.
33. van Vliet E, van Eijick C, de Krijger R, Nieveen van Dijkum E, Teunissen J, Kam B, et al. Neoadjuvant treatment of nonfunctioning pancreatic neuroendocrine tumors with [177Lu-DOTA0,Tyr3]Octreotate. J Nucl Med. 2015;56(11):1647–53.
34. Partelli S, Bertani E, Bartolomei M, Perali C, Muffati F, Maria Grana C, et al. Peptide receptor radionuclide therapy as neoadjuvant therapy for resectable or potentially resectable pancreatic neuroendocrine neoplasms. Surgery. 2018;163(4):761–7.
35. Xie H, Liu J, Yadav S, Keutgen X, Hobday T, Strosberg J, et al. The role of perioperative systemic therapy in localized pancreatic neuroendocrine neoplasms. Neuroendocrinology. 2020;110(3–4):234–45.
36. Wang Y, Chauhan A, Ramirez R, Beyer D, Stevens M, Woltering E, et al. Does the addition of adjuvant intraoperative tumor bed chemotherapy during midgut neuroendocrine tumor debulking procedures benefit patients? J Gastrointest Oncol. 2019;10(5) 928–34.
37. Barrett J, Rendell V, Pokrzywa C, Lopez-Aguilar A, Cannon J, Poultsides G, et al. Adjuvant therapy following resection of gastroenteropancreatic neuroendocrine tumors provides no recurrence or survival benefit. J Surg Oncol. 2020;121(7):1067–73.
38. Lamberti G, Manuzzi L, Maggio I, Campana D. Should we lose hope in adjuvant therapy for neuroendocrine tumors?-in response to: adjuvant therapy following resection of gastroenteropancreatic neuroendocrine tumors provides no recurrence or survival benefit. J Surg Oncol. 2020;122(3):570–1.
39. Nussbaum D, Speicher P, Gulack B, Hartwig M, Onaitis M, D'Amico T, et al. Defining the role of adjuvant chemotherapy after lobectomy for typical bronchopulmonary carcinoid tumors. Ann Thorac Surg. 2015;99:428–34.
40. Anderson K, Mulvihill M, Speicher P, D'Amico T, Berry M, Hartwig M, et al. Adjuvant chemotherapy does not confer superior survival in patients with atypical carcinoid tumors. Ann Thorac Surg. 2017;104(4):1221–30.
41. Howe J, Merchant N, Conrad C, Keutgen X, Hallet J, Drebin J, et al. The north American neuroendocrine tumor society consensus paper on the surgical Management of Pancreatic Neuroendocrine Tumors. Pancreas. 2020;49:1–33.

42. Pavel M, Oberg K, Falconi M, Krenning E, Sundin A, Perren A, et al. Gastroenteropancreatic neuroendocrine neoplasms: ESMO clinical practice guidelines for diagnosis, treatment and follow-up. Ann Oncol. 2020;31(7):844–60.
43. NCCN Guidelines Panel. Neuroendocrine and adrenal tumors. Available from: https://www.nccn.org/professionals/physician_gls/pdf/neuroendocrine.pdf.
44. Strosberg J, Haddad G, Wolin E, Hendifar A, Yao J, Chasen B, et al. Phase 3 trial of ^{177}Lu-Dotatate for midgut neuroendocrine tumors. N Engl J Med. 2017;376:125–35.
45. Kunz P, Catalano P, Nimeiri H, Fisher G, Longacre T, Suarez C, et al. A randomized study of temozolomide or temozolomide and capecitabine in patients with advanced pancreatic neuroendocrine tumors: A trial of the ECOGACRIN Cancer Research Group (E2211). J Clin Oncol. 2018;36(15_suppl):4004.
46. Jones G, Manchanda P, Pringle D, Zhang M, Kirschner L. Mouse models of endocrine tumors. Best Pract Res Clin Endocrinol Metab. 2011;24(3):451–60.

Carcinoid Crisis: History, Dogmas, and Data

6

Sarah M. Wonn and Rodney F. Pommier

Introduction

One aspect of operating on patients with neuroendocrine tumors (NETs) that is quite different from all other operations is that the patient may have an intraoperative event known as a carcinoid crisis. Carcinoid crisis has no strict definition, but is characterized by sudden, marked hemodynamic instability, sometimes accompanied by characteristics of carcinoid syndrome, such as flushing or bronchospasm. Carcinoid crisis has been reported to occur spontaneously, during abdominal examinations, procedures such as transesophageal echocardiography, colonoscopy and mammography, tumor biopsy, liver embolization, and operations, including at induction of anesthesia [1–7]. While hypertension and hypotension have been reported during crises, intraoperative crises usually manifests as profound hypotension. This presents a difficult and dangerous problem. The profound hypotension can result in hypoperfusion of vital organs that may lead to acute kidney injury, liver damage, stroke or myocardial infarction. In some instances, it can lead to complete circulatory collapse and death. Not surprisingly, the occurrence of intraoperative carcinoid crisis has been associated with increased risk of both minor and major postoperative complications [8, 9].

It is well known that NETs synthesize and release a variety of vasoactive compounds including serotonin, histamine, bradykinin, tachykinin, kallikrein and a host of others [10–13]. These compounds are associated with carcinoid syndrome. Early reports of carcinoid crisis involved patients with carcinoid syndrome and authors

S. M. Wonn
Department of Surgery, Oregon Health & Science University, Portland, OR, USA
e-mail: wonn@ohsu.edu

R. F. Pommier (✉)
Division of Surgical Oncology, Department of Surgery, Oregon Health & Science University, Portland, OR, USA
e-mail: pommierr@ohsu.edu

© Springer Nature Switzerland AG 2021
J. M. Cloyd, T. M. Pawlik (eds.), *Neuroendocrine Tumors*,
https://doi.org/10.1007/978-3-030-62241-1_6

assumed it was a severe manifestation of carcinoid syndrome [1]. These early reports hypothesized that the underlying mechanism of carcinoid crisis is a sudden, massive release of those hormones [1]. This theory has largely prevailed to the present day but has never been proven.

Based on this theory, various efforts have been made to reduce the incidence of intraoperative carcinoid crisis through administration of specific pharmacologic agents, such as anxiolytics and antihistamines, while avoiding administration of others, such as catecholamines which are believed to provoke endogenous release of hormones [14, 15]. Over time, however, the mainstay of management of carcinoid crisis has shifted to prophylactic administration of the somatostatin analog octreotide [16]. Recommendations for prophylactic use of octreotide abound but vary widely with respect to dose, route of administration, timing and duration of administration, and patient selection, detailed later in this chapter.

Data supporting the use of these prophylactic regimens are scant. The literature on the topic of carcinoid crisis, in general, is quite limited as these events are unpredictable and life-threatening. Much of it is in the form of single case reports which do not allow determinations of the incidence of or clinical risk factors for crisis and their comments about the etiology of crisis and effects or lack of effects of various treatments must be interpreted with great caution. Literature on intraoperative carcinoid crisis is also scant but, because some is in the form of case series, has provided some valuable information on incidence, risk factors, and outcomes. To date, seven single institution retrospective case series and one single institution prospective case series have been published [8, 9, 17–22].

Many statements about carcinoid crisis have been made within this body of literature. Some have become dogmas including: crisis is caused by massive release of carcinoid hormones (with serotonin being the chief suspect), crisis occurs only in patients with carcinoid syndrome, octreotide is the best treatment to prevent and treat crisis, antihistamines should also be used to prevent and treat crisis, and catecholamines worsen or provoke crisis and should not be given to patients with carcinoid syndrome.

This chapter will review the literature on carcinoid crisis, particularly intraoperative crisis during abdominal operations and provide the reader with a distillation of the data that have been published on this topic. In the course of review, it will seek out the origins of some of the dogmas and analyze whether they are actually supported or refuted by more recent findings.

History of Carcinoid Crisis

Carcinoid syndrome was first described in 1954 in a series of 16 patients with a diverse constellation of symptoms including patchy peculiar flushing, diarrhea, malar telangiectasia, right-sided heart failure, edema, abdominal pain, and bronchial asthma [23]. The authors implicated serotonin as the hormone responsible for many of these findings. Indeed, it was subsequently established that patients with carcinoid syndrome had a high prevalence of elevated levels of

5-hydroxyindolacetic acid (5-HIAA), the breakdown product of serotonin, in 24-hour collections of their urine and some patients also had elevated levels of urinary histamine [24]. However, reports soon followed which questioned the role of serotonin in flushing. Very few patients demonstrated elevation of serum serotonin or its metabolites in serum or urine after spontaneous flushing episodes [25–27]. Some patients with severe flushing had normal urinary 5-HIAA levels [25, 27]. Intravenous injection of serotonin into normal subjects and patients with carcinoid syndrome did not induce flushing [25, 26]. In addition, the serotonin antagonists cyproheptadine and methysergide were ineffective at controlling flushing [11, 27]. What could be shown was that patients with carcinoid flushing exhibited elevated levels of bradykinin and kallikrein in their hepatic venous blood and such elevations could be provoked with intravenous injections of epinephrine, which were accompanied by flushing. Thus, it wasn't clear which hormones were responsible for flushing, but data actually supported bradykinin and kallekrein rather than serotonin.

The first report of "carcinoid crisis" was published in 1964 [1]. It described a 41 year-old woman admitted to the hospital with liver metastases and carcinoid syndrome, including carcinoid heart disease, years after resection of an ileal primary tumor. On the 13th hospital day, she left to visit her family but, 15 minutes after returning to the ward, she had sudden onset of apprehension, oppressive chest pain, excruciating abdominal cramps, frequent diarrhea, facial flushing, pale cold extremities and cyanotic nail beds. Of note, although her apical cardiac impulse was strong and rapid, her peripheral pulses were absent and a blood pressure could not be recorded. She was not responsive to doses of metaraminol, an alpha-adrenergic agonist with some beta effect, nor the beta-adrenergic agonist norepinephrine. Over the next hour, her symptoms of apprehension, flushing, and burning and itching skin worsened. She was then given a single intravenous dose of cyproheptadine, after which there was dramatic relief of her chest and abdominal pain. A few minutes later, her femoral pulse became transiently palpable. Thirty minutes later, she had a normal blood pressure and peripheral pulses. Her symptoms (but not hypotension) returned twelve hours later but were again relieved with cyproheptadine. A norepinephrine infusion was continued for 15 hours, during which her blood pressure remained stable. The patient had been having daily measurement of her 24-hour urinary 5-HIAA levels and the level on the day of the crisis was higher than on any previous day.

While this may have been the first report of carcinoid crisis by that name, the authors point out as background in the first sentence of their manuscript that profound hypotension in patients with carcinoid syndrome had been noted during anesthesia and palpation of the tumor at operation; clear references to intraoperative carcinoid crises [28–31]. The authors point out that the mechanism of hypotension was not clear in those cases but an excessive amount of circulating serotonin was assumed to be a major causative factor. They did not know what triggered the crisis in their patient either, but noted the patient's consumption of tryptophan, a precursor to serotonin, had been changed from 300 to 1200 mg per day on the day of the crisis. They also thought it possible she had a surge of serotonin from tumor necrosis, but cite the literature described above reporting that a rise in patients' serum serotonin levels during flushing episodes were infrequent in previous research. They doubted histamine played a role. They found it interesting that the patient had relief of her symptoms with the serotonin antagonist cyproheptadine but her blood pressure did not respond to it nor to adrenergic vasopressors. They cited literature that patients with carcinoid syndrome had been reported to experience transient flushing and significant reductions in blood pressure when receiving intravenous norepinephrine and epinephrine [25, 26]. Therefore, they stated that when the need for vasopressor therapy arises in a patient with carcinoid syndrome, the use of norepinephrine and epinephrine should be avoided.

Although this first report is not an actual intraoperative crisis, it is similar in that it is a profound hypotensive crisis. This case report exemplified many of the dogmas listed earlier. This report likely contributed to the dogmas that persist to the present day including that patients in crisis do not respond to beta-adrenergic agonists like norepinephrine and epinephrine, that they worsen crises, and that they should not be administered to patients with carcinoid syndrome. This is curious given the fact that they administered a continuous intravenous infusion of norepinephrine to their patient for 15 hours with the result being stable blood pressure and no secondary hypotensive crises were triggered. Although they reported that her symptoms of apprehension and flushing, burning, and itching skin increased after norepinephrine, they did not report worsening of her hypotension.

It should also be noted that this patient had carcinoid heart disease, which could have significantly altered the interpretations of the events. Patients with carcinoid heart disease are very sensitive to loss of cardiac pre-load and can be extremely difficult to resuscitate from any hypotensive event, regardless of the etiology. The usual pattern of carcinoid heart disease consists of marked tricuspid insufficiency with the pulmonic valve exhibiting a combination of stenosis and regurgitation. This results in reflux of blood back out of the right heart into the venous circulation with each heartbeat and, as a result, the delivery of intravenous drugs to the systemic circulation can be significantly delayed. Therefore, apparent lack of responses and timing of responses to intravenous drugs administered in this case are all questionable. Although it appears the patient did have timely relief of symptoms and a transient return of pulses with the intravenous administration of the cyproheptadine, note that her pulses and blood pressure did not return to normal for another 30 minutes. So, it is difficult to know whether to ascribe their return to cyproheptadine, the norepinephrine given prior to it, or simply spontaneous recovery.

The elevated 24-hour urinary 5-HIAA level on the day of the crisis also seems to lend credence to the theory of massive release of hormones as the pathophysiologic origin of the crisis. However, examination of the graph published in their manuscript shows that while the level was about 550 mg per 24 hours on the day of the crisis, it had been typically above 400 mg per 24 hours and as high as 480 mg per 24 hours during the 12 preceding days without a crisis. Does that degree of rise support the theory of massive release? Also, if catecholamines trigger release of hormones like serotonin, then the urinary 5-HIAA levels would be expected to be higher on a day when the patient has received a continuous norepinephrine infusion for 15 hours.

In 1976, Mason and Steane published a comprehensive review of the literature on patients with carcinoid syndrome undergoing anesthesia. They found a total of 40 operations reported in nine papers. The incidence of intraoperative complications, including hypotension, bronchospasm, or hypertension was very high, occurring in 27 (54%) cases [32].

Treatment of Carcinoid Crisis with Octreotide

The first report of using octreotide to treat carcinoid crisis came from Kvols et al. at the Mayo Clinic in 1985, first as a letter to the editor of the New England Journal of Medicine and subsequently published in manuscript form [7, 33]. Dr. Kvols was investigating octreotide for treatment of carcinoid syndrome and had given lectures on its effects at the Mayo Clinic. A patient with small bowel NET causing stenosis of the ileum and liver metastases with carcinoid syndrome was taken to the operating room by Dr. Martin for primary tumor resection and ligation of the hepatic artery to induce necrosis of metastases to improve carcinoid syndrome symptoms. Minutes after induction of anesthesia as the abdominal skin was being prepared, the patient experienced flushing on the abdominal skin followed by profound, life-threatening hypotension. No blood pressure could be obtained and only the carotid pulse was palpable. The authors report the patient did not respond to intravenous fluids, intravenous calcium, nor intravenous conventional vasopressors, including neosynephrine and, eventually, epinephrine. Dr. Martin knew of the work Dr. Kvols was doing with octreotide and had him paged. When Dr. Kvols responded, Dr. Martin told him of the situation and asked if he could bring some octreotide to the operating room. Dr. Kvols sped to the investigational pharmacy, procured some octreotide and took it to the operating room. Several minutes after the onset of the crisis, the patient was given an intravenous dose of 50 µg of octreotide, which was repeated 15 seconds later. Thirty to 40 seconds later, the patient had bounding pulses and blood pressure returned to normal. About five minutes later, the flushing resolved. The authors state that the response to octreotide was dramatic and life-saving and recommended octreotide be kept available in the operating room during operations on patients with carcinoid syndrome.

Similar to the first case, interpretation of the timing of administration of pharmacologic agents and response are an issue in this case. In the graph of blood pressure versus time in the manuscript, a V-shaped dip of blood pressure is shown down to zero at the vertex and then rapid recovery. The graph indicates that octreotide was administered at the nadir of the blood pressure, which then immediately began to rise. It also indicates epinephrine was administered 3.5 minutes before the nadir and the octreotide administration. So, is the rise in blood pressure really an almost instantaneous effect of the octreotide administration, or was the epinephrine delivered earlier finally being distributed and taking effect? Or was it a combination of the two? This report further strengthened the dogma against the use of beta-adrenergic agonists.

The recommendation to treat crises with octreotide raises a very important question that is never answered. How would octreotide work to reverse an ongoing crisis? This is particularly difficult to explain in view of the theory that crisis is due to sudden massive release of hormones. Octreotide does inhibit the synthesis and release of vasoactive compounds from NET cells. But if a crisis is ongoing, then the hormones have already been released. Octreotide is not a hormone receptor blocker, so it cannot block the effects of hormones already released. It could be argued that crisis requires continued massive release of hormones to be sustained. Therefore, octreotide could inhibit the release of additional hormones and eventually relieve the crisis. But that doesn't adequately explain the rapid reversal of crises that has been reported [14, 33–35]. It would still take some time for hormones already released to be metabolized before the crisis would abate, let alone for the vascular system to reset itself to normal from whatever massive perturbation had occurred. Therefore, the dogma of octreotide reversing a crisis on the basis of inhibiting hormone release must be challenged.

The first publication of a large series of operations suggesting that octreotide administration might reduce the incidence of intraoperative carcinoid crisis also came from the Mayo Clinic in 2001 [17]. Kinney et al. reported their experience with 119 patients with metastatic carcinoid tumors undergoing abdominal operations between 1983 and 1996. Octreotide became available after Food and Drug Administration approval in 1988 and they began administering it both preoperatively and intraoperatively to some patients, likely spurred by their prior case report. Accordingly, some received no octreotide, some received a preoperative dose, and some received an intraoperative dose, either with or without a preoperative dose. Seventy percent of the patients had preoperative diarrhea and 64% had preoperative flushing.

They reviewed patients' records for what they termed as intraoperative complications, which included flushing, urticaria, ventricular dysrhythmias, bronchospasm, acidosis, hypoxemia, hypotension, systolic blood pressure (SBP) <80 mm Hg for >10 minutes, and total duration of sustained tachycardia. They also recorded perioperative complications and deaths. They found that 15 patients experienced a perioperative complication, including death in three. Among those 15 patients, eight had one or more intraoperative complications including flushing in four, sustained hypotension in two, and bronchospasm, acidosis, and ventricular tachycardia in one patient each. They found that eight of 73 patients (11%) who did not receive any octreotide and one of six patients (17%) who received only preoperative octreotide had an intraoperative complication. However, none of the 45 patients who received intraoperative octreotide had an intraoperative complication. The difference in intraoperative complications between the 45 patients who received intraoperative octreotide and the 73 who received none was statistically significant. They concluded that that the administration of intraoperative octreotide was associated with a decreased incidence of those intraoperative complications.

Octreotide Prophylaxis

Two years after the report by Kinney et al., two surgeons from the Mayo Clinic published a manuscript on hepatic surgery for NET metastases in which they claimed that preoperative preparation of patients with a dose of 150–500 µg of octreotide decreases the chance of carcinoid crisis [36]. However, no data supporting this claim were provided. Soon, numerous recommendations for prophylactic octreotide regimens also emerged within the literature. They varied widely in terms of dose, route of administration, timing and duration. A textbook of endocrine surgery stated that preoperative administration of octreotide LAR alone essentially eliminates the risk of crisis [37]. Others recommended a preoperative dose of 250–500 µg [36, 38]. Still others recommended subcutaneous administration of 100 µg of octreotide three times per day for two weeks prior to operation and then 100 µg administered intravenously at the induction of anesthesia [39]. The North American Neuroendocrine Tumor Society (NANETS) recommended continuous intravenous infusion at doses of 50–500 µg per hour [40]. Guidelines from the United Kingdom recommended beginning a continuous infusion of intravenous octreotide at a dose of 50 µg per hour for 12 hours prior to and continued at least 48 hours after operation [41]. Many authors recommended having additional vials of octreotide available for intravenous administration if crises still arose during the operation. Generally, these recommendations were made only for patients with carcinoid syndrome [39, 42]. However, data supporting any of these regimens were lacking. For example, the references supporting the NANETS guidelines of continuous infusion of octreotide were two single case reports in which infusions were given and no events occurred during those cases [16, 43].

Given that the claim about prophylactic octreotide reducing the incidence of carcinoid crisis came from the Mayo Clinic, it is logical to conclude that the concept arose from and is supported by the earlier report by Kinney et al. from the same institution. Indeed, it is quite common to see the report by Kinney et al. referenced as evidence for prophylactic octreotide on slides at conferences and in the literature. However, this single institution retrospective review should not be used as supportive evidence for the efficacy of prophylactic octreotide. An intraoperative complication still occurred in one of the six patients given only a preoperative dose, yielding a rate of intraoperative complications similar to that seen among the 73 who received none. Crises can occur with induction, yet no recommendation was made to administer it prior to induction. The doses of intraoperative octreotide given in their series ranged from 30–4000 µg. So, how much octreotide must be given to prevent a crisis? The timing of intraoperative doses was not specified, so when should it be given to prevent crisis?

Though this report is often used as evidence to support the use of prophylactic octreotide, their conclusions weakly support of the use of octreotide to treat an impending crisis before it progresses to the point of an intraoperative complication. No recommendation is made to give it before induction of anesthesia as it would only be given to those who began exhibiting a crisis at induction. It also explains why there is such a large range of intraoperative doses, as some patients received very little octreotide while others received massive doses for one or multiple impending events. It explains why there is no recommendation for when the dose should be given as it would only be given when there are indications of an impending crisis. The biggest argument against it is that the authors specifically state in the discussion that their study was not able to evaluate the efficacy of intraoperative octreotide to prevent intraoperative carcinoid crises. So, other than an occasional case report where preoperative octreotide was given and nothing occurred during that particular case, there were as yet no published data supporting the concept of octreotide prophylaxis [16, 43].

The Oregon Health & Science University Experience

Recognizing the lack of data on outcomes of various octreotide prophylaxis protocols being recommended, the senior author of this chapter decided to implement octreotide protocols in a somewhat systematic fashion, progressing through preoperative octreotide LAR, preoperative prophylactic doses, intraoperative doses, and eventually the use of continuous intravenous infusion, if necessary. The plan was to periodically analyze the outcomes of these various approaches and modify them accordingly. Based on recommendations in a consensus report in 2004, our initial prophylactic octreotide protocol was to prescribe octreotide LAR preoperatively and administer an additional preoperative dose of 250–500 μg of octreotide either subcutaneously or intravenously prior to induction of anesthesia [44]. Additional vials of octreotide would also be available for intraoperative intravenous administration as boluses of 250–500 μg for treatment of bronchospasm, flushing, or changes in blood pressure or heart rate not attributable to other causes such as blood loss or hypovolemia. At first, this was done only for syndromic patients, but, as will be seen shortly, it was soon discovered that patients without carcinoid syndrome could also have carcinoid crises and the protocol was extended to include all patients.

At Oregon Health & Science University, our first review of carcinoid crisis was published in 2013 on 97 patients undergoing operation [8]. Seventy-five patients (77%) had hepatic metastases and 57 (59%) carried a diagnosis of carcinoid syndrome. Seventy patients (72%) had received preoperative octreotide LAR and 87 (90%) received a preoperative bolus of octreotide, with a median dose of 500 μg. The principal procedure was hepatic resection in 50% of cases. Twenty-three patients (24%) had an intraoperative complication. This is a rate over three times higher than the overall rate of 7% reported at the Mayo Clinic. The most common intraoperative complication was SBP dropping to <80 mm Hg for ≥10 minutes not attributable to any other cause, such as blood loss or hypovolemia, by either the attending surgeon or attending anesthesiologist, which occurred in 18 patients (19%). Marked hemodynamic instability was reported to be a severe carcinoid crisis by either the attending anesthesiologist in the anesthesia record and/or by the attending surgeon in the operative report in an additional five cases (5%). Crises were statistically just as likely to occur in patients without carcinoid syndrome as in patients with syndrome. The only independent predictor of carcinoid crisis was the presence of hepatic metastases, as all crises occurred in patients with them.

Neither preoperative octreotide LAR administration nor a preoperative bolus of octreotide were associated with a statistically significant lower incidence of crises compared to no administration. Fifty-four patients (55%) received intraoperative boluses of octreotide to treat intraoperative hypotension. Despite previous reports of rapid, dramatic improvement in hypotension, 37 of those patients did not respond adequately and also required administration of intravenous vasopressors, including seven who required continuous intravenous infusion of vasopressors. Twenty-six percent of the patients who received intraoperative octreotide experienced another hypotensive event during the operation. Patients who had intraoperative complications were statistically significantly more likely to have postoperative complications. The overall 30-day postoperative complication rate for patients having an intraoperative event was 60.8%, with 39.1% having major complications.

The conclusions of this series were that the rate of intraoperative complications, or crises, is substantial at 23%, that a major risk factor is the presence of liver metastases, that they can occur in patients without carcinoid syndrome, and patients who have them are at markedly increased risk for both minor and major postoperative complications. The most important finding was that neither preoperative octreotide LAR nor preoperative bolus administration of octreotide showed any significant reduction in their occurrence compared to no octreotide therapy.

Following publication of this series, Woltering et al. hypothesized that a preoperative bolus of octreotide, with a half-life of 90–120 minutes, might not last long enough for protection against carcinoid crises during what are typically long operations and that this would be remedied by continuous intravenous infusion [18]. Their practice was to give a preoperative 500 µg bolus followed by an infusion at 500 µg per hour. They reviewed their experience with 179 operations, which had an average duration of 6.3 hours. They reviewed their records for instances of SBP <80 mm Hg for ≥10 minutes, hemodynamic instability, or either the attending surgeon or anesthesiologist having declared that a crisis occurred. They found an incidence of only 3.6%. Thus, this series showed a possible beneficial effect of a continuous octreotide infusion for reducing the incidence of intraoperative carcinoid crisis.

In the meantime, because of the lack of success with our original regimen, we modified it by adding a continuous intravenous infusion of octreotide at 500 µg per hour [19]. We also realized that we had to modify our criteria for declaring crises and initiating treatment of hypotension. Previously, it had been our practice to observe SBP <80 mm Hg for several minutes, to see if it spontaneously resolved, before declaring it to be a crisis and initiating therapy. However, our data showed that the mean time between initiating therapy and having SBP recover to >80 mm Hg was about nine minutes. Patients who were hypotensive for ≥10 minutes were significantly more likely to have postoperative complications. Therefore, we considered it unethical to observe hypotension for more than a minute without initiating therapy.

Our definition of carcinoid crisis was changed to be hemodynamic instability such as SBP <80 or >180 mm Hg, heart rate > than 120 beats per minute, or display of any physiology that, if sustained, would be expected to lead to end organ dysfunction, such as ventricular arrhythmias, or bronchospasm. It had to be unattributable to any other cause, such as hemorrhage, being behind on fluid resuscitation, or compression of the vena cava. Both attending surgeon and attending anesthesiologist had to agree there was no other plausible explanation before declaring a crisis. Upon declaration, therapy was begun immediately. These changes were applied prospectively to the next 150 operations, after which we published our results [19].

We found that the incidence of intraoperative events with continuous octreotide infusion was no lower, at 30%, than it had been without it. Crises again correlated with presence of liver metastases, older age, but also, with this larger sample, carcinoid syndrome and duration of anesthesia. They did not correlate with serum chromogranin A or 24-hour urinary 5-HIAA levels. Again, the predominant type of event was intraoperative hypotension, occurring in 23% of patients. However, immediate treatment had shortened the mean duration of crisis from our previous 19 minutes to 8.9 minutes and they no longer correlated with major postoperative complications, except among the 8% of patients where hypotension still persisted ≥10 minutes. Three operations were aborted due to medically refractory intraoperative carcinoid crises.

The results of our study using continuous infusion do not appear to agree with those of Woltering et al. But perhaps they actually do. Woltering et al. reviewed records only for episodes of hypotension lasting ≥10 minutes. Treatments for hypotension were not reported and events lasting <10 minutes with treatment would not have been captured by their methodology. In our series, hypotensive events lasting ≥10 minutes despite treatment occurred at a rate of 8%, similar to the 3.6% rate they reported. Although continuous infusion of octreotide was not the panacea we had hoped for, this study did show that prompt, aggressive treatment of hypotensive crises can shorten their duration and thereby reduce the rate of subsequent major postoperative complications as well as identify additional risk factors for crises.

Kinney et al. from the Mayo Clinic subsequently published a series in which they used prophylactic octreotide for some patients with liver metastases, a group now known to be high risk for crisis, undergoing partial hepatic resection [20]. The authors created a more stringent definition of carcinoid crisis rather than only hemodynamic instability not attributable to other causes, particularly hypotension, given that there could be multiple other causes for intraoperative hypotension during major operations. Accordingly, they changed their definition of crisis to be sudden or abrupt onset of at least two of the following: flushing or urticaria that is not explained by an allergic reaction, bronchospasm or bronchodilator administration, hypotension (SBP <80 mm Hg for >10 minutes and treated with vasopressors) not explained by volume status or hemorrhage, tachycardia ≥120 beats per minute. Among the 169 cases reviewed, 130 (77%) received a preoperative subcutaneous injection of 500 µg of octreotide and 39 did not, regardless of octreotide LAR use.

Using their new definition, they reported their incidence of intraoperative carcinoid crisis was 0%. It should be noted, however, that sustained hypotension occurred in 5.3% and sustained tachycardia occurred in another 8.9% of patients, but because none of those patients exhibited any other of their criteria, none of these events were declared to be crises. The authors do comment that their review is not able to evaluate the efficacy of octreotide to prevent or ameliorate intraoperative carcinoid crisis. Indeed, within their data set, no treatment with octreotide was statistically just as effective as octreotide at preventing crises when using their new definition. However, based on their clinical experience, the authors did recommend preoperative treatment with octreotide LAR, a preoperative dose of short acting octreotide to reduce hormone release during induction of anesthesia, and having additional octreotide available in the operating room to treat events for patients undergoing hepatic resection.

Another report on the outcomes of prophylactic octreotide was published by Kwon et al. at University of California, San Francisco [9]. They reported on 75 patients, 38 of whom underwent operation and 37 of whom received embolotherapy. They found that the incidence of carcinoid crisis or hemodynamic instability among all patients was 32%, but it was 42% among patients undergoing operation. Neither long acting somatostatin analog therapy, preoperative octreotide, intraoperative octreotide, nor any combination thereof was associated with a lower incidence of crisis or hemodynamic instability. Treatments of hypotension included additional octreotide and vasopressors, but norepinephrine and epinephrine were only rarely given. Patients who had events had a significantly higher incidence of postoperative complications.

Understanding Carcinoid Crisis Physiology

Having been disappointed by the lack of reduction of the incidence of carcinoid crisis by continuous infusion of octreotide, we concluded that determining proper pharmacologic intervention, let alone prophylaxis, for carcinoid crisis was severely hampered by lack of understanding of the actual pathophysiology and identification of the responsible hormones. There were three possible hormonally driven mechanisms for the hypotension. Hormones could cause pulmonary artery vasoconstriction, severely impeding cardiac output. They could constrict coronary vessels or directly affect heart muscle contractility resulting in cardiac failure or cardiogenic shock. Lastly, they could cause peripheral vasodilation.

In order to obtain data about what is actually occurring physiologically and hormonally during carcinoid crisis, we prospectively studied hemodynamic parameters and serum hormone levels during elective major operations on patients with carcinoid tumors [22]. To increase our odds of collecting data during crises, we intentionally selected patients at highest risk based on our previously identified risk factors. These included liver metastases, an anticipated long anesthesia time, and older age. Patients with carcinoid heart disease were excluded. To avoid introducing any new variables, all patients had the same octreotide prophylaxis protocol of preoperative octreotide LAR, a preoperative 500 μg bolus of octreotide, and continuous intravenous infusion of octreotide at 500 μg per hour, as used in our prior study.

Forty-six patients were enrolled and had pulmonary artery catheters inserted to obtain measurements of pulmonary artery pressure, cardiac output, and systemic vascular resistance. They also had transesophageal echocardiography probes inserted to monitor cardiac function. Patients had serial measurement of serum levels of the "usual suspect" carcinoid hormones serotonin, histamine, bradykinin, and kallikrein. Data sets were collected prior to incision, prior to closing, and during any crises declared. We used the same criteria for declaring crises as in the previous study. Seventeen patients experienced intraoperative hypotensive crises. Pulmonary artery pressures exhibited a statistically significant reduction, ruling out pulmonary vascular vasoconstriction as the mechanism. Echocardiography during crises was normal and unchanged from pre-incision parameters, ruling out coronary vasoconstriction or cardiac failure as the mechanism. However, cardiac hypovolemia was consistently observed. Systemic vascular resistance had a statistically significant reduction during crises. Thus the pathophysiology of hypotensive intraoperative carcinoid crisis was consistent with distributive shock.

Serum hormone levels prior to incision exhibited markedly diverse profiles; no two patient profiles looked alike (Fig. 6.1). Many patients had remarkably high serum hormone levels despite the preoperative octreotide LAR, octreotide bolus, and continuous infusion of octreotide and the hormone levels did not change with initiation of an octreotide infusion. The most significant finding was that the mean pre-incision serum serotonin level in patients who had crises was significantly

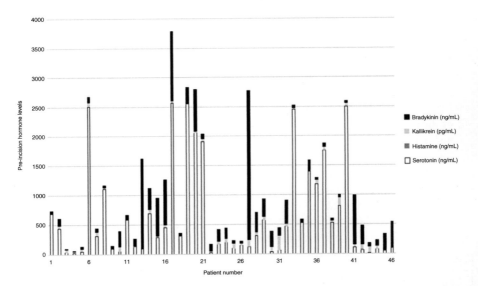

Fig. 6.1 Hormone Profile of Patients with Neuroendocrine Tumors. Levels of pre-incision serotonin, histamine, kallikrein, and bradykinin for 46 patients. (Data from the carcinoid crisis physiology study done at Oregon Health & Science University)

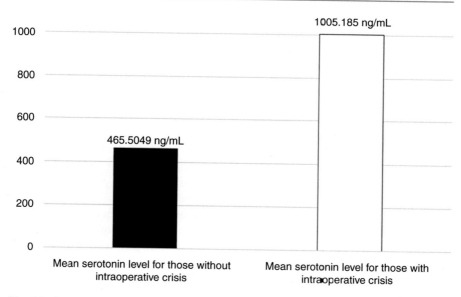

Fig. 6.2 Comparison of Mean Levels of Pre-incision Serotonin. The mean level of serotonin for those without intraoperative carcinoid crisis ($n = 29$) was 465.5 ng/mL and mean level of serotonin for those with intraoperative carcinoid crisis ($n = 17$) was 1005.185 ng/mL, $p < 0.05$. (Data from the carcinoid crisis physiology study done at Oregon Health & Science University)

higher at 1005 nanogram (ng) per milliliter (mL) compared to 496 ng per mL in patients who did not (Fig. 6.2). However, contrary to all expectations, there were no significant changes in the mean values of any of the four hormone levels during crises. In fact, all were somewhat lower. There were also highly significant negative linear correlations between individual pre-incision serotonin levels (and because they did not change during crisis, crisis serotonin levels) and the individual systemic vascular resistance values during crisis. Thus, the higher a patient's serum serotonin level, the lower their systemic vascular resistance was during a hypotensive crisis.

Conclusions drawn from this study were that there is no typical hormone profile for a carcinoid patient and that an elevated pre-incision serum serotonin level is a marker for increased risk of carcinoid crisis as well as the severity of a crisis. The most important conclusion was that, contrary to long standing popular theory, there was no evidence of any sudden massive release of hormones during a crisis. We also took the strong correlations we derived between serum serotonin levels and occurrence of crisis and between reductions in systemic vascular resistance to be strong evidence that the events we were calling hypotensive crises with our new definition were in fact crises and not due to other possible causes of intraoperative hypotension. Furthermore, given that the hormones causing flushing, urticaria, bronchospasm, and hypotension were unknown and given that no surge of any hormones was observed, it seems that requiring another manifestation such as flushing or urticarial to declare a crisis is not realistic. The results of this study greatly weakened the argument for efficacy of prophylactic octreotide. Anecdotally, we have made invasive physiologic observations in a few patients treated with intravenous octreotide during crisis. There was some increase in systemic vascular resistance and a return of some blood to the hypovolemic heart seen on echocardiography. We suspect these findings were due to the vasoconstrictive effect of octreotide on splanchnic vessels, which is well known and why it is used to treat gastrointestinal hemorrhage. So, it may have helped reverse crises in some reports simply because it is another vasopressor, not because it blocks hormone release. However, the treatment for distributive shock is fluids and vasopressors, so it makes more sense to use a vasopressor with wider systemic, not just splanchnic, effects. But if the dogma of not giving catecholamines to patients with carcinoid is to be followed, then the arsenal of available drugs is somewhat limited, particularly for patients in crisis not responding to vasopressin or alpha-adrenergic pressors.

Accordingly we also examined the dogma that beta-adrenergic agonists should be avoided due to the possibility of causing crises. Many doses of vasopressors have been given to treat hypotensive crises at our institution, and in some instances we had been forced to give beta-adrenergic agonists such as ephedrine, norepinephrine and epinephrine when patients failed to respond to other agents, such as vasopressin and phenylephrine. Reviewing our data, we analyzed the hemodynamic parameters for the 15 minute period after administration of over 800 doses of pressor agents [45]. We found that patients responded just as well to beta-adrenergic agonists as to other pressors. Blood pressure recovered quickly with their administration, usually under our 10 minute time limit, which is remarkable given that they were usually withheld until eight or nine minutes into a crisis. Furthermore, no worsening of crisis or secondary crises were ever observed after administration of beta-adrenergic agonists. Therefore, we believe that, contrary to dogma, beta-adrenergic agents should be administered when standard measures fail.

Conclusions

So, what do we really know about intraoperative carcinoid crisis? We know that it has no strict or universally accepted definition, but it is clear that a substantial percentage of patients (~25%) have sudden marked hemodynamic instability (ie profound hypotension) during anesthesia and operations. It may or may not be accompanied by other components of carcinoid syndrome. Risk factors for these events are the presence of liver metastases, carcinoid syndrome, long anesthesia time, and older age, but they can occur in any patient, even those without syndrome, at any point in an operation. These events are associated with increased risk of postoperative complications, particularly if they continue for ≥10 minutes. Prompt, aggressive treatment with fluids and vasopressors can shorten crisis duration and reduce postoperative complication rates. Despite numerous published recommendations and protocols, the data supporting prevention or reduction of carcinoid crisis by administration of prophylactic octreotide, as a whole, are weak or lacking. The theory that sudden massive release of hormones such as serotonin, histamine bradykinin and kallikrein occurs during crises is not supported by data. However, patients who have crises do have significantly higher pre-incision serum serotonin levels than patients who do not. High serum serotonin levels are a marker for increased risk and severity of crisis, but apparently not directly causative. The pathophysiology of crisis is one of distributive shock, for which the proper treatment is fluids and vasopressors agents and the effect of octreotide seen during treatment of crisis may be due to its effect as a splanchnic vasoconstrictor, not as an inhibitor of hormone release. Administration of beta-adrenergic agents like ephedrine, norepinephrine and epinephrine during crises is safe with rapid response of blood pressure, no worsening of crises and no triggering of secondary crises.

Based on our research, at Oregon Health & Science University, we have entirely stopped using octreotide during operations, relying instead on vasopressors, including beta-adrenergic agonists and a report on outcomes of 195 consecutive cases managed without octreotide is forthcoming. Our next line of research into this challenging but fascinating topic will be a clinical trial using preoperative doses of the serotonin converting enzyme inhibitor telotristat ethyl. One of the objectives will be to see if such treatment substantially lowers elevated pre-incision levels of serum serotonin toward the mean values we have associated with a lower risk of intraoperative crisis. If it does, it will be interesting to see if that change will also be associated with a lower incidence of intraoperative hypotensive carcinoid crisis.

References

1. Kahil ME, Brown H, Fred HL. The carcinoid crisis. Arch Intern Med. 1964;114:26–8.
2. Morrisroe K, Sim IW, McLachlan K, Inder WJ. Carcinoid crisis induced by repeated abdominal examination. Intern Med J. 2012;42(3):342–4.
3. Janssen M, Salm EF, Breburda CS, van Woerkens LJ, de Herder WW, v/d Zwaan C, et al. Carcinoid crisis during transesophageal echocardiography. Intensive Care Med. 2000;26(2):254.
4. Ozgen A, Demirkazik FB, Arat A, Arat AR. Carcinoid crisis provoked by mammographic compression of metastatic carcinoid tumour of the breast. Clin Radiol. 2001;56(3):250–1.
5. Magabe PC, Bloom AL. Sudden death from carcinoid crisis during image-guided biopsy of a lung mass. J Vasc Interv Radiol. 2014;25(3):484–7.
6. Fujie S, Zhou W, Fann P, Yen Y. Carcinoid crisis 24 hours after bland embolization: a case report. Biosci Trends. 2010;4(3):143–4.
7. Kvols LK, Martin JK, Marsh HM, Moertel CG. Rapid reversal of carcinoid crisis with a somatostatin analogue. N Engl J Med. 1985;313(19):1229–30.
8. Massimino K, Harrskog O, Pommier S, Pommier R. Octreotide LAR and bolus octreotide are insufficient for preventing intraoperative complications in carcinoid patients. J Surg Oncol. 2013;107(8):842–6.
9. Kwon DH, Paciorek A, Mulvey CK, Chan H, Fidelman N, Meng L, et al. Periprocedural management of patients undergoing liver resection or embolotherapy for neuroendocrine tumor metastases. Pancreas. 2019;48(4):496–503.
10. Mason DT, Melmon KL. New understanding of the mechanism of the carcinoid flush. Ann Intern Med. 1966;65(6):1334–9.
11. Oates JA, Melmon K, Sjoerdsma A, Gillespie L, Mason DT. Release of a kinin peptide in the carcinoid syndrome. Lancet. 1964;1(7332):514–7.
12. Goedert M, Otten U, Suda K, Heitz PU, Stalder GA, Obrecht JP, et al. Dopamine, norepinephrine and serotonin production by an intestinal carcinoid tumor. Cancer. 1980;45(1):104–7.

13. Oates JA, Pettinger WA, Doctor RB. Evidence for the release of bradykinin in carcinoid syndrome. J Clin Invest. 1966;45(2):173–8.
14. Miller R, Patel AU, Warner RR, Parnes IH. Anaesthesia for the carcinoid syndrome: a report of nine cases. Can Anaesth Soc J. 1978;25(3):240–4.
15. Marsh HM, Martin JK Jr, Kvols LK, Gracey DR, Warner MA, Warner ME, et al. Carcinoid crisis during anesthesia: successful treatment with a somatostatin analogue. Anesthesiology. 1987;66(1):89–91.
16. Parris WC, Oates JA, Kambam J, Shmerling R, Sawyers JF. Pre-treatment with somatostatin in the anaesthetic management of a patient with carcinoid syndrome. Can J Anaesth. 1988;35(4):413–6.
17. Kinney MA, Warner ME, Nagorney DM, Rubin J, Schroeder DR, Maxson PM, et al. Perianaesthetic risks and outcomes of abdominal surgery for metastatic carcinoid tumours. Br J Anaesth. 2001;87(3):447–52.
18. Woltering EA, Wright AE, Stevens MA, Wang YZ, Boudreaux JP, Mamikunian G, et al. Development of effective prophylaxis against intraoperative carcinoid crisis. J Clin Anesth. 2016;32:189–93.
19. Condron ME, Pommier SJ, Pommier RF. Continuous infusion of octreotide combined with perioperative octreotide bolus does not prevent intraoperative carcinoid crisis. Surgery. 2016;159(1):358–65.
20. Kinney MAO, Nagorney DM, Clark DF, O'Brien TD, Turner JD, Marienau ME, et al. Partial hepatic resections for metastatic neuroendocrine tumors: perioperative outcomes. J Clin Anesth. 2018;51:93–6.
21. Fouché M, Bouffard Y, Le Goff MC, Prothet J, Malavieille F, Sagnard P, et al. Intraoperative carcinoid syndrome during small-bowel neuroendocrine tumour surgery. Endocr Connect. 2018;7(12):1245–50.
22. Condron ME, Jameson NE, Limbach KE, Bingham AE, Sera VA, Anderson RB, et al. A prospective study of the pathophysiology of carcinoid crisis. Surgery. 2019;165(1):158–65.
23. Thorson A, Biorck G, Bjorkman G, Waldenstrom J. Malignant carcinoid of the small intestine with metastases to the liver, valvular disease of the right side of the heart (pulmonary stenosis and tricuspid regurgitation without septal defects), peripheral vasomotor symptoms, bronchoconstriction, and an unusual type of cyanosis; a clinical and pathologic syndrome. Am Heart J. 1954;47(5):795–817.
24. Pernow B, Waldenstrom J. Determination of 5-hydroxytryptamine, 5-hydroxyindole acetic acid and histamine in thirty-three cases of carcinoid tumor (argentaffinoma). Am J Med. 1957;23(1):16–25.
25. Robertson JI, Peart WS, Andrews TM. The mechanism of facial flushes in the carcinoid syndrome. Q J Med. 1962;31:103–23.
26. Levine RJ, Sjoerdsma A. Pressor amines and the carcinoid flush. Ann Intern Med. 1963;58:818–28.
27. Sjoerdsma A, Melmon KL. The carcinoid spectrum. Gastroenterology. 1964;47:104–7.
28. Jones WP. Serotonin release from carcinoid tumours. Can Anaesth Soc J. 1962;9:42–50.
29. Snow PJ, Lennard-Jones JE, Curzon G, Stacey RS. Humoral effects of metastasising carcinoid tumours. Lancet. 1955;269(6898):1004–9.
30. Bean WB, Funk D. The vasculo-cardiac syndrome of metastatic carcinoid. AMA Arch Intern Med. 1959;103(2):189–99.
31. Daugherty GW, Manger WM, Roth GM, Flock EV, Childs DS Jr, Waugh JM. Malignant carcinoid with hyperserotonemia occurring spontaneously or induced by palpation of the tumor or by intravenous histamine: report of a case. Proc Staff Meet Mayo Clin. 1955;30(25):595–601.
32. Mason RA, Steane PA. Carcinoid syndrome: its relevance to the anaesthetist. Anaesthesia. 1976;31(2):228–42.
33. Kvols LK, Moertel CG, O'Connell MJ, Schutt AJ, Rubin J, Hahn RG. Treatment of the malignant carcinoid syndrome. Evaluation of a long-acting somatostatin analogue. N Engl J Med. 1986;315(11):663–6.

34. Veall GR, Peacock JE, Bax ND, Reilly CS. Review of the anaesthetic management of 21 patients undergoing laparotomy for carcinoid syndrome. Br J Anaesth. 1994;72(3):335–41.
35. Warner RR, Mani S, Profeta J, Grunstein E. Octreotide treatment of carcinoid hypertensive crisis. Mt Sinai J Med. 1994;61(4):349–55.
36. Sarmiento JM, Que FG. Hepatic surgery for metastases from neuroendocrine tumors. Surg Oncol Clin N Am. 2003;12(1):231–42.
37. Thompson GB. Textbook of endocrine surgery. Mayo Clin Proc. 1998;73(1):102.
38. Phan AT, Oberg K, Choi J, Harrison LH Jr, Hassan MM, Strosberg JR, et al. NANETS consensus guideline for the diagnosis and management of neuroendocrine tumors: well-differentiated neuroendocrine tumors of the thorax (includes lung and thymus). Pancreas. 2010;39(6):784–98.
39. Vaughan DJ, Brunner MD. Anesthesia for patients with carcinoid syndrome. Int Anesthesiol Clin. 1997;35(4):129–42.
40. Boudreaux JP, Klimstra DS, Hassan MM, Woltering EA, Jensen RT, Goldsmith SJ, et al. The NANETS consensus guideline for the diagnosis and management of neuroendocrine tumors: well-differentiated neuroendocrine tumors of the Jejunum, Ileum, Appendix, and Cecum. Pancreas. 2010;39(6):753–66.
41. Ramage JK, Davies AH, Ardill J, Bax N, Caplin M, Grossman A, et al. Guidelines for the management of gastroenteropancreatic neuroendocrine (including carcinoid) tumours. Gut. 2005;54(Suppl 4):iv1–16.
42. Dierdorf SF. Carcinoid tumor and carcinoid syndrome. Curr Opin Anaesthesiol. 2003;16(3):343–7.
43. Quinlivan JK, Roberts WA. Intraoperative octreotide for refractory carcinoid-induced bronchospasm. Anesth Analg. 1994;78(2):400–2.
44. Oberg K, Kvols L, Caplin M, Delle Fave G, de Herder W, Rindi G, et al. Consensus report on the use of somatostatin analogs for the management of neuroendocrine tumors of the gastroenteropancreatic system. Ann Oncol. 2004;15(6):966–73.
45. Limbach KE, Condron ME, Bingham AE, Pommier SJ, Pommier RF. B-Adrenergic agonist administration is not associated with secondary carcinoid crisis in patients with carcinoid tumor. Am J Surg. 2019;217(5):932–6.

Part II

Primary GEP-NETs

Gastroduodenal NETs

7

David A. Mahvi and Thomas E. Clancy

Introduction

Gastroduodenal neuroendocrine tumors (NETs) have seen a steady rise in incidence concurrent with the increasing prevalence of upper endoscopy. When lesions are small and asymptomatic and with favorable histology, the tumors can typically be treated endoscopically. The role and extent of surgery is dependent on tumor location and staging. The following chapter will describe the epidemiology, diagnosis, treatment, and follow-up for gastroduodenal NETs.

Gastric NETs

Gastric neuroendocrine tumors (gNETs) arise from enterochromaffin-like cells (ECLs) in the gastric mucosa. They are generally indolent slow-growing tumors, though a subset can also be very aggressive with early metastasis. ECLs are stimulated by gastrin to release histamine, which promotes acid secretion from neighboring parietal cells in the stomach. Since gastrin has trophic effects on ECLs, hypergastrinemic states can lead to ECL hyperplasia with subsequent neoplastic transformation that leads to formation of the majority of gNETs.

Epidemiology and Classification

The incidence of gNETs has increased 15-fold from 1973 to 2012 according to the SEER (Surveillance, Epidemiology, and End Results) database [1]. This increased incidence is likely due to a combination of increased number of endoscopic

D. A. Mahvi · T. E. Clancy (✉)
Department of Surgery, Brigham and Women's Hospital, Boston, MA, USA
e-mail: dmahvi@partners.org; tclancy@bwh.harvard.edu

© Springer Nature Switzerland AG 2021
J. M. Cloyd, T. M. Pawlik (eds.), *Neuroendocrine Tumors*,
https://doi.org/10.1007/978-3-030-62241-1_7

Table 7.1 Types of gastric neuroendocrine tumors

	Type 1	Type 2	Type 3
Percentage of gNETs	70–80%	5–10%	10–20%
Associated pathology	Atrophic gastritis, pernicious anemia	ZES, MEN1	n/a
Number of lesions	Multiple	Multiple	Solitary
Location	Fundus, body	Fundus, body, antrum	Fundus, antrum
Acid level	Low	High	Normal
Gastrin level	High	High	Normal
Underlying mucosa	Atrophic	Hypertrophic	Normal
Prognosis	Excellent	Good	Poor

procedures, increased awareness of the disease itself, and possibly also the long-term use of proton pump inhibitors (PPIs) [2]. The stomach is the primary site of 6.9–8.7% of all gastrointestinal NETs, and gNETs represent 0.3–1.8% of all gastric tumors [3]. The median age of diagnosis is approximately 65 years old and there is a slight female predominance [4].

There are three distinct subtypes of gNETs (Table 7.1). Type 1 gNETs are the most common, accounting for 70–80%. They are associated with pernicious anemia and chronic atrophic gastritis and are further characterized by hypergastrinemia and low gastric acid levels. Type 2 gNETs represent 5–10% of lesions and are also characterized by high gastrin levels though they also have high gastric acid levels. Type 2 gNETs are associated with Zollinger-Ellison syndrome and multiple endocrine neoplasia (MEN) type 1. Both type 1 and type 2 gNETs have relatively favorable prognoses and typically present with multiple lesions. In contrast, type 3 gNETs normally present as solitary lesions and have a greater propensity to metastasize. Gastrin and stomach acid levels are normal in patients with type 3 gNETs, which represent 10–20% of gNETs. Neuroendocrine carcinomas are rare, poorly differentiated tumors that behave like adenocarcinoma but have an endocrine phenotype; these are sometimes referred to as type 4 gNETs [5].

Clinical Presentation, Diagnosis, and Staging

The cornerstone for diagnosis is esophagogastroduodenoscopy (EGD). Similar to other gastric polyps, gNETs are typically diagnosed incidentally on endoscopic workup for nonspecific upper gastrointestinal symptoms such as epigastric pain, dyspepsia, nausea, and early satiety or as part of workup for unexplained anemia (Fig. 7.1). Unlike other gastroenteropancreatic NETs, gNETs are rarely functional. Carcinoid syndrome is seen in less than 1% of patients, almost exclusively in type 3 gNETs with liver metastases [6]. For type 1 and type 2 gNETs, the associated

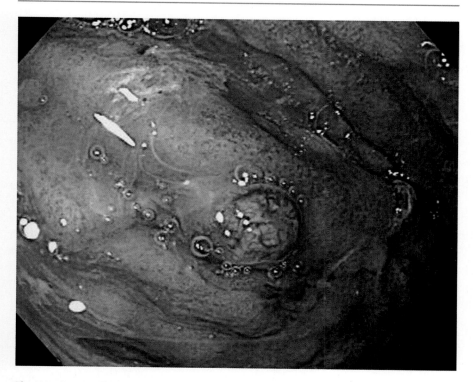

Fig. 7.1 Gastric NET. A typical gastric subcentimeter gastric neuroendocrine tumor seen on surveillance endoscopy. (Photo courtesy of Kunal Jajoo, MD, Brigham and Women's Hospital, Boston)

atrophic gastritis and gastrinoma, respectively, may lead to symptoms, but the gNET itself is typically small in size and unlikely to be symptomatic itself. Type 3 gNETs may present as larger lesions and are thus more likely to cause symptoms from the primary lesion. Lesions are broad-based and submucosal in appearance endoscopically.

At time of endoscopy, biopsy is recommended. Due to the submucosal location of gNETs, standard mucosal biopsy may be insufficient for diagnosis; endoscopic snare polypectomy are ultrasound-guided needle biopsy are higher yield [7]. Histologic tissue staining for chromogranin A and synaptophysin should be performed. Additionally, random biopsies of the surrounding fundic and antral mucosa should be taken to assess for underlying atrophic gastritis, ECL hyperplasia, and *H. pylori* status. Gastric pH should also be measured, ideally off PPIs if possible. Type 1 gNETs are associated with high gastric pH (>4) and type 2 with low pH (<2) [8]. A fasting serum gastrin level while the patient is off PPIs should be measured to help differentiate types 1 and 2 (elevated) from type 3 (normal). Baseline serum chromogranin A levels should also be obtained. Patients with *H. pylori* infection should be treated with triple or quadruple therapy based on local resistance rates and patient allergies. Vitamin B12 levels should be checked in type 1 tumors given their association with pernicious anemia [9].

Table 7.2 WHO classification and grading criteria for neuroendocrine neoplasms, 2019

	Differentiation	Grade	Mitoses per 10 HPF	Ki-67 index
G1	Well	Low	<2	<3
G2	Well	Intermediate	2–20	3–20
G3	Well	High	>20	>20
NEC	Poorly	High	>20	>20

WHO World Health Organization, *NEC* neuroendocrine carcinoma, *HPF* High-power field

For NETs, both the mitotic rate and Ki-67 proliferation index should be measured to allow for tumor grade assessment [10]. Tumor grade is measured in the area with greatest mitotic activity as there is often intra-tumoral heterogeneity. Types 1 and 2 gNETs are typically grade 1, with a mitotic count of <2 per 10 high-power field and Ki-67 index <3. In contrast, type 3 gNETs are often grade 2 or 3, with higher mitotic count and Ki-67 indices (Table 7.2). Tumor differentiation refers to the extent to which the tumor cells histologically resemble normal tissue and should also be assessed. Well-differentiated NETs consist of trabeculae with typical "salt and pepper" chromatin staining, while poorly differentiated NETs display sheets of pleomorphic cells with significant necrosis [11].

TNM staging classification is shown in Table 7.3. Per AJCC eighth edition guidelines, T1 tumors are 1 cm or less and confined to the lamina propria and submucosa. T2 tumors either are larger than 1 cm or invade the muscularis propria. T3 tumors invade into the subserosa without penetrating the serosa, and T4 tumors invade the serosa or other organs. For N stage, any regional lymph node involvement is N1. Distant metastases qualify for M1 stage, with M1a being confined to the liver, M1b involving extrahepatic site(s), and M1c having both liver and extrahepatic disease.

A full staging workup is typically only indicated for type 3 gNETs or type 1 and 2 gNETs with worrisome features. In type 1 gNETs smaller than 1 cm, no further imaging tests are recommended. For type 1 gNETs that are 1 cm to 2 cm in size, endoscopic ultrasound (EUS) may be helpful to delineate depth of gastric wall involvement prior to resection. For the rare type 1 gNETs >2 cm in size, multiphasic CT or MRI should also be performed to assess for metastatic spread [9]. Patients with type 2 gNETs may require additional imaging with computed tomography (CT), magnetic resonance imaging (MRI), and/or somatostatin receptor scintigraphy. Further, functional imaging with 68-gallium DOTATATE PET/CT may be considered for patients with concern for occult metastatic disease as it is felt to be the most accurate imaging modality for staging and identification of small gastrinomas [8].

Patients with type 3 gNETs or type 1 or 2 gNETs with worrisome features (size >2 cm, high grade) should undergo multiphasic abdominal imaging with either CT or MRI [9] as well as 68-gallium DOTATATE PET/CT.

The World Health Organization (WHO) has updated its classification system for gastric NETs based on tumor grade and tumor differentiation as described above (Table 7.2). A prior classification system published in 2010 was based only on tumor grade; this was modified to reflect the fact that while almost all poorly

Table 7.3 TNM staging of gastric and duodenal neuroendocrine tumor

T stage gastric	
Tx	Primary tumor cannot be assessed
T0	No evidence of primary tumor
T1	Tumor invades lamina propria or submucosa and is ≤1 cm
T2	Tumor invades the muscularis propria or is ≥1 cm
T3	Tumor invades into subserosa without penetrating serosa
T4	Tumor invades the serosa or other organs
T stage duodenal	
Tx	Primary tumor cannot be assessed
T0	No evidence of primary tumor
T1	Tumor invades mucosa or submucosa only and is ≤1 cm
T2	Tumor invades the muscularis propria or is ≥1 cm
T3	Tumor invades the pancreas or peripancreatic adipose tissue
T4	Tumor invades the serosa or other organs
N stage (both)	
Nx	Regional lymph nodes cannot be assessed
N0	No regional lymph node involvement
N1	Regional lymph node involvement
M stage (both)	
M0	No distant metastasis
M1a	Metastasis confined to the liver
M1b	Metastasis in at least one extrahepatic site
M1c	Both hepatic and extrahepatic metastases

	T stage	N stage	M stage
Stage I	T1	N0	M0
Stage II	T2–T3	N0	M0
Stage III	T4	N0	M0
	Any T	N1	M0
Stage IV	Any T	Any N	M1

AJCC 8th edition

differentiated tumors were high grade, not all high-grade tumors were poorly differentiated [12]. In 2019, the WHO published updated grading classification separating well- and poorly differentiated high-grade tumors. Well-differentiated tumors are categorized as low (G1), intermediate (G2), and high (G3) grades based on mitotic count and Ki-67 index. All poorly differentiated tumors are considered neuroendocrine carcinomas and behave like adenocarcinomas.

Management

Type 1

Type 1 gNETs typically follow a benign and indolent course, with only 5–10% of patients developing lymph node involvement and 2–5% developing liver metastases [3]. Tumors are typically 5–8 mm in size, polypoid, multicentric, and located in the fundus [5]. A multicenter retrospective series compared 20 patients with metastatic type 1 gNET (12 lymph node, 8 liver) to 234 patients without metastases. The mean follow-up period was 83 months. Greater size of largest tumor (20.1 vs. 7.9 mm), higher Ki-67 index (6.8% vs. 1.9%), symptomatic disease (90% vs. 44%), and higher serum gastrin levels (2138 vs. 898) were all significantly associated with metastatic type 1 gNETs [13]. All patients remained alive during the follow-up period.

Chronic atrophic gastritis is an autoimmune disease characterized by antibodies against parietal cells and intrinsic factor, affecting the mucosa of the stomach's fundus and corpus. This mucosal inflammatory infiltration causes intestinal metaplasia or atrophy, achlorhydria, hypergastrinemia, and enterochromaffin cell hyperplasia [14]. There is a 3:1 female predominance and a high association with other autoimmune diseases, especially thyroid disease. *H. pylori* is also associated with atrophic gastritis which can be multifocal throughout the stomach. Patients with atrophic gastritis can develop type 1 gNET related to hypergastrinemia. In addition to gNETs, patients with atrophic gastritis can develop pernicious anemia and neurologic symptoms related to cobalamin deficiency. Atrophic gastritis is also associated with an increased risk for developing intestinal-type gastric adenocarcinoma. A large longitudinal study of over 10,000 patients in Korea found the incidence of gastric neoplasm was 0.1% without atrophic gastritis, 1.6% with mild disease, 5.2% with moderate disease, and 12.0% with severe atrophic gastritis ($r = 0.184$, $p < 0.001$) [15].

Small type 1 gNET, particularly lesions <1 cm in size, can typically be managed without surgical intervention given their excellent prognosis. The 5-year disease-specific survival approaches 100% for both endoscopic and surgical treatment [16]. Management options include either endoscopic polypectomy or endoscopic surveillance. One series of 11 patients underwent endoscopic surveillance with a median follow-up of 54 months; four patients had an increased number of lesions, but no patient developed a lesion over 1 cm or evidence of metastatic disease [17]. Regular endoscopic surveillance is recommended to monitor both for further or growing gNETs and for gastric adenocarcinoma given that atrophic gastritis is a risk factor for this more malignant disease [5].

For type 1 tumors ≤2 cm in size without nodal or distant metastases, endoscopic resection is considered adequate therapy (Fig. 7.2). There are two primary modalities of endoscopic resection: endoscopic mucosal resection (EMR) and endoscopic submucosal dissection (ESD). EMR is performed by injecting saline with epinephrine in the submucosal plane immediately underneath the lesion to raise the tumor. After injection, a snare is placed around the lesion and pressed into the mucosa with resection performed with or without electrocautery. EMR utilizes adjuncts such as ligation or precutting to increase the likelihood of complete resection. Ligation involves applying suction to the lesion and then deploying a band to create a pseudopolyp followed by using an electrocautery snare to retrieve the lesion. Precutting entails using an endoscopic knife or snare tip to make a circumferential incision around the lesion followed by snare retrieval. For ESD, following submucosal injection, an endoscopic knife is used to circumferentially cut around the lesion. Subsequently, a variety of endoscopic knives are available to carefully dissect the

Fig. 7.2 Gastric NET resected with NET. A small submucosal gastric neuroendocrine tumor is resected with endoscopic mucosal resection. An endoscopic clip has been placed in the resection bed for hemostasis, and the tumor is seen to the right of the photo. (Photo courtesy of Kunal Jajoo, MD, Brigham and Women's Hospital, Boston)

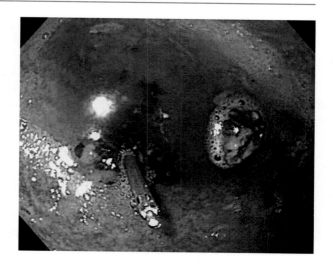

lesion en bloc in the submucosal plane [18]. In experienced hands, ESD may offer higher complete resection rates compared to EMR. For example, ESD had a 94% complete resection rate versus 83% for EMR in a 62-patient series of patients with type 1 gNET [19]. In a smaller series, four out of six patients with EMR had a positive vertical margin, whereas none of the seven patients had a positive margin treated with ESD [20]. However, ESD does have reported higher complication rates, specifically with bleeding and perforation. Recurrence after endoscopic resection can be as high as 65% within the first year; thus, continued endoscopic surveillance is imperative [3]. Recurrent lesions are typically indolent and typically small-sized with no negative impact on prognosis [21].

The National Comprehensive Cancer Network (NCCN) guidelines recommend consideration of surgery for tumors 2 cm or larger, invading the muscularis propria, or tumors with metastases [9]. Similarly, the European Neuroendocrine Tumor Society (ENETS) guidelines recommend surgical resection for tumors extending beyond the submucosa, lymph node or other metastatic disease, or poorly differentiated tumors [22]. Other potential surgical indications are positive margins after endoscopic resection and angioinvasion [3] or when there are six or more lesions with at least three being larger than 1 cm in size [5]. A recent meta-analysis focusing on lymph node metastasis rates found that tumors at least 1 cm in size had a 15.3% chance of lymph node disease compared to 0.8% if less than 1 cm. Additionally, tumors which invaded the muscularis propria had a 29.4% lymph node positivity rate compared to 3.1% without [14].

The extent of surgical resection should be tailored to each particular patient. Historically, antrectomy was standardly offered as this removes the gastrin-producing G cells, thus removing the source of hypergastrinemia for this subtype of gNET. Antrectomy has been shown to induce regression of tumors in approximately 70–80% of cases, with the remainder likely having developed metaplasia allowing for gastrin-independent growth [3]. However, increasingly, more limited resections are being performed given the relatively benign disease prognosis. When tumor location allows, gastric wedge resection alone can be performed if all lesions can be completely resected. In patients with persistent or recurrent type 1 gNETs after endoscopic or more limited resection, antrectomy or partial gastrectomy should be performed [6]. Total gastrectomy is very rarely indicated, as residual tumors in the gastric fundus or body often regress postoperatively. Regardless of the operation performed, regional lymphadenectomy should be carried out.

There is no standardized post-procedure surveillance regimen after endoscopic or surgical resection. ENETS guidelines recommend endoscopy at least every 2 years [22]. The NCCN recommends history and physical examination with upper endoscopy every 6–12 months for the first 3 years and then annually thereafter [9].

Type 2

Treatment of type 2 gNETs differs somewhat from that of type 1 gNETs given their association with MEN1 syndrome as well as the slightly higher malignant and invasive potential of the tumors [3]. Serum gastrin levels are elevated in most patients, with levels greater than 1000 pg/mL commonly seen [5]. All patients with type 2 gNET should undergo genetic MEN1 testing to look for a mutation on chromosome 11q13. The clinical diagnosis of MEN1 requires two or more of the following: multigland parathyroid hyperplasia (98%), pancreatic NET (50%), or pituitary tumor (35%) [9]. Genetic testing for *MEN1* gene mutations can also be performed, and referral to genetic counseling should be considered. Diagnostic workup should be tailored and can include serum calcium and 25-OH vitamin D (with ultrasound and sestamibi scan as needed) for the parathyroids, biochemical evaluation as indicated and multiphasic CT or MRI to assess for pancreatic NETs, pituitary MRI, and chest CT for bronchus/thymus NETs. Approximately 23% of patients with MEN1 will develop type 2 gNETs, which is more than 70-fold more frequent than patients with sporadic Zollinger-Ellison syndrome [10].

Management of concomitant gastrinoma is covered in greater detail elsewhere in this textbook. Patients should be initially treated medically with proton pump inhibitors or H2 blockers. If acid blockade is unable to control symptoms, somatostatin analogs such as octreotide can be considered. In cases of sporadic gastrinoma, surgery to resect the gastrinoma should be offered with the goal of removing at least ten lymph nodes. Conversely, most patients with MEN1 can be well-controlled with only medical therapy [23].

Including the need to address hypergastrinemia, the management of the type 2 gNET itself is similar to the management of type 1 gNETs. Type 2 gNETs have a slightly higher malignant potential with 10–20% metastasizing to lymph nodes and ~ 10% to the liver [3] but have overall similar outcomes relative to type 1. As a result, smaller tumors can be resected endoscopically, with surgical resection recommended for tumors larger than 2 cm or with other worrisome features such as high tumor grade, local invasion, or metastasis. Tumors <1 cm can undergo either endoscopic resection or surveillance [24]. If surgical resection is being planned, then consideration should be made for concurrent gastrinoma resection depending on the necessary extent for each procedure.

Type 3

Type 3 gNETs are also referred to as "sporadic" and occur in the absence of atrophic gastritis, Zollinger-Ellison syndrome, or hypergastrinemia. These tumors are much more aggressive than type 1 or 2 lesions, with 22–75% of patients having liver metastases at presentation [3]. Type 3 gNETs are therefore managed similarly to gastric adenocarcinoma in most cases. Patients typically present with tumors larger than 2 cm, and the lesions are more commonly located in the antrum. Type 3 gNETs more often produce 5-hydroxytryptophan (as opposed to serotonin) [10]. Some authors describe a type 4 lesion as consisting of a poorly differentiated lesion arising from serotonin cells or of mixed endocrine-exocrine etiology [5]; this point is mostly academic as these tumors are managed similarly to type 3 lesions.

All patients diagnosed with type 3 gNET should undergo a full staging workup, including EUS, CT/MRI, and consideration of somatostatin-based imaging. Treatment decisions should be made by a multidisciplinary team. Most patients with type 3 gastric NETs without metastatic disease should undergo partial or total gastrectomy with local lymph node dissection. There is presently no standard role for neoadjuvant or adjuvant systemic chemotherapy in patients with upfront resectable disease.

Those with resectable liver metastases who are otherwise reasonable surgical candidates should be offered surgical resection of their primary tumor and liver metastases for curative intent. For unresectable liver disease, local therapy (i.e., radiofrequency ablation) aimed at dominant hepatic metastases and/or resection of the primary tumor could also be considered as adjuncts to decrease hormone secretion to improve symptoms.

Some evidence suggests that endoscopic resection can be considered selectively for the few patients who present with early disease. One series of 50 patients with type 3 gNETs less than 2 cm in size managed endoscopically was reported, including 41 treated with EMR and 9 with ESD. All tumors were confined to the submucosal layer and had no evidence of lymphovascular invasion. The complete resection rate was 80%. At median follow-up of 43 months, no patients had evidence of recurrent disease and there were no mortalities reported [25]. These results suggest that select patients with type 3 gNET with low-risk features could be candidates for less aggressive therapy, but more data is needed before this becomes standard practice.

Advanced Disease

In the presence of metastatic disease, resection or debulking of metastases can be considered. The most common site of metastasis is the liver, and the incidence of liver metastases are 2–5% for type 1 gNETs, 10% for type 2 gNETs, and 22–75% for type 3 gNETs [3]. Liver-directed options include metastasectomy, ablation, and transarterial embolization. Liver metastases can be resected either via anatomic hepatectomy or nonanatomic wedge resection. If the primary gNET is symptomatic, patients can be offered a palliative resection or bypass to alleviate symptoms. A retrospective study of patients with stage IV gNETs in the National Cancer Database

(NCDB) compared 114 patients who underwent primary tumor resection to 869 patients who did not; none of the patients had surgery on their metastatic disease. Patients undergoing primary tumor resection had a prolonged overall survival compared to those who did not (21.2 months vs. 7.0 months, $p < 0.001$). Patients who were younger and had distal stomach primary tumors and grade 1 or 2 differentiation were more likely to have undergone primary resection on multivariable analysis [26].

Patients who are not candidates for curative resection for either medical or oncologic reasons should be referred for systemic therapy. If patients are asymptomatic and have low tumor burden, either observation with tumor markers and serial imaging every 3–12 months or utilization of somatostatin analogs (most commonly octreotide or lanreotide) can be performed [9]. If there is disease progression on somatostatin analog therapy, cytotoxic chemotherapy (i.e., etoposide with carboplatin or cisplatin), everolimus, or interferon-alpha can be given as second-line agents [9].

Other systemic options are limited for gNET. Netazepide is an oral antagonist of the gastrin/cholecystokinin-2 receptor that has been investigated specifically for patients with type 1 gNETs. A non-randomized trial of 16 patients showed that daily administration of netazepide reduced the number and size of tumors and normalized chromogranin A levels when given for 12 weeks; however, tumors regrew once treatment was stopped. Of the original 16 patients, 13 underwent another 52 weeks of treatment. Five patients had complete tumor eradication and one had eradication of all but one tumor. The remaining seven patients had reduction in the number of lesions and size of the largest lesion [27].

Peptide receptor radionuclide therapy (PRRT) delivers radiation therapy via binding of the somatostatin receptor by 177-Lu-DOTATATE and may be considered in locally advanced or metastatic NET. Treatment decisions for patients with advanced or metastatic disease should be made in a multidisciplinary fashion.

A suggested algorithm for management of gastric NET is shown in Fig. 7.3.

Duodenal NETs

Neuroendocrine tumors of the duodenum have traditionally been grouped together with those of the stomach or small intestine. However, duodenal neuroendocrine tumors (dNETs) are increasingly being recognized as a distinct clinical entity. As more is learned about the clinical behavior of these rare tumors, the recommended workup and therapeutic interventions are shifting. The epidemiology, clinical features, and management of dNET are reviewed.

Epidemiology and Classification

Duodenal neuroendocrine tumors comprise approximately 3% of all NETs and up to 3% of all duodenal neoplasms [10]. There is a slight male predominance, and the median age at time of diagnosis is approximately 60 years old. The incidence of

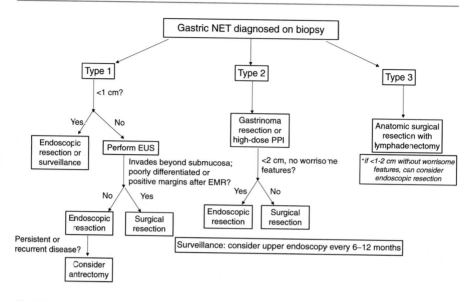

Fig. 7.3 Algorithm for gastric NET. (National Comprehensive Cancer Network: Neuroendocrine Tumors [9]; Delle Fave et al. [22]; Falconi et al. [23])

dNETs has increased in recent years, concurrent with the increasing utilization of upper endoscopy. According to SEER data, there have been 1258 patients diagnosed with duodenal carcinoid tumors between 1983 and 2010. The incidence in 1983 was 0.027 per 100,000 and climbed to 1.1 per 100,000 in 2010 [28]. The majority of dNETs are located in the duodenal bulb (40–60%) and descending duodenum (~20%). Approximately 10–30% of dNETs are periampullary.

There are multiple subtypes of dNET. The majority of dNETs are nonfunctional (70–90%). Nonfunctional tumors may stain for calcitonin or serotonin on pathology. Gastrinomas are the most common functional NET in the duodenum, centered within what is traditionally described as Passaro's (gastrincma) triangle. Less commonly, functional somatostatinomas and glucagonomas have been described in the duodenum. Duodenal gangliocytic paragangliomas represent less than 2% of dNETs and follow a benign course. Finally, poorly differentiated neuroendocrine carcinomas are seen in less than 3% of cases but have higher malignant potential [6]. Approximately 10% of patients will present with multiple dNETs, which should raise suspicion for an associated genetic component. Multiple endocrine neoplasia 1 is associated with multiple duodenal gastrinomas presenting with Zollinger-Ellison syndrome. Approximately 20–30% of patients with duodenal somatostatinomas and 20% with periampullary dNETs have neurofibromatosis type 1 [6].

Clinical Presentation and Diagnosis

Nonfunctional dNETs are most commonly diagnosed in patients undergoing upper endoscopy for nonspecific GI symptoms. Epigastric pain is the most common presenting symptoms. Less commonly, nausea, bleeding, diarrhea, and duodenal obstruction can be seen. In obstructing periampullary tumors, patients can present with jaundice [29]. Carcinoid syndrome secondary to liver metastases (flushing, diarrhea, and rarely heart failure or bronchoconstriction) is seen in less than 4% of dNETs. Similar to gNETs, it is likely that the symptoms which prompted the upper endoscopy are often unrelated to the dNET itself, as most are diagnosed at a median of just over 1 cm in size. The serum tumor marker chromogranin A should be drawn prior to resection to allow for surveillance.

Endoscopy with tissue biopsy remains the gold standard for diagnosis of dNETs [22]. The tumors arise in the deep duodenal mucosa and will invade into the submucosa. The tumors typically appear as hemispherical with a pink or yellow color. The differential diagnosis includes other submucosal lesions, including GIST, Brunner's gland hyperplasia, schwannomas, and adenocarcinomas. The addition of endoscopic ultrasound can aid in assessing depth of invasion and more accurately measure tumor size. In patients with suspected or proven advanced disease based on endoscopic findings, additional preoperative staging imaging should be obtained with either a CT or MRI. Somatostatin receptor scintigraphy or ^{68}Ga-PET-DOTANOC scans can also be considered, but currently there currently is no definitive evidence to suggest one staging scan over another.

Histologically, dNETs typically stain positive for synaptophysin and chromogranin A (similar to gNETs). Mitotic count and Ki-67 levels should also be assessed for grading purposes. Grade 1 tumors have Ki-67 $\leq$ 2% or < 2 mitoses/10 high-power field (HPF). Grade 2 tumors have either Ki-67 of 3–20% or 2–20 mitoses/HPF, and grade 3 tumors have >20% Ki-67 or > 20 mitoses/HPF. Low-grade tumors are more common, with 65–77% of patients presenting with G1 primary tumors, 10–31% with G2, and 3–14% with G3 [30–32].

Staging

Duodenal NETs have a slightly different tumor staging system than gNETs that considers the relationship with the pancreas and peripancreatic tissue in the T staging. Per AJCC eighth edition guidelines, T1 tumors are 1 cm or less and confined to the mucosa and submucosa. T2 tumors are either larger than 1 cm or invade the muscularis propria. T3 tumors invade the pancreas or peripancreatic adipose tissue, and T4 tumors invade the visceral peritoneum or other organs. N and M staging are identical to that of gNETs (Table 7.3). Notably, coinciding with the increasing incidence of dNETs, patients are being diagnosed at an earlier stage. While 57.5% of patients presented with stage I disease between 1983 and 2005 in the SEER database, 69.9% were diagnosed at this earlier stage between 2005 and 2010 [28].

Management

Treatment of dNETs varies depending on their size, grade, stage, location, and histologic subtype. No standardized management algorithm has gained consensus. Options for curative-intent treatment include endoscopic and/or surgical approaches depending on tumor and patient characteristics. Similar to gNETs, there are two primary endoscopic techniques. Endoscopic mucosal resection (EMR) can be used for early-stage tumors by dissecting in the mucosal plane. Endoscopic submucosal dissection (ESD) has the ability to completely resect dNETs that invade slightly deeper; however, ESD is associated with higher risks of bleeding and perforation [29].

Similarly, there are a number of potential surgical approaches. Tumor location and characteristics dictate the extent of resection required. Depending on these factors, transduodenal resection, partial duodenectomy, segmental duodenectomy, or pancreaticoduodenectomy could be performed. Pancreaticoduodenectomy is typically indicated for periampullary tumors if a transduodenal or segmental resection is not technically possible. Pancreaticoduodenectomy is associated with a higher lymph node yield and R0 resection rate, at the cost of significantly increased morbidity.

The European Neuroendocrine Tumor Society (ENETS) published updated management guidelines in 2016 [22]. For dNETs that are ≤1 cm, confined to the submucosa (T1) and without evidence of spread to the lymph nodes or adjacent organs, endoscopic resection is recommended. For tumors between 1 and 2 cm without worrisome features, there is no consensus on treatment and either surgical or endoscopic approaches could be employed. For tumors greater than 2 cm in size, formal staging workup is recommended followed by surgical resection or medical therapy if metastatic disease is identified.

To date, no prospective trials have been performed regarding therapeutic options for dNETs, but a number of groups have published retrospective series. A multicenter series from Italy included 108 patients with dNETs [30]. Stage IV disease was present at diagnosis in 17 patients and another 37 had stage III disease. Gastrinoma (23.1%) and somatostatinoma (4.6%) were the only functional tumors, and 22% of patients had multiple dNETs. Younger age, higher tumor grade, and functioning tumors were significantly more likely to develop metastatic disease on multivariable regression. Higher tumor grade and older age were the only factors significantly predictive of worse overall survival (OS). When comparing the 57 patients who underwent surgery to the 16 patients who had an endoscopic resection, no difference was seen in either overall survival (OS) or progression-free survival (PFS). The median OS was 15.6 years.

Memorial Sloan-Kettering published a series of 75 patients undergoing curative resection for dNETs between 1983 and 2011 [31]. Pancreaticoduodenectomy was performed in 29 patients, 34 had a local resection (either duodenotomy with tumor resection and closure, segmental duodenal resection, or distal gastrectomy including a portion of the duodenum), and 12 patients underwent EMR. Ampullary tumors were significantly more likely to be intermediate or high grade (50% vs. 11% for non-ampullary, $p < 0.001$). High-grade tumors and larger tumor size were associated with recurrence on univariate analysis. When comparing low- and intermediate-grade tumors, the type of resection was not significantly correlated with recurrence. However, it is notable that the EMR group had a 67% rate of positive margins, significantly smaller median tumor size (0.6 cm versus 1.8 cm), and a median follow-up of only 9 months. The overall 5-year recurrence-free survival (RFS) was 81%.

The Johns Hopkins Hospital reviewed 101 patients between 1996 and 2012 with dNETs (including 16 patients with incidental dNET undergoing pancreaticoduodenectomy for other indications) [33]. For primary dNET, 35 patients underwent pancreaticoduodenectomy, 12 had a local resection, and 38 had endoscopic resection. The 5-year OS was 79%, with no significant difference seen based on extent of resection. In the surgical patients, the probability of lymph node involvement was significantly correlated with primary tumor size (4.5% in tumors <1 cm, 72% for 1–2 cm, and 81% for >2 cm, $p = 0.029$), adding to the justification that lymphadenectomy is not necessary in tumors amenable to endoscopic resection under 1 cm in size.

Two large multi-institutional studies have been published in the USA with some overlap in centers included. Margonis et al. described management of 146 patients with dNET treated between 1993 and 2015 [34]. Local surgical resection was done in 39.1%, pancreaticoduodenectomy in 34.3%, and endoscopic resection in 26.7%. Five-year OS for the entire cohort was 78.3% and 5-year RFS was 66.8%. Metastatic disease at presentation and higher-grade tumors were associated with recurrence on multivariable analysis. Tumor size >1.5 cm was predictive of lymph node positivity and moderate- to high-grade tumors on univariate regression ($p = 0.04$ for both). Type of procedure was again not predictive of recurrence.

The second study included 162 patients undergoing curative dNET resection between 1997 and 2016 [32]. The 5-year OS was 84.7%, with only G2/G3 tumor grade being associated with worse OS on multivariable analysis. Interestingly, unlike the Hopkins group, 40% of patients with tumors ≤1 cm who underwent a lymphadenectomy had at least one positive lymph node. A receiver operating characteristic (ROC) analysis to identify the optimal number of lymph nodes to harvest found that eight was the most predictive cutoff for identifying lymph node metastases, though the sensitivity was only 67%.

The NCDB has also been queried for dNETs [35]. Between 2004 and 2014, 3954 patients underwent a resection for nonmetastatic dNET; 61% had a local resection and 39% an anatomic resection. In patients undergoing lymphadenectomy, 41% had a positive lymph node. For patients that underwent a resection, neither the type of resection, addition of lymphadenectomy, lymph node positivity, nor margin status correlated with OS regardless of tumor size.

The liver is the most common site of metastatic disease for gastroduodenal NETs, yet less than 10% of patients with dNETs develop liver metastases [10]. The presence of limited liver metastases does not necessarily rule out the potential for curative-intent treatment. Various forms of liver-directed therapy may be employed for symptom management and potentially increase disease-specific survival. In patients with limited or unilobar metastases that are candidates for hepatic resection, either wedge or anatomic resection can be performed. For example, one large single-center cohort of 649 patients with NETs metastatic to the liver found that hepatic resection was significantly associated with improved OS [36]. Bilobar involvement may necessitate preoperative portal vein embolization or concurrent use of liver-directed therapy (i.e., radiofrequency ablation, transarterial chemoembolization) with hepatic resection. Extrahepatic metastases are not an absolute contraindication to hepatectomy; however, oncologic outcomes are worse [37]. Interestingly, in one study, the presence of unresectable primary tumor was not associated with worse oncologic outcomes in patients undergoing hepatic resection for NETs [37]. For poor surgical candidates, liver-directed therapies alone can be considered and have been shown to improve outcomes. A recent series of patients with unresectable liver metastases comparing transarterial chemoembolization to transarterial radioembolization showed similar long-term oncologic outcomes (progression-free survival of 15.9 months versus 19.9 months, $p = 0.37$) [38]. In a very select subset of patients (age under 60, liver metastases not amenable to surgical resection, no evidence of extrahepatic disease, nonpoorly differentiate tumor), liver transplantation can be considered as well.

Areas of controversy in the management of dNET are the expanding roles of endoscopic and local resection and, relatedly, the need for lymphadenectomy. Given the indolent nature of most dNETs as well as the morbidity of pancreaticoduodenectomy, there is interest in shifting toward less radical resections if similar oncologic outcomes can be obtained. None of the series cited previously have shown a survival difference based on type of resection, though these series may be biased by smaller-sized tumors in the endoscopic cohorts, shorter follow-up periods, and selection bias. The higher margin positivity seen with endoscopic resection has not led to short-term local recurrences, though follow-up time for most series is limited. Increased expertise with more advanced endoscopic techniques will hopefully improve R0 resection rates without increasing complication rates. The shorter length of stay and lower complication rates associated with endoscopic resection are also important factors in treatment decision. In centers with appropriate advanced endoscopic capabilities, current consensus guidelines suggest that tumors 1–2 cm in size can be resected either endoscopically when technically feasible or surgically [22]. Prospective studies will be critical to determine the optimal oncologic therapy for these patients.

Retrospective data also points toward a limited role for full lymphadenectomy in the management of dNETs. Multiple large studies [31, 32, 34] have shown that lymph node positivity had no impact on survival, and the abovementioned NCDB study [35] showed that lymph node retrieval also did not affect survival. Furthermore, no study showed that type of resection (endoscopic, local, or anatomic) was associated with recurrence or survival. Again, selection bias in retrospective studies should be considered before any definitive recommendations can be made. A propensity-matched or prospective comparison between receipt of lymphadenectomy and not could potentially illuminate if lymph node dissection is beneficial in select patient populations (i.e., high-grade primary tumors or suspicious lymph nodes seen on staging workup).

Surveillance

There is no validated follow-up regimen for dNETs following curative resection. Guideline proposals for follow-up after endoscopic resection include endoscopy, serum chromogranin A, and either ultrasound or CT at 6 months, 24 months, and 36 months. After surgical resection, CT and serum chromogranin A is recommended at 6, 12, 24, and 36 months [29]. Given the risk of late recurrences, there should also be consideration for subsequent biennial follow-up [22].

Advanced Disease

Patients who are not candidates for curative resection should be referred for systemic therapy options. Given the rarity of dNETs and their typically indolent nature, no studies focusing specifically on this patient population have been performed. Somatostatin analogs (i.e., octreotide, lanreotide) have shown significantly improved progression-free survival for patients with advanced gastroenteropancreatic NETs and are typically used as first-line therapy. Cytotoxic chemotherapy agents such as carboplatin with etoposide, FOLFIRI, and FOLFIRINOX have shown antiproliferative activity in patients with poorly differentiated NETs. Everolimus (mTOR inhibitor) can be considered as second- or third-line therapy. Peptide receptor radionuclide therapy (PRRT) can be considered after failure of medical therapy. The most commonly used PRRT is 177-Lu-DOTATATE, which delivers radiation therapy to the NET via binding of the somatostatin receptor. Given the paucity of data specific for patients with advanced dNETs, treatment decisions for patients with advanced disease should ideally be made in a multidisciplinary tumor board.

A suggested algorithm for the management of duodenal NET is shown in Fig. 7.4.

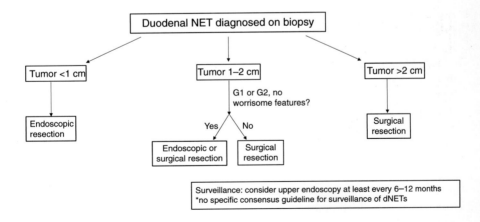

Fig. 7.4 Algorithm for duodenal NET. (National Comprehensive Cancer Network: Neuroendocrine Tumors [9]; Delle Fave et al. [22])

Summary and Conclusions

Gastroduodenal neuroendocrine tumors are being diagnosed with increasing frequency, and management strategies are evolving. Ultimately, the cornerstone of diagnosis is esophagogastroduodenoscopy with tissue biopsy which helps determine the necessary staging workup prior to appropriate definitive management. Figure 7.3 summarizes the diagnostic algorithm and management of gastric NETs, and Fig. 7.4 summarizes the diagnostic algorithm and management of duodenal NETs based on the most recent consensus guidelines from the NCCN [9], the North American Neuroendocrine Tumor Society [24], and the European Neuroendocrine Tumor Society [22].

References

1. Dasari A, Shen C, Halperin D, et al. Trends in the incidence, prevalence, and survival outcomes in patients with neuroendocrine tumors in the United States. JAMA Oncol. 2017;3(10):1335–42.
2. Nandy N, Hanson JA, Strickland RG, McCarthy DM. Solitary gastric carcinoid tumor associated with long-term use of omeprazole: a case report and review of the literature. Dig Dis Sci. 2016;61(3):708–12.
3. Grozinsky-Glasberg S, Alexandraki KI, et al. Gastric Carcinoids. Endocrinol Metab Clin N Am. 2018;47:645–60.
4. Yao JC, Hassan M, Phan A, et al. One hundred years after "carcinoid": epidemiology of and prognostic factors for neuroendocrine tumors in 35,825 cases in the United States. J Clin Oncol. 2008;26(18):3063–72.
5. Corey B, Chen H. Neuroendocrine tumors of the stomach. Surg Clin N Am. 2017;97:333–43.
6. Sato Y, Hashimoto S, Mizuno KI, et al. Management of gastric and duodenal neuroendocrine tumors. World J Gastroenterol. 2016;22(30):6817–28.
7. Christopoulos C, Papavassiliou E. Gastric neuroendocrine tumors: biology and management. Ann Gastroenterol. 2005;18(2):127–40.
8. Gluckman CR, Metz DC. Gastric neuroendocrine tumors (carcinoids). Curr Gastroenterol Rep. 2019;21(4):1–7.
9. National Comprehensive Cancer Network: Neuroendocrine Tumors, Version 3, 2017;399–437.
10. O'Toole D, Delle Fave G, Jensen RT. Gastric and duodenal neuroendocrine tumours. Best Pract Res Clin Gastroenterol. 2012;26(6):719–35.
11. Cives M, Strosberg JR. Gastroenteropancreatic neuroendocrine tumors. CA Cancer J Clin. 2018;68(6):471–87.
12. Coriat R, Walter T, Terris B, et al. Gastroenteropancreatic well-differentiated grade 3 neuroendocrine tumors: review and position statement. Oncologist. 2016;21(10):1191–9.
13. Grozinsky-Glasberg S, Thomas D, Strosberg JR, et al. Metastatic type 1 gastric carcinoid: a real threat or just a myth? World J Gastroenterol. 2013;19(46):8687–95.
14. Massironi S, Zilli A, Elvevi A, Invernizzi P. The changing face of chronic autoimmune atrophic gastritis: an updated comprehensive perspective. Autoimmun Rev. 2019;18(3):215–22.
15. Song JH, Kim SG, Jin EH, et al. Risk factors for gastric tumorigenesis in underlying gastric mucosal atrophy. Gut Liver. 2017;11(5):612–9.
16. Tsolakis AV, Ragkousi A, Vujasinovic M, et al. Gastric neuroendocrine neoplasms type 1: a systematic review and meta-analysis. World J Gastroenterol. 2019;25(35):5376–87.
17. Ravizza D, Fiori G, Trovato C, et al. Long-term endoscopic and clinical follow-up of untreated type 1 gastric neuroendocrine tumours. Dig Liver Dis. 2007;39(6):537–43.
18. Matsui N. Endoscopic submucosal dissection for removal of superficial gastrointestinal neoplasms: a technical review. World J Gastrointest Endosc. 2012;4(4):123–36.

19. Kim HH, Kim GH, Kim JH, et al. The efficacy of endoscopic submucosal dissection of type I gastric carcinoid tumors compared with conventional endoscopic mucosal resection. Gastroenterol Res Pract. 2014;2014:253860.
20. Sato Y, Takeuchi M, Hashimoto S, et al. Usefulness of endoscopic submucosal dissection for type I gastric carcinoid tumors compared with endoscopic mucosal resection. Hepato-Gastroenterology. 2013;60(126):1524–9.
21. Sato Y. Endoscopic diagnosis and management of type I neuroendocrine tumors. World Journal of Gastrointestinal Endoscopy. 2015;7(4):346–53.
22. Delle Fave G, O'Toole D, Sundin A, et al. ENETS consensus guidelines update for gastroduodenal neuroendocrine neoplasms. Neuroendocrinology. 2016;103(2):119–24.
23. Falconi M, Eriksson B, Kaltsas G, et al. Consensus guidelines update for the management of functional p-NETs (F-p-NETs) and non-functional p-NETs (NF-p-NETs). Neuroendocrinology. 2016;103(2):153–71.
24. Kunz PL, Reidy-Lagunes D, Anthony LB, et al. Consensus guidelines for the management and treatment of neuroendocrine tumors. Pancreas. 2013;42(4):557–77.
25. Kwon YH, Jeon SW, Kim GH, et al. Long-term follow up of endoscopic resection for type 3 gastric NET. World J Gastroenterol. 2013;19(46):8703–8.
26. Tierney JF, Chivukula SV, Wang X, et al. Resection of primary tumor may prolong survival in metastatic gastroenteropancreatic neuroendocrine tumors. Surgery. 2019;165(3):644–51.
27. Boyce M, Moore AR, Sagatun L, et al. Netazepide, a gastrin/cholecystokinin-2 receptor antagonist, can eradicate gastric neuroendocrine tumours in patients with autoimmune chronic atrophic gastritis. Br J Clin Pharmacol. 2017;83(3):466–75.
28. Fitzgerald TL, Dennis SO, Kachare SD, et al. Increasing incidence of duodenal neuroendocrine tumors: incidental discovery of indolent disease? Surgery. 2015;158(2):466–71.
29. Rossi RE, Rausa E, Cavalcoli F, et al. Duodenal neuroendocrine neoplasms: a still poorly recognized clinical entity. Scand J Gastroenterol. 2018;53(7):835–42.
30. Massironi S, Campana D, Partelli S, et al. Heterogeneity of duodenal neuroendocrine tumors: an Italian multi-center experience. Ann Surg Oncol. 2018;25(11):3200–6.
31. Untch BR, Bonner KP, Roggin KK, et al. Pathologic grade and tumor size are associated with recurrence-free survival in patients with duodenal neuroendocrine Tumors. J Gastrointest Surg. 2014;18(3):457–63.
32. Zhang XF, Wu XN, Tsilimigras DI, et al. Duodenal neuroendocrine tumors: impact of tumor size and total number of lymph nodes examined. J Surg Oncol. 2019;120(8):1302–10.
33. Dogeas E, Cameron JL, Wolfgang CL, et al. Duodenal and ampullary carcinoid tumors: size predicts necessity for lymphadenectomy. J Gastrointest Surg. 2017;21:1262–9.
34. Margonis GA, Samaha M, Kim Y, et al. A multi-institutional analysis of duodenal neuroendocrine tumors: tumor biology rather than extent of resection dictates prognosis. J Gastrointest Surg. 2016;20(6):1098–105.
35. Gamboa AC, Liu Y, Lee RM, et al. Duodenal neuroendocrine tumors: somewhere between the pancreas and small bowel? J Surg Oncol. 2019;120(8):1293–301.
36. Fairweather M, Swanson R, Wang J, et al. Management of Neuroendocrine Tumor Liver Metastases: long-term outcomes and prognostic factors from a large prospective database. Ann Surg Oncol. 2017;24:2319–25.
37. Xiang JX, Zhang XF, Beal EW, et al. Hepatic resection for non-functional neuroendocrine liver metastasis: does the presence of unresected primary tumor or extrahepatic metastatic disease matter? Ann Surg Oncol. 2018;25:3928–35.
38. Egger ME, Armstrong E, Martin RC 2nd, et al. Transarterial chemoembolization vs radioembolization for neuroendocrine liver metastases: a multi-institutional analysis. J Am Coll Surg. 2020;230(4):363–70.

Non Functional Pancreatic Neuroendocrine Tumors

8

Francesca Muffatti, Valentina Andreasi, Stefano Partelli, and Massimo Falconi

Epidemiology

Pancreatic neuroendocrine neoplasia (PanNEN) are rare tumors accounting for 2% of all pancreatic neoplasms. Their incidence in the United States has been rising in the last decades, reaching an estimated incidence in 2012 of 0.8:100,000 inhabitants [1]. Although they may manifest at any age, they most often occur in the fourth to sixth decades of life. They tend to present slightly more in male (55%) than in women (45%) and are more frequently discovered in White patients, whereas Blacks and Asians seem to be less frequently affected. The majority of NF-PanNEN are sporadic; however, nearly 10% of them are associated with a hereditary syndrome, such as von Hippel Lindau disease (VHL), neurofibromatosis type I (NF1) multiple endocrine neoplasia type I (MEN1), or tuberous sclerosis.

Preoperative Evaluation

An accurate diagnosis is crucial for choosing the most appropriate treatment of NF-PanNEN. The majority of patients are asymptomatic, and the rate of incidental diagnoses is increasing due to the widespread use of radiological examinations [2]. On the other hand, patients with advanced disease may present with non-specific symptoms such as pain, weight loss, anorexia, nausea and/or jaundice.

F. Muffatti (✉) · V. Andreasi · S. Partelli · M. Falconi
Pancreas Translational & Clinical Research Center, Pancreatic Surgery IRRCS San Raffaele Hospital Vita-Salute San Raffaele University, Milan, Italy
e-mail: muffatti.francesca@hsr.it; andreasi.valentina@hsr.it; partelli.stefano@hsr.it; falconi.massimo@hsr.it

© Springer Nature Switzerland AG 2021
J. M. Cloyd, T. M. Pawlik (eds.), *Neuroendocrine Tumors*,
https://doi.org/10.1007/978-3-030-62241-1_8

Laboratory

Chromogranin A (CgA) is the most used biomarker for diagnosis and follow-up of NF-PanNEN, especially for metastatic forms [3]. Several factors affect the sensitivity of CgA. In particular, CgA may be increased by several conditions (i.e. Parkinson's disease, hypertension, pregnancy, endocrine disorders and chronic gastritis type A) as well as different drugs (i.e. steroids and protein pump inhibitor) [4]. Other biomarkers such as Pancreatic Polypeptide, Neuron-Specific Enolase, and Pancreastatin have been advocated as possible biomarkers for NF-PanNEN but no robust evidence on their routine use in clinical practice have been provided [5]. In recent years some novel promising biomarkers emerged. These include microRNAs (miRNAs), long non-coding RNAs (lncRNAs), circulating tumor cells, blood gene expression of RNA transcript (NEtest) [2]. Despite initial promising results, all these new tools need to be further validated in prospective studies.

Radiology

High-quality imaging is crucial for an accurate definition of NF-PanNEN primary tumor features as well as for disease staging. Diagnostic work-up should include an anatomic high-resolution imaging with a quadruple-phase computed tomography (CT) scan with contrast enhancement and/or a Magnetic Resonance imaging (MRI). NF-PanNEN appear usually as small and well-delineated lesions, highly vascularized during the arterial inflow phase. Necrosis can be present, especially in large lesions. CT also delineates the relationship between the tumor and the nearby organs with a high accuracy in determining possible vascular infiltration. Moreover, the presence of distant metastases or enlarged and hypervascularized lymph nodes can be assessed [6] (Fig. 8.1). MRI has also a good accuracy in the diagnosis of NF-PanNEN and it can be useful for a better definition of liver metastasis (LM) when it is performed with liver-specific contrast agent.

Panel A   **Panel B**

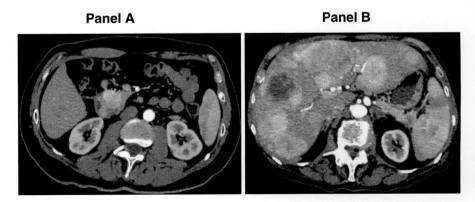

Fig. 8.1 CT scan appearance of NF-PanNEN in *Panel A:* NF-PanNEN of the uncinate process of the pancreas; in *Panel B:* NF-PanNEN of the pancreatic tail with liver metastases

Several lesions such as solid serous cystadenoma, metastases from renal cell carcinoma, acinar carcinoma, and accessory spleen may mimic NF-PanNET having similar radiological features. The differential diagnosis may be challenging since most of these conditions are positive also on functional imaging and preoperative biopsy may not be always diagnostic.

Nuclear Medicine Imaging

Functional imaging plays an essential role in the diagnosis and staging of NF-PanNEN. Somatostatin receptor (SSTR) Positron Emission Tomography (PET) with ^{68}Gallium-labeled somatostatin analogs (^{68}Ga-PET) is highly accurate in detecting primary NF-PanNEN and the presence of distant metastases and is considered the gold standard for well- and moderately-differentiated NF-PanNEN. In general, the higher the grade of the tumor, the lower the SSTR expression and, consequently, the tumor uptake on somatostatin receptor imaging. On the other hand, high-grade or poorly differentiated NF-PanNEN tend to be positive on ^{18}F-FDG PET [6].

The role of dual tracer PET (^{68}Galllium + ^{18}F-FDG) in clinical practice is still debated, but it seems to be useful for achieving a better staging and driving the treatment choice in patients with metastatic diseases [7].

Combined PET/CT scan with contrast-enhancement improves the diagnostic accuracy when compared to PET alone and can be recommended in all patients with a suspicious NF-PanNEN in order to define possible vascular involvement. PET/MRI is a novel modality with simultaneous acquisition of PET and MRI that can define precisely hepatic burden at baseline and during follow up (Fig. 8.2).

Endoscopic Ultrasound

Endoscopic ultrasound of the pancreas (EUSP) is essential to evaluate the relationship between the nodule and the main pancreatic duct, to assess the presence of multifocal NF-PanNEN, and to provide additional information on possible vascular

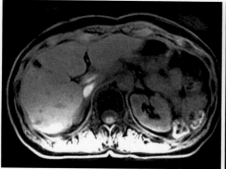 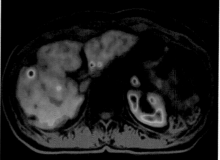

Fig. 8.2 ^{68}Ga-PET/MRI of NF-PanNEN showing hepatic lesions

infiltration or nodal involvement. EUSP is also important for achieving a cytological/histological diagnosis with a Fine Needle Aspiration/Biopsy (FAN/B). The accuracy of EUS depends by the experience of the endoscopic team and it should be performed in highly specialized institutions.

Staging

In 2017, the World Health Organization (WHO) published the latest classification for pancreatic NEN, dividing NF-PanNEN in three different categories, based on the Ki67 proliferation index and mitotic count: well differentiated PanNEN (Grade 1 [G1] with Ki67 index <3%, Grade 2 [G2] with Ki67 index between 3 and 20%, Grade 3 [G3] with Ki67 index >20%), poorly differentiated pancreatic carcinoma (PanNEC)-G3 and mixed neuroendocrine-non neuroendocrine neoplasia (Table 8.1) [8].

The two staging systems of NF-PanNEN have been proposed by the European Neuroendocrine Tumor Society (ENETS) [9] and the American Joint Cancer Committee (AJCC)/Union for International Cancer Control (UICC) (Table 8.2) [10].

Surgical Management

The surgical approach of NF-PanNEN should consider several factors including tumor size, grading, stage and the heterogeneity of disease. Since the potential complexity of most of surgical indications, each patient affected by NF-PanNEN should be referred to and managed by a dedicated tumor board in highly specialized centers (Table 8.3).

Table 8.1 2017 WHO classification of pancreatic neuroendocrine neoplasms (PanNENs) [8]

Well-differentiated PanNENs: Pancreatic Neuroendocrine Tumor (PanNET)		
	Mitotic count	Ki67 index
PanNEN G1	<2	<3%
PanNEN G2	≥2 ≤20	≥ 3% ≤ 20%
PanNEN G3	>20	>20%
Poorly differentiated PanNENs: Pancreatic Neuroendocrine Carcinoma (PanNEC)		
	Mitotic count	Ki67 index
PanNEC (G3)	>20	>20%
Small cell type		
Large cell type		
Mixed neuroendocrine-non-neuroendocrine tumor		

Note: The Ki-67 proliferation index is based on the evaluation of ≥500 cells in areas of higher nuclear labelling (so-called hotspots). The mitotic index is based on the evaluation of mitoses in 50 high-power fields (0.2 mm2 each) in areas of higher density and is expressed as mitoses per 10 high-power fields (2.0 mm2). The final grade is determined based on whichever index (Ki-67 or mitotic) places the tumour in the highest grade category. For assessing Ki-67, casual visual estimation (eyeballing) is not recommended; manual counting using printed images is advocated

Table 8.2 Staging system of AJCC/UICC and ENETS [9, 10]

	AJCC/UICC staging system	ENETS staging system
T1	Limited to the pancreas, <2 cm in greatest dimension	Tumor limited to the pancreas <2 cm
T2	Tumor limited to the pancreas 2–4 cm	Tumor limited to the pancreas 2–4 cm
T3	Tumour limited to pancreas, more than 4 cm in greatest dimension or tumour invading duodenum or bile duct.	Tumor limited to the pancreas >4 cm, or invading the duodenum or common bile duct
T4	Tumour perforates visceral peritoneum (serosa) or invades other organs or adjacent structures	Tumor invades adjacent structures
N0	No regional lymph node metastasis	No regional lymph node metastasis
N1	Regional lymph node metastasis	Regional lymph node metastasis
M0	No distant metastasis	No distant metastasis
M1	Distant metastasis M1a Hepatic metastasis(is) only M1b Extrahepatic metastasis(is) only M1c Hepatic and extrahepatic metastases	Distant metastasis

ENETS

Stage	T	N	M
I	T1	N0	M0
IIA	T2	N0	M0
IB	T3	N0	M0
IIIA	T4	N0	M0
IIIB	Any T	N1	M0
IV	Any T	Any N	M1

AJCC/UICC

Stage	T	N	M
I	T1	N0	M0
II	T2-T3	N0	M0
III	T4	N0	M0
	Any T	N1	M0
IV	Any T	Any N	M1

Abbreviations: *AJCC* American Joint Cancer Committee, *UICC* Union for International Cancer Control, *ENETS* European Neuroendocrine Tumor Society, *M* distant metastasis, *N* lymph nodes, *T* primary tumor

Active Surveillance

The widespread use of high-quality imaging has led to a dramatic increase in the diagnosis of small, asymptomatic, incidentally discovered, NF-PanNEN. It has been estimated that the incidence of NF-PanNEN <2 cm has increased more than 700% in the last 20 years [11]. Moreover, the frequency of incidental histological diagnosis of PanNEN is around 4%, suggesting that their real prevalence is probably underestimated [12].

Table 8.3 Nonfunctioning pancreatic Neuroendocrine neoplasms algorithm for diagnosis, therapy and follow-up

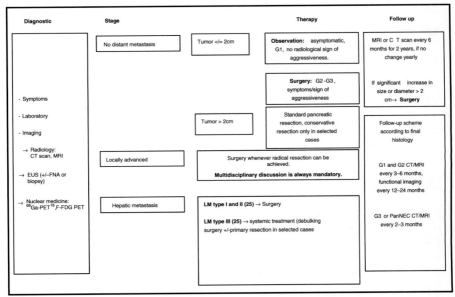

CT computed tomography, *MRI* Magnetic resonance imaging, *EUS* endoscopic ultrasound, *FNA* Fine needle aspiration, *68Ga-PET* 68Gallium Positron Emission Tomography, *18F-FDG PET* 18F-fluorodeoxyglucose Positron Emission Tomography, *G1* grade 1, *G2* Grade 2, *PanNEC* pancreatic neuroendocrine carcinoma, *LM* Liver metastases

Several retrospective studies [13, 14] demonstrated that these forms are generally indolent and tend to remain stable during active surveillance confirming that a watchful strategy can be advocated for the majority of patients. Based on these assumptions, both the ENETS and the North American Neuroendocrine Tumor Society (NANETS) guidelines consider conservative management for selected NF-PanNEN <2 cm to be appropriate [15, 16]. Nevertheless, the rational management of these small lesions should be always tailored according to specific criteria such as patients' expectations, tumor growth over time, tumor grade, extent and possible risks of surgical resection according to tumor location and radiological signs of aggressiveness such as pancreatic duct infiltration [17].

The most appropriate follow-up scheme is still unknown although it seems reasonable to recommend for the first two years after diagnosis a high quality imaging (CT scan or MRI) every six months and yearly thereafter if NF-PanNEN remains stable (Table 8.3).

Active surveillance should be interrupted in favor of surgical resection if the following conditions occur: significant enlargement of the lesion (>20% of initial size), dilatation of the main pancreatic or biliary duct, appearance of tumor-related symptoms.

Surgery

Surgical resection is the cornerstone of the treatment of localized NF-PanNEN and the only available curative treatment. Surgery also plays an important role in the treatment of metastatic disease (Table 8.3).

Surgical Management of Localized NF-PanNEN

Surgical treatment should be individualized considering several factors such as the size and the location of the nodule, as well as patients' age and comorbidities.

Standard pancreatic resection [pancreaticoduodenectomy (PD) or distal pancreatectomy (DP)] with lymphadenectomy should be always preferred to parenchyma sparing surgery (enucleation, central pancreatectomy, middle preserving pancreatectomy) for NF-PanNEN >2 cm, given the risk of nodal involvement [15, 18]. The number of minimum harvested lymph nodes for a proper staging during pancreaticoduodenectomy is 12 [19]. Indications for atypical resection for NF-PanNEN is therefore limited to very selected cases of NF-PanNEN < 2 cm. These procedures are associated with a higher risk of pancreatic fistula compared to standard resection although the low risk of developing pancreatic endocrine and exocrine insufficiency is lower [16, 20, 21]. Intraoperative nodal sampling and frozen sections during parenchyma-sparing procedures is always recommended [22].

NF-PanNEN represent ideal entities for a minimally invasive approach (laparoscopic or robotic) for neoplasms located in the pancreatic body or tail, or for those amenable of enucleation or central pancreatectomy. Laparoscopic distal pancreatectomy in high-volume center is considered safe and feasible in selected patients, with similar postoperative and oncological outcome if compared to traditional approach, with the well-known benefits of minimally invasive surgery [17, 22].

Surgical Management of NF-PanNEN-G3

Surgical indications for NF-PanNEN-G3 should be carefully evaluated since the aggressiveness of these forms. It is important to preoperatively assess the tumor differentiation according to the 2017 WHO classification [23]. Radical surgical resection of well-differentiated PanNEN G3 (PanNET G3) is associated with an improved survival especially when the Ki67 value is < 55% although available studies are retrospective and based on small series [19, 24]. The possible benefit of surgery in patients with poorly differentiated PanNEN G3 (pancreatic neuroendocrine carcinoma – PanNEC G3) is more controversial. In patients affected by NF-PanNEC-G3 the choice of performing upfront surgical resection in the rare cases of localized disease, should be carefully weighted with the high risk of postoperative recurrence that could be improved by preoperative or postoperative platinum based chemotherapy.

Surgical Management of Locally Advanced NF-PanNEN

In the presence of locally advanced disease, radical resection for well differentiated NF-PanNEN G1 and G2 should be attempted whenever possible, surgical approach may include multivisceral and vascular resection [22]. A preoperative treatment with PRRT may reduce the size of the tumor and improve the outcomes after surgery when curative resection is achieved [25].

Surgical Management of Metastatic NF-PanNEN

Surgery plays an important role even for metastatic disease. Before planning a possible surgical resection, various elements should be considered. These include: tumor grade, localization, progression-free interval during systemic treatment, SSTR expression and the burden and distribution of metastatic disease.

The most common site of distant metastasis of NF-PanNEN is the liver. In particular, 3 patterns of distribution of liver metastases (LM) have been described: type I with a single LM, type II isolated metastatic bulk accompanied by smaller deposits, with bilobar involvement, type III disseminated metastatic spread, with both liver lobes always involved, single lesion of varying size and virtually no normal liver parenchyma [26]. Type I and II LM are resectable or potentially resectable, whereas type III is unresectable. Surgery is generally recommended for those patients with type I and II LM since it is associated with an improved survival [27, 28].

In the presence of type III LM, systemic therapy remains the backbone of patients' management, although primary tumor resection could be an option in selected cases. On this specific issue, there is still no consensus in literature as only retrospective studies are available [19]. It seems that primary NF-PanNEN resection in the presence of unresectable LM, it is associated with an improved survival compared to systemic treatments alone [19]. Primary tumor resection may improve survival outcomes also by enhancing the efficacy of specific treatment such as PRRT [24]. Moreover, resection of the primary tumor may prevent local complications such as jaundice, duodenal obstruction or bleeding. The surgical evaluation of patients affected by NF-PanNEN with LM should consider the localization of the primary lesion in the pancreatic gland. Distal pancreatectomy for NF-PanNEN of the pancreatic body-tail is associated with a relatively low risk of severe complications and mortality. On the other hand, pancreaticoduodenectomy is affected by a high risk of postoperative complications and the presence of a bilio-enteric anastomosis may increase the risk of liver abscess after locoregional treatment of LM (i.e. embolization or radiofrequency ablation) [29].

Regarding the treatment of type III LM, some retrospective studies demonstrated a possible benefit of hepatic cytoreductive surgery by removing 70 to 90% of the tumor mass [30, 31].

Another surgical option for very selected patients with unresectable LM that may be taken into account is liver transplantation [32, 33].

Patients with LM from NF-PanNEN may be eligible for liver transplantation under strict criteria that include [34]:

- histological confirmation of low-grade neuroendocrine tumor (Ki67 < 10%),
- primary tumor drained by the portal system previously removed with all the extrahepatic deposits,
- involvement of less than 50% of liver parenchyma,
- stable disease/response to therapies for ≥6 months during the pre-transplantation period,
- Age < 60 years old (relative criteria).

Follow-up

Due to the indolent and the slow rate of growing of PanNEN the advised follow up should last lifelong or at least for 20 years.

For NF-PanNEN G1 and G2 resected conventional high quality imaging (CT scan or MRI) should be scheduled every 3–6 months, whereas functional imaging every 12–24 months or when relapse/progression is suspected, whereas for G3 or PanNEC follow up must be intensified every 2–3 months for morphological imaging. EUS is advised only in case of relapse or progression [35, 36]. Interval between investigations can be increased after 5 years, for G1 or indolent neoplasm (Table 8.3).

Acknowledgments Francesca Muffatti research fellowship and Valentina Andreasi studentship were supported by Gioja Bianca Costanza legacy donation.

References

1. Dasari A, Shen C, Halperin D, Zhao B, Zhou S, Xu Y, et al. Trends in the incidence, prevalence, and survival outcomes in patients with neuroendocrine tumors in the United States. JAMA Oncol. 2017;3(10):1335–42.
2. Partelli S, Andreasi V, Muffatti F, Schiavo Lena M, Falconi M. Circulating Neuroendocrine Gene Transcripts (NETest): a postoperative strategy for early identification of the efficacy of radical surgery for pancreatic neuroendocrine tumors. Ann Surg Oncol. 2020;27(10):3928–36.
3. Lawrence B, Gustafsson BI, Kidd M, Pavel M, Svejda B, Modlin IM. The clinical relevance of chromogranin A as a biomarker for gastroenteropancreatic neuroendocrine tumors. Endocrinol Metab Clin N Am. 2011;40(1):111–34.
4. Oberg K, Couvelard A, Delle Fave G, Gross D, Grossman A, Jensen RT, et al. ENETS consensus guidelines for the standards of care in neuroendocrine tumors: biochemical markers. Neuroendocrinology. 2017;105(3):201–11.
5. Nobels FRE, Kwekkeboom DJ, Coopmans W, Schoenmakers CHH, Lindemans J, De Herder WW, et al. Chromogranin A as serum marker for neuroendocrine neoplasia: comparison with neuron-specific enolase and the α-subunit of glycoprotein hormones. J Clin Endocrinol Metab. 1997;82(8):2622–8.
6. Sundin A, Arnold R, Baudin E, Cwikla JB, Eriksson B, Fanti S, et al. ENETS consensus guidelines for the standards of care in neuroendocrine tumors: radiological, nuclear medicine and hybrid imaging. Neuroendocrinology. 2017;105(3):212–44.

7. Muffatti Francesca, Partelli Stefano, Cirocchi Roberto, Andreasi Valentina, Mapelli Paola, Picchio MAria GL& FM. Combined 68Ga-DOTA-peptides and 18F-FDG PET in the diagnostic work-up of neuroendocrine neoplasms (NEN). Clin Transl Imaging. 2019;7:181–87.
8. Lloyd RV, Osamura YR, Kloppel G, Rosai J. WHO classification of tumours of endocrine organs: WHO Press; 2017.
9. Klöppel G, Rindi G, Perren A, Komminoth P, Klimstra DS. The ENETS and UICC TNM classification of neuroendocrine tumors of the gastrointestinal tract and the pancreas: comment. Pathologe. 2010;31(5):353–4.
10. Brierley JD, Gospodarowicz MK. Wittekind C. TNM classification of malignant tumours – 8th edition. Union for International. Cancer Control. 2017.
11. Kuo EJ, Salem RR. Population-level analysis of pancreatic neuroendocrine tumors 2 cm or less in size. Ann Surg Oncol. 2013;20(9):2815–21.
12. Partelli S, Giannone F, Schiavo Lena M, Muffatti F, Andreasi V, Crippa S, et al. Is the real prevalence of pancreatic neuroendocrine tumors underestimated? A retrospective study on a large series of pancreatic specimens. Neuroendocrinology. 2019;109(2):165–70.
13. Partelli S, Cirocchi R, Crippa S, Cardinali L, Fendrich V, Bartsch DK, et al. Systematic review of active surveillance versus surgical management of asymptomatic small non-functioning pancreatic neuroendocrine neoplasms. Br J Surg. 2017;104(1):34–41.
14. Sallinen V, Le Large TYS, Galeev S, Kovalenko Z, Tieftrunk E, Araujo R, et al. Surveillance strategy for small asymptomatic non-functional pancreatic neuroendocrine tumors – a systematic review and meta-analysis. HPB. 2017;19(4):310–20.
15. Partelli S, Javed AA, Andreasi V, He J, Muffatti F, Weiss MJ, et al. The number of positive nodes accurately predicts recurrence after pancreaticoduodenectomy for nonfunctioning neuroendocrine neoplasms. Eur J Surg Oncol. 2018;44(6):778–83.
16. Hüttner FJ, Koessler-Ebs J, Hackert T, Ulrich A, Büchler MW, Diener MK. Meta-analysis of surgical outcome after enucleation versus standard resection for pancreatic neoplasms. Br J Surg. 2015;102(9):1026–36.
17. Howe JR, Merchant NB, Conrad C, Keutgen XM, Hallet J, Drebin JA, et al. The North American neuroendocrine tumor society consensus paper on the surgical management of pancreatic neuroendocrine tumors. Pancreas. 2020;49(1):1–33.
18. Parekh JR, Wang SC, Bergsland EK, Venook AP, Warren RS, Kim GE, et al. Lymph node sampling rates and predictors of nodal metastasis in pancreatic neuroendocrine tumor resections: the UCSF experience with 149 patients. Pancreas. 2012;41(6):840–4.
19. Partelli S, Cirocchi R, Rancoita PMV, Muffatti F, Andreasi V, Crippa S, et al. A systematic review and meta-analysis on the role of palliative primary resection for pancreatic neuroendocrine neoplasm with liver metastases. HPB. 2018;20(3):197–203.
20. Chua TC, Yang TX, Gill AJ, Samra JS. Systematic review and meta-analysis of enucleation versus standardized resection for small pancreatic lesions. Ann Surg Oncol. 2016;23(2):592–9.
21. Heeger K, Falconi M, Partelli S, Waldmann J, Crippa S, Fendrich V, et al. Increased rate of clinically relevant pancreatic fistula after deep enucleation of small pancreatic tumors. Langenbeck's Arch Surg. 2014;399(3):315–21.
22. Partelli S, Bartsch DK, Capdevila J, Chen J, Knigge U, Niederle B, et al. ENETS consensus guidelines for standard of care in neuroendocrine tumours: surgery for small intestinal and pancreatic neuroendocrine tumours. Neuroendocrinology. 2017;105(3):255–65.
23. Klimstra DS, Kloppell G, La Rosa S RG. The 2019 WHO classification of tumours of the digestive system. 5 th. International Agency for Research on Cancer, editor. Lyon; 2020 Jan;76(2):182–88.
24. Bertani E, Fazio N, Radice D, Zardini C, Spinoglio G, Chiappa A, et al. Assessing the role of primary tumour resection in patients with synchronous unresectable liver metastases from pancreatic neuroendocrine tumour of the body and tail. A propensity score survival evaluation. Eur J Surg Oncol. 2017;43(2):372–79.
25. Partelli S, Bertani E, Bartolomei M, Perali C, Muffatti F, Grana CM, et al. Peptide receptor radionuclide therapy as neoadjuvant therapy for resectable or potentially resectable pancreatic neuroendocrine neoplasms. Surg (United States). 2018;163(4):761–67.

26. Frilling A, Li J, Malamutmann E, Schmid KW, Bockisch A, Broelsch CE. Treatment of liver metastases from neuroendocrine tumours in relation to the extent of hepatic disease. Br J Surg. 2009;96(2):175–84.
27. Frilling A, Modlin IM, Kidd M, Russell C, Breitenstein S, Salem R, et al. Recommendations for management of patients with neuroendocrine liver metastases. Lancet Oncol. 2014 Jan;15(1):e8–21.
28. Tierney JF, Chivukula SV, Wang X, Pappas SG, Schadde E, Hertl M, et al. Resection of primary tumor may prolong survival in metastatic gastroenteropancreatic neuroendocrine tumors. Surg (United States). 2019;165(3):644–51.
29. Scoville SD, Xourafas D, Ejaz AM, Tsung A, Pawlik T, Cloyd JM. Contemporary indications for and outcomes of hepatic resection for neuroendocrine liver metastases. World J Gastrointest Surg. 2020;12(4):159–70.
30. Maxwell JE, Sherman SK, O'Dorisio TM, Bellizzi AM, Howe JR. Liver-directed surgery of neuroendocrine metastases: what is the optimal strategy? Surgery (United States). 2016;159(1):320–33.
31. Morgan RE, Pommier SEJ, Pommier RF. Expanded criteria for debulking of liver metastasis also apply to pancreatic neuroendocrine tumors. Surg (United States). 2018;163(1):218–25.
32. Mazzaferro V, Sposito C, Coppa J, Miceli R, Bhoori S, Bongini M, et al. The long-term benefit of liver transplantation for hepatic metastases from neuroendocrine tumors. Am J Transplant. 2016;16(10):2892–902.
33. Moris D, Tsilimigras DI, Ntanasis-Stathopoulos I, Beal EW, Felekouras E, Vernadakis S, et al. Liver transplantation in patients with liver metastases from neuroendocrine tumors: a systematic review. Surg (United States). 2017;162(3):525–36.
34. Mazzaferro V, Pulvirenti A, Coppa J. Neuroendocrine tumors metastatic to the liver: how to select patients for liver transplantation? J Hepatol. 2007;47(4):460–6.
35. Knigge U, Capdevila J, Bartsch DK, Baudin E, Falkerby J, Kianmanesh R, et al. ENETS consensus recommendations for the standards of care in neuroendocrine neoplasms: follow-up and documentation. Neuroendocrinology. 2017;105(3):310–19.
36. Zaidi MY, Lopez-Aguiar AG, Switchenko JM, Lipscomb J, Andreasi V, Partelli S, et al. A novel validated recurrence risk score to guide a pragmatic surveillance strategy after resection of pancreatic neuroendocrine tumors: an international study of 1006 patients. Ann Surg. 2019;270(3):422–33.

Functional Pancreatic Neuroendocrine Tumors

9

Sean Alexander Bennett, Calvin How Lim Law,
Angela Assal, Sten Myrehaug, and Julie Hallet

Introduction

Eight years after the discovery of insulin in 1921, in the same Toronto hospital, the first successful resection of a pancreatic insulinoma was performed by Dr. Roscoe Graham, who would later go on to describe the omental patch procedure that bears his name [1–3]. Dr. Graham performed abdominal exploration for a 54-year-old patient with a 6-year history of sporadic convulsions and coma, found a lesion on the anterior body of the pancreas, enucleated it, and cured the patient of her hypoglycemia [2]. Since this early description of what was a functional pancreatic

S. A. Bennett
Department of Surgery, University of Toronto, Toronto, ON, Canada
e-mail: seana.bennett@sunnybrook.ca

C. H. L. Law · J. Hallet (✉)
Department of Surgery, University of Toronto, Toronto, ON, Canada

Susan Leslie Clinic for Neuroendocrine Tumors, Sunnybrook Health Sciences Centre, Toronto, ON, Canada
e-mail: calvin.law@sunnybrook.ca; Julie.hallet@sunnybrook.ca

A. Assal
Susan Leslie Clinic for Neuroendocrine Tumors, Sunnybrook Health Sciences Centre, Toronto, ON, Canada

Department of Medicine, University of Toronto, Toronto, ON, Canada
e-mail: angela.assal@sunnybrook.ca

S. Myrehaug
Susan Leslie Clinic for Neuroendocrine Tumors, Sunnybrook Health Sciences Centre, Toronto, ON, Canada

Department of Radiation Oncology, University of Toronto, Toronto, ON, Canada
e-mail: sten.myrehaug@sunnybrook.ca

© Springer Nature Switzerland AG 2021
J. M. Cloyd, T. M. Pawlik (eds.), *Neuroendocrine Tumors*,
https://doi.org/10.1007/978-3-030-62241-1_9

neuroendocrine tumor (pNET) nearly 100 years ago, much has been discovered about these rare tumors; however, owing largely to their rarity, much is still left to be understood.

Pancreatic neuroendocrine tumors (pNETs) are classified as functional if they are hormonally active and result in symptoms that can be attributed to this hormone activity. Some pNETs may produce excess hormones without associated symptoms, and these are typically considered as non-functional [4–6]. Functional pNETs have an added element of complexity to their management, as the clinician must manage both the oncologic consequences of the tumor as well as the associated endocrinopathy. They represent a group of heterogeneous tumors with regard to biological and endocrine behavior. However, they are generally associated with a more favorable prognosis [4, 7, 8]. This chapter will review the epidemiology, pathology, clinical work-up, and management of primary sporadic functional pNETs.

Epidemiology

The incidence of pNETs has increased to reach 8 per 1,000,000 in North America [4, 9], attributed mainly to improvements in diagnostic imaging and endoscopic techniques [10]. The proportion of functional pNETs among all pNETs is traditionally estimated at 9% [4, 9, 11]. However, it is difficult to estimate from population-based registries due to classification errors, and some have suggested the true proportions of functional pNETs may be up to 25% [5, 6].

Of the subtypes of functional pNETs, insulinomas are the most common (70–75%), followed by gastrinomas (20%) [5]. The remainder of functional pNETs is grouped together as rare functional pNETs, including those secreting glucagon, vasoactive intestinal polypeptide (VIP), somatostatin, adrenocorticotropic hormone (ACTH), calcitonin, growth hormone-releasing factor, and parathyroid hormone-related peptide. Prognosis depends on the malignant potential of the pNETs which varies by subtype. In all functional pNETs, median overall survival is reported at 14.3 years [7].

The details of each entity will be discussed in further detail below. This includes the manner in which patients present, the pathologic appearance and oncologic aggressiveness of their tumor, and the necessary steps in clinical management.

Pathology

The neuroendocrine cells of the pancreas are the islets cells, which make up roughly 1–2% of the pancreatic volume. They are scattered throughout the pancreatic parenchyma and are typically found in clusters of mixed populations of endocrine cells. The clusters consist of about 70% beta cells which produce insulin, 20% alpha cells which produce glucagon, and the remaining 10% of cells produce a number of other hormones and peptides [12]. Interestingly, the normal adult pancreas does not contain any gastrin-producing G-cells, which are found in the gastric antrum or duodenum. Gastrinomas do occur in both the duodenum and pancreas however, and some interesting work has been done identifying embryonic and neonatal gastrin-producing cells in the pancreas that appear to be progenitors for islet cells and could represent the tumor cells of origin [13].

The World Health Organization (WHO) grading system for pNETs includes well-differentiated neuroendocrine tumors subdivided into G1, G2, and G3 based on Ki-67 proliferation index and differentiation, similarly to other NETs [14]. There is also a category of poorly differentiated G3 pNETs. Functional pNETs are typically well-differentiated low-grade (G1 or G2) tumors with preservation of cell differentiation associated with the endocrine activity.

Clinical Presentation and Work-Up

Functional pNETs can have as heterogeneous a presentation as their type and level of endocrine activity. While some tumors will be sought out and identified following a diagnosis of endocrine-related syndrome (such as insulinoma or gastrinoma clinical manifestations), others may present as incidental imaging findings with clinical endocrine manifestations being identified upon further clinical history and work-up. Therefore, it is crucial to understand clinical, biochemical, and imaging features of pNETs and obtain comprehensive detailed assessments prior to devising a management plan.

The work-up can be divided into:

1. Tumor staging: identification of primary tumor site and extent of disease via imaging including computerized tomography (CT) scan, magnetic resonance imaging (MRI), and endoscopy;
2. Histology diagnosis and grading, via tissue diagnosis and functional imaging such as somatostatin-receptor based Positron emmission tomography (PET) (SSTR-PET) imaging;
3. Endocrine staging, via clinical evaluation for functional syndrome and biochemical assessment to confirm such syndrome.

Tumor Staging

Cross-Sectional Imaging: CT Scan and MRI

The best overall imaging modality for the primary tumor is a pancreas-protocol CT scan [6], with arterial and portal venous phases and thin-cuts through the pancreas. This allows for lesion detection in the majority of cases. pNETs can be characterized on multi-phasic cross-sectional imaging by their unique enhancement and growth patterns. On CT scan, they appear isodense on pre-contrast phases, become very hyperenhancing on the arterial phase, and retain hyperenhancement, though to a lesser degree, in the venous phase. They are typically homogeneous without any distortion of the pancreatic contour [15]. Thin-sliced high-resolution MRI (1.5 T) can be useful when diagnostic uncertainty remains. pNETs typically present as lesions that are hypodense on T1, hyperdense on T2, hyperdense in fat-suppressing phases, and have homogeneous enhancement after injection of gadolinium [15]. While there has been some suggestion that use of MRI diffusion-weighted imaging (DWI) could help determine grade of pNET, such findings have not been validated and histology examination remains the method of choice to establish grade [6, 16]. In addition to establishing an imaging diagnosis of pNETs, cross-sectional imaging allows for an assessment of resectability of the primary tumor and identification of aberrant anatomy.

In addition to imaging the primary tumor, CT scan of the chest, abdomen, and pelvis is recommended for staging of distant disease [17]; it provides detailed imaging of the regional and distant lymph nodes, liver, peritoneal cavity, and chest. Of note, the pancreatic protocol used for assessment of the primary tumor does not interfere with the assessment of intra-abdominal metastases [18]. MRI with hepatobiliary phase contrast agents is the modality of choice to assess for liver metastases. This modality is superior to CT scan with superior sensitivity of detecting metastases, ruling out lesions seen on CT as non-metastatic, and ability to improve the consistency of images on repeated tests over time [19–21].

Minimum imaging for the evaluation of both the primary tumor and metastatic disease for pNETs should include multi-phasic CT of the abdomen and pelvis, liver MRI with hepatobiliary phase contrast agents, and CT of the chest.

SSTR-PET Imaging

SSTR-PET imaging (68Ga-DOTATATE or 68GA-DOTATOC receptor-PET) has largely replaced traditional 111In-Pentetreotide Scintigraphy (octreotide scan) [6]. The use of the original octreotide scan should be limited to settings where there is no access to DOTATATE/TOC.

The role of SSTR-PET imaging is primarily for the detection of metastatic disease or disease recurrence [22]. This modality has limited ability to characterize pancreatic masses beyond cross-sectional imaging and endoscopic ultrasound (EUS). For example, if there is diagnostic doubt on CT scan and/or MRI, PET imaging cannot distinguish between a splenule and a pNET. Furthermore, physiologic uptake in the pancreas may happen in 50% of patients undergoing SSTR-PET, especially in the uncinate process and the pancreatic tail, which is associated with risks of false-positives [23, 24]. SSTR-PET uptake in the pancreas must be confirmed by detecting an associated lesion on CT [6]. Therefore, cross-sectional imaging and EUS with biopsy is considered superior to PET imaging for evaluation of the primary tumor [6]. One potential use may be in the patient diagnosed with metastatic NET with an unidentifiable primary on traditional imaging modalities. In a series of 40 such patients, 68Ga-DOTATOC-PET/CT was able to identify the primary tumor in 15 patients (6 pancreatic, 8 small bowel, 1 retrorectal) [25].

The best test for the detection of metastatic disease in pNETs is SSTR-PET with either ^{68}Ga-DOTATATE or ^{68}Ga-DOTATOC [6]. Benefits of SSTR-PET over octreotide scan include improved sensitivity, lower radiation dose, shorter scan time, and the ability to quantify uptake [6]. If the diagnosis of additional metastatic disease would change management, then SSTR-PET is indicated.

Endoscopic Ultrasound (EUS)

Used as an imaging modality alone, EUS does have a select role in imaging of the primary tumor in sporadic pNETs. Studies have demonstrated increased detection of pancreatic lesions not appreciated by CT, MRI, and somatostatin-receptor scintigraphy [26, 27]. It can also identify multifocal pNETs in patients with tumors associated with hereditary syndromes Multiple endocrine neoplasia type 1 (e.g., MEN-1). The use of EUS for determining surgical resectability has not been evaluated in pNETs specifically, but is comparable to CT and MRI for pancreatic adenocarcinoma [28, 29]. Therefore, EUS is used selectively for identification of sporadic pNETs when there is potential added benefit to cross-sectional and functional imaging, but is not necessary for assessment of resectability [6].

The Non-localized Primary Tumor

One of the more challenging clinical scenarios in the realm of functional pNETs is that of the unidentifiable primary tumor. In this scenario, the clinician has made the clinical and biochemical diagnosis of an endocrine syndrome associated with a functional pNET, but imaging shows no abnormality. It is important that the clinical endocrine diagnosis be confirmed by an experienced endocrinology team; false-positive diagnoses may put patients through unnecessary invasive testing and interventions. For example, serum gastrin level is frequently falsely elevated in patients under proton pump inhibitor therapy, such that a finding of hypergastrinemia should not lead to a diagnosis of gastrinoma without careful endocrinology confirmation.

Providing that the endocrine syndrome is confirmed biochemically, the search for the primary tumor follows a stepwise approach from non-invasive to invasive testing. Comprehensive imaging including pancreas-protocol CT scan, MRI pancreas, EUS, and SSTR-PET should be performed prior to concluding an unidentified primary functional pNET. Further steps to undertake, such as interventional radiology sampling or surgical exploration, depend on the clinical endocrine syndrome and will be discussed below for each entity. Of note, most of the literature regarding the management of unidentified primary functional pNETs relies on non-contemporary data from patients treated prior to the availability of high-resolution CT scan, MRI, EUS, and SSTR-PET.

Histology Diagnosis and Grading

In the setting of a localized, resectable pNET with clinical and biochemical confirmation that it is functional, and typical imaging characteristics, there is no need for a tissue biopsy prior to surgical resection. Unlike non-functional pNETs there is no role to observe small functional pNETs, and therefore no need to establish tumor grade prior to planned observation. In unresectable, metastatic functional pNETs there would be a role for biopsy in order to confirm the diagnosis pathologically, as well as grade the tumor to determine which systemic therapies may be indicated. This biopsy could be obtained either through EUS from the primary or preferably percutaneously from an accessible metastatic deposit.

Endocrine Staging

Routine testing for hypersecretion of pancreatic hormones is not recommended for all pNETs. The assessment of a patient with suspected functional pNET should begin with a clinical evaluation of the potential for endocrinopathy in addition to the general medical history and physical exam, with a thorough review of medication and drug use, family history of endocrine tumors, prior diagnostic tests, and previous operations. This information should guide the use of biochemical tests to confirm the suspected diagnosis. Importantly, hormone levels should be checked at a fasting state, as secretion is stimulated post-prandially. Furthermore, hormone levels need to be interpreted in the context of the clinical situation; an elevated value may represent an appropriate physiologic response and is not necessarily pathologic [30]. Specific details for each entity are discussed below and summarized in Table 9.1.

Insulinoma

Symptoms related to an insulinoma derive mainly from neuroglycopenia (fatigue, confusion, blurred vision, seizures, AND/OR coma) and from the catecholamine surge secondary to the hypoglycemia (sweating, tremor, anxiousness, weakness, and palpitations) [31]. Given their persistent need to try to maintain normoglycemia, patients will often describe a history of weight gain. The classic Whipple's triad of hyperinsulinemia consists of symptoms of hypoglycemia, with documented low plasma glucose, and the resolution of symptoms with the administration of glucose. The Endocrine Society recommends only pursuing evaluation of

Table 9.1 Clinical and biochemical diagnoses of endocrine syndromes associated with functional pNETs

Type of functional pNET	Hormone	Clinical syndrome	Biochemical diagnosis
Insulinoma	Insulin	Whipple's triad: Documented hypoglycemia (blood glucose <55 mg/dL or 3.0 mmol/L) associated with symptoms of hypoglycemia (confusion, sweating, weakness, unconsciousness), and immediate relief with administration of glucose Weight gain	Inappropriately elevated insulin (>3.0 µU/mL or 20 pmol/L) and C-peptide (>0.6 ng/ml or 200 pmol/L) when hypoglycemic (blood glucose <55 mg/dL or 3.0 mmol/L) 48–72 hours supervised fasting test: glucose, insulin, C-peptide, pro-insulin, beta-hydroxybutyrate, sulfonylurea screen, drawn at the time of hypoglycemia Response to glucagon may also be assessed

Table 9.1 (continued)

Type of functional pNET	Hormone	Clinical syndrome	Biochemical diagnosis
Gastrinoma	Gastrin	Zollinger-Ellison syndrome (ZES): • Multiple ulcers • Diarrhea (may resolve with proton pump inhibitor – PPI) Gastroscopy: Document peptic ulcer disease	Elevated fasting serum gastrin (off PPI for one week, can use H2 blockers during this period) • Usually >200 pg/mL • If >1000 pg/mL: diagnostic of ZES unless hypochlorhydria present • If <1000 pg/mL: confirm with secretin or calcium simulated gastrin or acidic gastric acid Gastroscopy: measure gastric pH < 2 (perform off PPI to avoid false negatives)

Glucagonoma	Glucagon	"Sweet" syndrome: 4Ds:
		• Dermatosis (necrolytic migratory erythema)
		• Depression
		• Deep venous thrombosis
		  Diabetes: 40–90% will have glucose intolerance
		  Weight loss
			Fasting serum glucagon >500 pg/ml (normal ≤ 50) (check with a blood glucose to rule out a physiologic response to hypoglycemia)

VIPoma	Vasoactive intestinal peptide (VIP)	Verner-Morrison syndrome: • Watery, secretory diarrhea (>700 ml/day) • Hypokalemia • Hypochlorhydria • Hypercalcemia	Elevated serum VIP
Somatostatinoma	Somatostatin	• Secretory diarrhea that persists with fasting • Possible steatorrhea (secondary to somatostatin inhibition of digestive enzymes) • Cholelithiasis • Diabetes • Hypochlorhydria	Elevated fasting serum somatostatin

Adapted from: Khorasani M, Law C, Myrehaug S, Singh S, Assal A, Hiseh E, Cukier M, Hallet J. Neuroendocrine tumors (gastroenteropancreatic). In: Wright FC, Escallon J, editors. Surgical Oncology Manual, 3rd edition. Toronto (Canada). Springer. 2020; In Press hypoglycemia in patients with documented Whipple's triad [32]. Hypoglycemia (blood glucose <55 mg/dL or 3.0 mmol/L) while the patient is experiencing symptoms and relieved by administration of glucose should be documented first. Endogenous hyperinsulinemia is then confirmed with inappropriately elevated insulin and C-peptide, while the patient is hypoglycemic. If such an episode of hypoglycemia cannot easily be observed, a confirmation test during 48–72 h of supervised fasting is necessary [32].

Gastrinoma

Elevation in serum gastrin levels, and the subsequent gastric acid hypersecretion, results in peptic ulcer disease (PUD) in about 90% of patients with gastrinoma [33]. This will typically manifest in dyspepsia, anemia, or complications of PUD such as perforation, gastric outlet obstruction, or significant upper GI bleeding. Patients may have a history of PUD refractory to proton pump inhibition proton pump inhibitor (PPI), or with early recurrence after cessation of PPI. Recurrent PUD in the absence of H. pylori infection should strongly raise the suspicion of gastrinoma [34]. Other symptoms that gastrinoma patients may present with include diarrhea, heartburn, nausea/vomiting, and weight loss. The classic Zollinger-Ellison syndrome (ZES) from gastrinomas, described in 1955, consists of gastric acid hypersecretion, PUD, and diarrhea [35]. Patients may also present with multifocal gastric carcinoids (type 2), which develop secondary to hypergastrinemia.

Testing to confirm hypergastrinemia typically begins with a fasting serum gastrin level. If this level is not elevated on two separate measurements, this rules out ZES with a negative predictive value (NPV) of 97% [36]. If gastrin level is elevated, further testing is required along with a measurement of gastric pH to confirm that the hypergastrinemia is, in fact, inappropriate. This requires stopping any PPI medications for one week, because PPI therapy is associated with high rates of falsely elevated serum gastrin level, which can be a challenge in some patients with severe symptoms. While off PPI, patients can take anti-H2 medication for symptom control. A gastric pH ≤ 2 and a gastrin level of ≥ 1000 pg/mL is diagnostic of ZES [36]. If the gastrin level is below this, a confirmatory secretin test is required which is 94% sensitive and 100% specific for ZES [37].

The difficulty of taking patients off PPI treatment, combined with the unreliability of certain serum gastrin assays, has resulted in some advocating for the use of SSTR-PET for the diagnosis of ZES, rather than just its localization, in suspected patients [36]. While increasing access to this imaging modality may lead to its integration in gastrinoma diagnosis algorithms, it remains limited by false-positive physiologic uptake in the pancreas and is yet to be validated. Therefore, biochemical confirmation of inappropriate hypergastrinemia remains required to establish a diagnosis of gastrinoma.

Glucagonoma

The classic signs and symptoms of glucagonoma are the four Ds: diabetes, dermatitis, depression, and deep vein thrombosis (DVT), first described in 1942 [38]. The presence of diabetes mellitus can be easily understood, as glucagon plays a key role in promoting gluconeogenesis and glycogenolysis. The dermatitis observation is necrolytic migratory erythema (NME), which consists of eruptions of irregular red patches containing vesicles. There is no unifying explanation for the pathophysiology of NME, but it likely is a combination of nutritional deficiencies leading to inflammation in the epidermis [39]. Similarly, the pathophysiology of depression and increased risk of DVT in glucagonoma are not well explained. As glucagon prevents glucose uptake and storage, and promotes glycogenolysis and lipolysis, it results in decreased levels of amino acids [40]. Patients can present in profound catabolic states with prolonged exposure to elevated glucagon levels, which can manifest by weight loss, progressive neurological symptoms including cognitive dysfunction, incontinence, muscle weakness, and ataxia. Such effects can be reversible with treatment to normalize glucagon levels [41].

The biochemical test for glucagonoma is simply a fasting serum glucagon level. If not already established, testing for the presence for diabetes mellitus would be important at this time also.

VIPoma

The excess secretion of VIP will result in surplus secretions of fluids and electrolytes into the intestinal lumen [33]. This is what leads to the WDHA syndrome – watery diarrhea, hypokalemia, and achlorhydria, otherwise known as the Verner-Morrison syndrome. The main presenting symptoms are that of ongoing, large volume watery diarrhea and its sequelae – dehydration, muscle weakness, cramping, and lethargy.

Confirmatory tests begin with serum electrolytes to assess for hypokalemia and a stool analysis showing secretory diarrhea. It is important to rule out other causes of secretory diarrhea such as infections, laxative abuse, and colitis. Serum VIP levels, if markedly elevated, confirm the diagnosis. Of note, mild elevation of serum VIP can be seen in chronic renal failure, inflammatory bowel disease, or with previous bowel resection [42].

Somatostatinoma

Somatostatin is primarily an inhibitory hormone that has both endocrine and paracrine functions. It exerts its paracrine effects by inhibiting insulin, glucagon, and cholecystokinin. Clinical sequelae of a somatostatinoma are diabetes, cholelithiasis, and pancreatic exocrine insufficiency manifesting as malabsorption and steatorrhea [33]. A suspected diagnosis of somatostatinoma can be confirmed with an elevated fasting serum somatostatin level.

Other Biochemical Markers

Serum Chromogranin A

Chromogranin A (CgA) is a useful histopathological marker for NETs on biopsy or surgical pathology. It has also been found to be elevated in the serum in pNET and used as a biomarker [43]. It can be elevated in a number of other scenarios, such as PPI use, chronic renal or hepatic insufficiency, and other cancers [43], and therefore shouldn't be used as a diagnostic test. Because of low sensitivity and specificity, the use of CgA for both diagnosis and surveillance of pNETs is limited [44].

Urinary 5-Hydroxyindoleacetic Acid (5-HIAA)

5-HIAA is a by-product of serotonin breakdown, and can be measured in the urine, typically collected over 24 hours. The associated carcinoid syndrome has been reported in 50 cases of pNETs, and emerging evidence suggests there may be serotonin secretion in both functional and non-functional pNETs [45, 46]. It is not routinely recommended to measure urinary 5-HIAA for functional pNETs, unless typical signs and symptoms of carcinoid syndrome are noted.

Management

Goals of Treatment

The goals of therapy for sporadic functional PNETs are (1) management of the endocrinopathy for symptom control and (2) tumor control for oncologic management to improve survival. Depending on the clinical scenario, treatment of the endocrinopathy may come in the form of surgical resection of the localized primary tumor, surgical cytoreduction or complete metastasectomy, liver-directed therapies, hormone-specific medical therapy such as a PPI, or systemic therapy with somatostatin analogs or cytotoxic chemotherapy. Regarding oncologic management, though typically indolent, pNETs can have the potential to metastasize. The risk of malignancy is however heterogeneous between and within subtypes of functional pNETs (Table 9.2). We will herein focus on the management of loco-regional sporadic functional pNETs, with specific nuances for each tumor type.

Endocrine Therapy

One of the mainstays of NETs treatment in general are somatostatin analogs (SSAs). While there are many other therapies available to treat functional pNETs, most patients will find themselves on an SSA at some point in their treatment. SSAs mimic somatostatin, and consequently have an inhibitory function, blocking the release of insulin, glucagon, gastrin, cholecystokinin (CCK), and pancreatic enzymes. Therefore, it can be used to control symptoms due to hormonal hypersecretion for insulinoma, gastrinoma, glucagonoma, VIPomas, and somatostatinoma [47].

SSAs may be indicated in the newly diagnosed functional pNET to improve symptom control while work-up and treatment planning are being conducted. This treatment should continue until surgery and likely during the perioperative period.

Table 9.2 Malignant potential and management of loco-regional functional pNETs

Type of functional pNET	Location	Malignant potential	Management — endocrine medical management for symptom control	Surgery for loco-regional tumor	Perioperative considerations
Insulinoma	100% pancreas (equal throughout)	5–15%	Small frequent meals Diazoxide Short and long-acting SSA	R0 resection: • Parenchymal-sparing if possible (e.g., enucleation and central pancreatectomy) • No routine LND.	Glucose monitoring
Gastrinoma	90% within "gastrinoma triangle": junction of second and third duodenum, pancreatic neck, cystic duct/common bile duct	60–90%	Control acid secretion with PPI Short and long-acting SSA Assess and manage potential anemia from PUD Monitor B12 levels	R0 resection: • Formal pancreatectomy • LND	Continue PPI therapy
Glucagonoma	100% pancreas (equal throughout)	50–80%	Short and long-acting SSA Manage consequences of catabolic state, such as weight loss, malnutrition, electrolytes disturbances, cutaneous breakdown Screen for deep vein thrombosis	R0 resection: • Formal pancreatectomy • LND	Short and long-acting SSA Nutritional support
VIPoma	90% pancreas (75% tail)	40–70%	Short and long-acting SSA Manage consequences of high-volume watery diarrhea, such as hypovolemia, acute kidney injury, and electrolytes disturbance	R0 resection: • Formal pancreatectomy • LND	Short and long-acting SSA Monitoring of electrolytes
Somatostatinoma	2/3 pancreas (2/3 head)	60–70%	Short and long-acting SSA	R0 resection: • Formal pancreatectomy • LND	Short and long-acting SSA

SSA somatostatin analogs, LND lymph node dissection (recommended 11–15 nodes), PPI proton pump inhibitors, PUD peptic ulcer disease

Surgical Resection

Complete resection is the mainstay of treatment for localized, resectable disease, for both oncologic and symptom control. There is typically no role for neoadjuvant or adjuvant therapies.

Given the malignant potential of functional pNETs other than insulinomas, most should undergo a formal pancreatectomy. Compared to parenchymal-sparing resections, benefits of a formal resection include increased likelihood of negative resection margins, increased lymph node retrieval, and decreased postoperative pancreatic fistula rates [48, 49]. A negative resection margin has been shown to be associated with improved ten-year recurrence-free survival, but no improvement in overall survival [50]. Overall survival is primarily determined by tumor biology (differentiation, grade, perineural, and vascular invasion) rather than margin status.

Central Pancreatectomy

A parenchymal-sparing technique that can be considered for central pancreatic lesions is the central pancreatectomy. This involves the resection of the central portion of the gland, near the pancreatic neck, without any formal lymphadenectomy. Reconstruction is usually performed by oversewing or stapling the pancreas to the right of the resection and anastomosing the pancreatic tail to either the posterior stomach or a Roux limb of jejunum [51]. Benefits of this procedure include the preservation of exocrine and endocrine pancreatic function but may result in higher operative morbidity and fistula rates than distal pancreatectomy [52]. Central pancreatectomy is ideally suited for an insulinoma near the pancreatic neck that is too close to the pancreatic duct to safely perform enucleation.

Lymphadenectomy

The need and extent of lymphadenectomy in functional pNETs is unclear. The two preoperative predictors of lymph node metastases are tumor size and location [53]. The likelihood of having lymph node metastases increases with increasing tumor size, with those over 1.5 cm having over a 40% nodal positivity rate. While less likely to have nodal metastases, tumors smaller than 1.5 cm still have a nodal positivity rate of 15–30% [53–55]. Tumors located in the head of the pancreas are associated with about a 50% nodal positivity rate, while those in the body/tail only about 25% [53]. Tumor grade is also associated with the presence of nodal metastases; however, this is not reliably known prior to resection.

The impact of lymphadenectomy on survival in pNETs is not fully established. Large cancer database studies did not show a difference in the likelihood of nodal positivity between functional and non-functional pNETs [53, 56]. While some studies have demonstrated an association between nodal metastases and worse survival, such retrospective analyses are limited by nodal sampling and stage migration [55–58]. Other large database studies have not shown a survival benefit based on the extent of lymphadenectomy [54, 56]. Nevertheless, to adhere to oncologic and disease control principles, it is recommended to perform a formal lymphadenectomy for functional pNETs, other than insulinomas, both for complete treatment of the endocrinopathy and potential for improved survival, with retrieval of 11–15 nodes as per the expert consensus statement from the North American Neuroendocrine Tumor Society (NANETS) [6].

Insulinoma

Insulinomas are benign in about 90% of cases, and therefore parenchymal-sparing resection is often a consideration and lymphadenectomy is not routinely needed [33].

Symptoms from insulinoma can be effectively managed by dietary changes and medication with diazoxide, a potassium channel activator that prevents the pancreatic release of insulin, with control of hyperglycemia in 50–60% of patients, as well as short and long-acting SSA with up to 50% hormonal control [59, 60]. For patient undergoing surgery, control of hypoglycemia episodes should be achieved prior to surgery if feasible and blood glucose monitored in the perioperative period [6].

Complete resection of a localized insulinoma has a 98% biochemical cure rate with 6% ten-year recurrence rate [61]. If technically possible, enucleation can be performed for insulinoma. Enucleation is better suited for small tumors (less than 3 cm), located in the head or central body of the pancreas and away from the main pancreatic duct. Distal tail lesions are often better managed with distal pancreatectomy due to the proximity to the pancreatic duct in that area. While associated with better endocrine and exocrine function, reduced blood loss, and shorter operating room time and length of stay compared to pancreatectomy [48, 49, 62], enucleation presents an increased risk of postoperative pancreatic fistula [48, 49].

In some cases, a diagnosis of insulinoma is made clinically and biochemically but no pancreatic tumor can be identified despite comprehensive work-up. Of note, SSTR-PET imaging is limited for insulinomas, with specificity, sensitivity, and accuracy of approximately 25% [63]. Traditionally, it was reported that 20% of insulinomas could not be identified on imaging; however, this information is based on older imaging modalities and the rate of truly unidentified insulinomas is likely much lower in current times. If the insulinoma is not localized despite pancreas-protocol CT scan, MRI, and EUS, further attempt at localization can be done with selective arterial calcium stimulation test (SACS). SACS takes advantage of the fact that intravenous calcium stimulates insulin release from insulinomas but not normal islet cells. This procedure requires arterial catheterization of the splenic, superior mesenteric, and gastroduodenal arteries where calcium is sequentially injected, while at the same time a separate catheter measures insulin levels from the hepatic veins. An increase of two- to threefold in the insulin concentration is highly sensitive for insulinoma in the injected territory [61]. A 2014 meta-analysis of localization techniques found that the SACS was used in 6.2% of published cases, with 84.7% of cases being localized correctly [61].

While surgical exploration was traditionally considered for non-localized insulinoma, it is not recommended anymore [6]. Indeed, there is considerable morbidity associated with exploration and complete mobilization of the pancreatic gland, and despite such exploration, 10% of tumors can remain unidentified [33, 64]. The risks of surgical exploration outweigh the low-risk presented by a truly non-localized tumor. In particular, blind resection of the pancreatic tail should not be performed since a primary tumor may be present throughout the pancreatic gland [6]. For non-localized insulinomas, symptoms can be managed medically with interval re-imaging recommended, as outlined in the NANETS expert consensus statement [6].

Gastrinoma

The risk of malignancy for gastrinoma is the highest among functional pNETs at 60–90 [57, 65]. Importantly, gastrinomas have a high rate of nodal metastases ranging from 43% to 75% [4, 57, 59, 65].

Symptoms from Zollinger-Ellison syndrome resulting from a gastrinoma can be managed with PPI therapy to control the gastric hyperacidity and PUD and with short and long-acting SSA to control the gastrin hypersecretion [59, 60, 66].

Resection of sporadic gastrinomas leads to 60% immediate and 30–40% five-year biochemical cure rate. Formal pancreatectomy is recommended and associated with improved disease-free survival to 98% compared to 74% without resection [6, 67]. Biochemical cure rate with surgery is 51% immediately and goes down to 41% in the long-term [67, 68]. Because of the common occurrence of nodal metastases, lymphadenectomy is crucial both for tumor control and to achieve lasting biochemical response [57, 67, 68].

In case of non-localized gastrinoma despite complete imaging work-up including pancreas-protocol CT scan, MRI, EUS, and SSTR-PET, further attempt at localization can be done with selective arterial infusion of secretin. This technique is similar to SACS described above for insulinoma, but with selective arterial infusion of secretin and measurement of gastrin levels in the hepatic veins.

For non-localized gastrinomas, surgical exploration is not routinely recommended. The data supporting traditional surgical exploration with duodenotomy rely on patients treated in the 1980s and 1990s when imaging's sensitivity was limited [67–71]. The majority of gastrinomas identified during surgical exploration were small duodenal lesions with low gastrin levels that portend excellent biochemical and oncologic prognosis even without surgery [72, 73]. Indeed, patients who die of gastrinoma most often present with high gastrin levels, large pancreatic primary tumors, and metastases [72]. Of note, of patients with gastrinoma who died during a median follow-up of nine years, no death was related to hyperacidity events. Considering that medical therapy with PPI can provide long-term control of symptoms for up to 20 years, especially with low gastrin levels, surgical exploration with duodenotomy is not routinely recommended. Patients with non-localized gastrinoma and symptoms that cannot be controlled with medical therapy should be referred to centers with expertise in gastrinoma management. Surgical exploration should not be undertaken outside of such centers [6].

Other Functional pNETs

Cure has rarely been reported for other rare functional pNETs, including gluca-gonoma, VIPoma, somatostatinoma, and tumors secreting PTHrP or ectopic ACTH [46, 74–76]. The recommendation for resection of localized primary tumors is based on expert opinions [6, 77]. Symptoms can initially be managed with short and long-acting SSA. For patients undergoing surgery, every effort should be made to control the endocrinopathy and their repercussions prior to surgery. For example, this includes treatment of the consequences of the catabolic state for glucagonoma and correction of dehydration and electrolytes disturbances for VIPoma. It is important to mention that medical therapy may have a time-limited effect in those circumstances; therefore, surgery should be undertaken as soon as possible following symptom control to avoid the development of resistance to SSA [6].

Non-resectable Loco-Regional Functional pNETs

While vascular invasion with or without tumor thrombus should not be an absolute contra-indication to resection for functional pNETs [6], there may be some instances when functional pNETs do not harbor distant metastases but are locally unresectable. In some patients, surgery may not be medically feasible or not aligned with patients' wishes, despite the tumor being resectable.

In those cases, non-surgical therapy may be needed to both manage the endocrinopathy and provide tumor control. In addition to providing hormonal control, long-acting SSA can be used as a cytostatic agent, prolonging time to tumor progression [78, 79]. The two trials examining long-acting SSA (octreotide LAR and lanreotide) for unresectable or metastatic low-grade NETs have included a majority of non-functional tumors. The CLARINET trial is the only study that enrolled pNETs, including four patients with gastrinomas [79]. Therefore, the use of long-acting SSA for tumor control in functional pNETs is extrapolated from data in other types of NETs. Other local tumor ablation treatments have also been proposed for both endocrine and tumor control. Stereotactic body radiation therapy has been reported to result in biochemical, clinical, and radiological response in functional NETs [80, 81]. EUS-guided ablation has also been suggested for non-operable functional pNETs [82, 83]. While not standard of care and still the subject of investigations, these therapies represent possible alternatives for patients with unresectable or inoperable tumors and uncontrolled symptoms despite medical therapy. Such approaches should be considered in NETs centers of expertise by an experienced multidisciplinary team.

Conclusion

It is crucial that patients with functional pNETs be treated by a multidisciplinary team of experienced clinicians with expertise in surgery, medical oncology, interventional radiology, gastroenterology, and endocrinology. The management of non-metastatic sporadic functional pNETs should be aimed at both endocrine and tumor control. Proper management relies on the identification and confirmation of the biochemical diagnosis of an endocrine syndrome and localization of a pancreatic lesion typical for pNET. With the exception of insulinoma, the majority of functional pNETs have malignant potential. Patients with a localized and biochemically confirmed functional pNET should undergo pancreatic resection. Patients for whom a biochemical diagnosis cannot be established or with non-localized functional pNETs would benefit from referral to specialized NETs centers. Routine surgical exploration should not be undertaken for non-localized functional pNETs. Finally, patients with functional pNETs planned for surgery should undergo preoperative preparation and perioperative monitoring tailored to their diagnosed endocrine syndrome.

References

1. Howland G, Campbell WR, Maltby EJ, Robinson WL. Dysinsulinism: convulsions and coma due to islet cell tumor of the pancreas with operation and cure. JAMA. 1929;93:674.
2. Istl AC, Gray DK. Roscoe R. Graham. J Trauma Acute Care Surg. 2017;82(1):216–20.
3. Graham RR. Treatment of perforated duodenal ulcers. Surg Gynec Obst. 1937;64:235–8.
4. Halfdanarson TR, Rabe KG, Rubin J, Petersen GM. Pancreatic neuroendocrine tumors (PNETs): incidence, prognosis and recent trend toward improved survival. Ann Oncol. 2008;19(10):1727–33.
5. Zerbi A, Falconi M, Rindi G, Delle Fave G, Tomassetti P, Pasquali C, et al. Clinicopathological features of pancreatic endocrine tumors: a prospective multicenter study in Italy of 297 sporadic cases. Am J Gastroenterol. 2010;105(6):1421–9.
6. Howe JR, Merchant NB, Conrad C, Keutgen XM, Hallet J, Drebin JA, et al. The North American Neuroendocrine Tumor Society consensus paper on the surgical management of pancreatic neuroendocrine tumors. Pancreas. 2020;49(1):1–33.
7. Roland CL, Bian A, Mansour JC, Yopp AC, Balch GC, Sharma R, et al. Survival impact of malignant pancreatic neuroendocrine and islet cell neoplasm phenotypes. J Surg Oncol. 2012;105(6):595–600.
8. Bilimoria KY, Talamonti MS, Tomlinson JS, Stewart AK, Winchester DP, Ko CY, et al. Prognostic score predicting survival after resection of pancreatic neuroendocrine tumors: analysis of 3851 patients. Ann Surg. 2008;247(3):490–500.
9. Hallet J, Law CHL, Cukier M, Saskin R, Liu N, Singh S. Exploring the rising incidence of neuroendocrine tumors: a population-based analysis of epidemiology, metastatic presentation, and outcomes. Cancer. 2015;121(4):589–97.
10. Zárate X, Williams N, Herrera MF. Pancreatic incidentalomas. Best Pract Res Clin Endocrinol Metab. 2012;26(1):97–103.
11. Dasari A, Shen C, Halperin D, Zhao B, Zhou S, Xu Y, et al. Trends in the incidence, prevalence, and survival outcomes in patients with neuroendocrine tumors in the United States. JAMA Oncol. 2017;3(10):1335–42.
12. Da Silva Xavier G. The cells of the islets of Langerhans. J Clin Med. 2018;7(3):54. https://doi.org/10.3390/jcm7030054.
13. Bonnavion R, Teinturier R, Jaafar R, Ripoche D, Leteurtre E, Chen Y-J, et al. Islet cells serve as cells of origin of pancreatic gastrin-positive endocrine tumors. Mol Cell Biol. 2015;35(19):3274–83.
14. Nagtegaal ID, Odze RD, Klimstra D, Paradis V, Rugge M, Schirmacher P, et al. The 2019 WHO classification of tumors of the digestive system. Histopathology. 2020;76(2):182–8.

15. Noone TC, Hosey J, Firat Z, Semelka RC. Imaging and localization of islet-cell tumours of the pancreas on CT and MRI. Best Pract Res Clin Endocrinol Metab. 2005;19(2):195–211.
16. Lotfalizadeh E, Ronot M, Wagner M, Cros J, Couvelard A, Vullierme M-P, et al. Prediction of pancreatic neuroendocrine tumour grade with MR imaging features: added value of diffusion-weighted imaging. Eur Radiol. 2017;27(4):1748–59.
17. Shah MH, Goldner WS, Halfdanarson TR, Bergsland E, Berlin JD, Halperin D, et al. NCCN guidelines insights: neuroendocrine and adrenal tumors, version 2.2018, Journal of the National Comprehensive Cancer Network, vol. 16; 2018. p. 693–702.
18. Kambadakone AR, Fung A, Gupta RT, Hope TA, Fowler KJ, Lyshchik A, et al. LI-RADS technical requirements for CT, MRI, and contrast-enhanced ultrasound. Abdom Radiol (NY). 2018;43(1):56–74.
19. Balthazar P, Shinagare AB, Tirumani SH, Jagannathan JP, Ramaiya NH, Khorasani R. Gastroenteropancreatic neuroendocrine tumors: impact of consistent contrast agent selection on radiologists' confidence in hepatic lesion assessment on restaging MRIs. Abdom Radiol (NY). 2018;43(6):1386–92.
20. Tirumani SH, Jagannathan JP, Braschi-Amirfarzan M, Qin L, Balthazar P, Ramaiya NH, et al. Value of hepatocellular phase imaging after intravenous gadoxetate disodium for assessing hepatic metastases from gastroenteropancreatic neuroendocrine tumors: comparison with other MRI pulse sequences and with extracellular agent. Abdom Radiol (NY). 2018;43(9):2329–39.
21. Morse B, Jeong D, Thomas K, Diallo D, Strosberg JR. Magnetic resonance imaging of neuroendocrine tumor hepatic metastases: does Hepatobiliary phase imaging improve lesion conspicuity and interobserver agreement of lesion measurements? Pancreas. 2017;46(9):1219–24.
22. Hope TA, Bergsland EK, Bozkurt MF, Graham M, Heaney AP, Herrmann K, et al. Appropriate use criteria for Somatostatin receptor PET imaging in neuroendocrine tumors. J Nucl Med. 2018;59(1):56–74.
23. Jacobsson H, Larsson P, Jonsson C, Jussing E, Grybäck P. Normal uptake of 68Ga-DOTA-TOC by the pancreas uncinate process mimicking malignancy at somatostatin receptor PET. Clin Nucl Med. 2012;37(4):362–5.
24. Al-Ibraheem A, Bundschuh RA, Notni J, Buck A, Winter A, Wester H-J, et al. Focal uptake of 68Ga-DOTATOC in the pancreas: pathological or physiological correlate in patients with neuroendocrine tumours? Eur J Nucl Med Mol Imaging. 2011;38(11):2005–13.
25. Menda Y, O'Dorisio TM, Howe JR, Schultz M, Dillon JS, Dick D, et al. Localization of unknown primary site with 68Ga-DOTATOC PET/CT in patients with metastatic neuroendocrine tumor. J Nucl Med. 2017;58(7):1054–7.
26. Barbe C, Murat A, Dupas B, Ruszniewski P, Tabarin A, Vullierme M-P, et al. Magnetic resonance imaging versus endoscopic ultrasonography for the detection of pancreatic tumours in multiple endocrine neoplasia type 1. Dig Liver Dis. 2012;44(3):228–34.
27. van Asselt SJ, Brouwers AH, van Dullemen HM, van der Jagt EJ, Bongaerts AHH, Kema IP, et al. EUS is superior for detection of pancreatic lesions compared with standard imaging in patients with multiple endocrine neoplasia type 1. Gastrointest Endosc. 2015;81(1):159–67.
28. Dewitt J, Devereaux BM, Lehman GA, Sherman S, Imperiale TF. Comparison of endoscopic ultrasound and computed tomography for the preoperative evaluation of pancreatic cancer: a systematic review. Clin Gastroenterol Hepatol. 2006;4(6):717–25
29. Ahmad NA, Lewis JD, Siegelman ES, Rosato EF, Ginsberg GG, Kochman ML. Role of endoscopic ultrasound and magnetic resonance imaging in the preoperative staging of pancreatic adenocarcinoma. Am J Gastroenterol. 2000;95(8):1926–31.
30. Khorasani M, Law C, Myrehaug S, Singh S, Assal A, Hiseh E, et al. Neuroendocrine tumors (gastroenteropancreatic). In: Wright FC, Escallon J, editors. Surgical oncology manual. 3rd ed. Toronto: Springer; 2020; In Press.
31. Grant CS. Insulinoma. Best Pract Res Clin Gastroenterol. 2005;19(5):783–98.
32. Cryer PE, Axelrod L, Grossman AB, Heller SR, Montori VM, Seaquist ER, et al. Evaluation and management of adult hypoglycemic disorders: an endocrine society clinical practice guideline. J Clin Endocrinol Metab. 2009;94(3):709–28.

33. O'Grady HL, Conlon KC. Pancreatic neuroendocrine tumours. Eur J Surg Oncol. 2008;34(3):324–32.
34. Jensen RT, Niederle B, Mitry E, Ramage JK, Steinmuller T, Lewington V, et al. Gastrinoma (duodenal and pancreatic). Neuroendocrinology. 2006;84(3):173–82.
35. Zollinger RM, Ellison EH. Primary peptic ulcerations of the jejunum associated with islet cell tumors of the pancreas. Ann Surg. 1955;142(4):709–23.
36. Metz DC, Cadiot G, Poitras P, Ito T, Jensen RT. Diagnosis of Zollinger-Ellison syndrome in the era of PPIs, faulty gastrin assays, sensitive imaging and limited access to acid secretory testing. Int J Endocr Oncol. 2017;4(4):167–85.
37. Berna MJ, Hoffmann KM, Long SH, Serrano J, Gibril F, Jensen RT. Serum gastrin in Zollinger-Ellison syndrome: II. Prospective study of gastrin provocative testing in 293 patients from the National Institutes of Health and comparison with 537 cases from the literature. Evaluation of diagnostic criteria, proposal of new criteria, and correlations with clinical and tumoral features. Medicine (Baltimore). 2006;85(6):331–64.
38. Becker SW, Khan D, Rothman S. Cutaneous manifestations of internal malignant tumours. Arch Dermatol Syphilol. 1942;45:1069–80.
39. Tierney EP, Badger J. Etiology and pathogenesis of necrolytic migratory erythema: review of the literature. Medscape Gen Med. 2004;6(3):4.
40. Klein S, Jahoor F, Baba H, Townsend CM, Shepherd M, Wolfe RR. In vivo assessment of the metabolic alterations in glucagonoma syndrome. Metab Clin Exp. 1992;41(11):1171–5.
41. Mozell E, Stenzel P, Woltering EA, Rösch J, O'Dorisio TM. Functional endocrine tumors of the pancreas: clinical presentation, diagnosis, and treatment. Curr Probl Surg. 1990;27(6):301–86.
42. Koch TR, Michener SR, Go VL. Plasma vasoactive intestinal polypeptide concentration determination in patients with diarrhea. Gastroenterol. 1991;100(1):99–106.
43. Singh S, Law C. Chromogranin A: a sensitive biomarker for the detection and post-treatment monitoring of gastroenteropancreatic neuroendocrine tumors. Expert Rev Gastroenterol Hepatol. 2012;6(3):313–34.
44. Strosberg JR, Halfdanarson TR, Bellizzi AM, Chan JA, Dillon JS, Heaney AP, et al. The North American Neuroendocrine Tumor Society consensus guidelines for surveillance and medical management of midgut neuroendocrine tumors. Pancreas. 2017;46(6):707–14.
45. Mirakhur B, Pavel ME, Pommier RF, Fisher GA, Phan AT, Massien C, et al. Biochemical responses in symptomatic and asymptomatic patients with neuroendocrine tumors: pooled analysis of 2 phase 3 trials. Endocr Pract. 2018;24(11):948–62.
46. Chiruvella A, Kooby DA. Surgical management of pancreatic neuroendocrine tumors. Surg Oncol Clin N Am. 2016;25(2):401–21.
47. Angeletti S, Corleto VD, Schillaci O, Marignani M, Annibale B, Moretti A, et al. Use of the somatostatin analogue octreotide to localise and manage somatostatin-producing tumours. Gut. 1998;42(6):792–4.
48. Pitt SC, Pitt HA, Baker MS, Christians K, Touzios JG, Kiely JM, et al. Small pancreatic and periampullary neuroendocrine tumors: resect or enucleate? J Gastrointest Surg. 2009;13(9):1692–8.
49. Hüttner FJ, Koessler-Ebs J, Hackert T, Ulrich A, Büchler MW, Diener MK. Meta-analysis of surgical outcome after enucleation versus standard resection for pancreatic neoplasms. Br J Surg. 2015;102(9):1026–36.
50. Zhang X-F, Wu Z, Cloyd J, Lopez-Aguiar AG, Poultsides G, Makris E, et al. Margin status and long-term prognosis of primary pancreatic neuroendocrine tumor after curative resection: results from the US Neuroendocrine Tumor Study Group. Surgery. 2019;165(3):548–56.
51. Iacono C, Bortolasi L, Facci E, Nifosì F, Pachera S, Ruzzenente A, et al. The Dagradi-Serio-Iacono operation central pancreatectomy. J Gastrointest Surg. 2007;11(3):364–76.
52. Xiao W, Zhu J, Peng L, Hong L, Sun G, Li Y. The role of central pancreatectomy in pancreatic surgery: a systematic review and meta-analysis. HPB. 2018;20(10):896–904.
53. Hashim YM, Trinkaus KM, Linehan DC, Strasberg SS, Fields RC, Cao D, et al. Regional lymphadenectomy is indicated in the surgical treatment of pancreatic neuroendocrine tumors (PNETs). Ann Surg. 2014;259(2):197–203.

54. Gratian L, Pura J, Dinan M, Roman S, Reed S, Sosa JA. Impact of extent of surgery on survival in patients with small nonfunctional pancreatic neuroendocrine tumors in the United States. Ann Surg Oncol. 2014;21(11):3515–21.
55. Postlewait LM, Ethun CG, Baptiste GG, Le N, McInnis MR, Cardona K, et al. Pancreatic neuroendocrine tumors: preoperative factors that predict lymph node metastases to guide operative strategy. J Surg Oncol. 2016;114(4):440–5.
56. Conrad C, Kutlu OC, Dasari A, Chan JA, Vauthey J-N, Adams DB, et al. Prognostic value of lymph node status and extent of lymphadenectomy in pancreatic neuroendocrine Tumors confined to and extending beyond the pancreas. J Gastrointest Surg. 2016;20(12):1966–74.
57. Krampitz GW, Norton JA, Poultsides GA, Visser BC, Sun L, Jensen RT. Lymph nodes and survival in pancreatic neuroendocrine tumors. Arch Surg. 2012;147(9):820–7.
58. Tomassetti P, Campana D, Piscitelli L, Casadei R, Santini D, Nori F, et al. Endocrine pancreatic tumors: factors correlated with survival. Ann Oncol. 2005;16(11):1806–10.
59. Ito T, Igarashi H, Jensen RT. Pancreatic neuroendocrine tumors: clinical features, diagnosis and medical treatment: advances. Best Pract Res Clin Gastroenterol. 2012;26(6):737–53.
60. Mansour JC, Chen H. Pancreatic endocrine tumors. J Surg Res. 2004;120(1):139–61.
61. Mehrabi A, Fischer L, Hafezi M, Dirlewanger A, Grenacher L, Diener MK, et al. A systematic review of localization, surgical treatment options, and outcome of insulinoma. Pancreas. 2014;43(5):675–86.
62. Hackert T, Hinz U, Fritz S, Strobel O, Schneider L, Hartwig W, et al. Enucleation in pancreatic surgery: indications, technique, and outcome compared to standard pancreatic resections. Langenbeck's Arch Surg. 2011;396(8):1197–203.
63. Sharma P, Arora S, Karunanithi S, Khadgawat R, Durgapal P, Sharma R, et al. Somatostatin receptor based PET/CT imaging with 68Ga-DOTA-Nal3-octreotide for localization of clinically and biochemically suspected insulinoma. Q J Nucl Med Mol Imaging. 2016;60(1):69–76.
64. Norton JA, Alexander HR, Fraker DL, Venzon DJ, Gibril F, Jensen RT. Does the use of routine duodenotomy (DUODX) affect rate of cure, development of liver metastases, or survival in patients with Zollinger-Ellison syndrome? Ann Surg. 2004;239(5):617–25.
65. Tsutsumi K, Ohtsuka T, Mori Y, Fujino M, Yasui T, Aishima S, et al. Analysis of lymph node metastasis in pancreatic neuroendocrine tumors (PNETs) based on the tumor size and hormonal production. J Gastroenterol. 2012 Jun;47(6):678–85.
66. Nightingale KJ, Davies MG, Kingsnorth AN. Glucagonoma syndrome: survival 24 years following diagnosis. Dig Surg. 1999;16(1):68–71.
67. Bartsch DK, Waldmann J, Fendrich V, Boninsegna L, Lopez CL, Partelli S, et al. Impact of lymphadenectomy on survival after surgery for sporadic gastrinoma. Br J Surg. 2012;99(9):1234–40.
68. Norton JA, Fraker DL, Alexander HR, Gibril F, Liewehr DJ, Venzon DJ, et al. Surgery increases survival in patients with gastrinoma. Ann Surg. 2006;244(3):410–9.
69. Norton JA, Fraker DL, Alexander HR, Venzon DJ, Doppman JL, Serrano J, et al. Surgery to cure the Zollinger-Ellison syndrome. NEJM. 1999;341(9):635–44.
70. Fraker DL, Norton JA, Alexander HR, Venzon DJ, Jensen RT. Surgery in Zollinger-Ellison syndrome alters the natural history of gastrinoma. Ann Surg. 1994;220(3):320–8.
71. Fishbeyn VA, Norton JA, Benya RV, Pisegna JR, Venzon DJ, Metz DC, et al. Assessment and prediction of long-term cure in patients with the Zollinger-Ellison syndrome: the best approach. Ann Intern Med. 1993;119(3):199–206.
72. Yu F, Venzon DJ, Serrano J, Goebel SU, Doppman JL, Gibril F, et al. Prospective study of the clinical course, prognostic factors, causes of death, and survival in patients with long-standing Zollinger-Ellison syndrome. JCO. 1999;17(2):615–30.
73. Norton JA, Fraker DL, Alexander HR, Jensen RT. Value of surgery in patients with negative imaging and sporadic Zollinger-Ellison syndrome. Ann Surg. 2012;256(3):509–17.
74. Knigge U, Hansen CP. Surgery for GEP-NETs. Best Pract Res Clin Gastroenterol. 2012;26(6):819–31.
75. Falconi M, Eriksson B, Kaltsas G, Bartsch DK, Capdevila J, Caplin M, et al. ENETS consensus guidelines update for the management of patients with functional pancreatic neuroen-

docrine tumors and non-functional pancreatic neuroendocrine tumors. Neuroendocrinology. 2016;103:153–71.

76. O'Toole D, Salazar R, Falconi M, Kaltsas G, Couvelard A, de Herder WW, et al. Rare functioning pancreatic endocrine tumors. Neuroendocrinology. 2006;84:189–95.

77. Jensen RT, Cadiot G, Brandi ML, de Herder WW, Kaltsas G, Komminoth P, et al. ENETS consensus guidelines for the management of patients with digestive neuroendocrine neoplasms: functional pancreatic endocrine tumor syndromes. Neuroendocrinology. 2012;95(2):98–119.

78. Caplin ME, Pavel M, Ćwikła JB, Phan AT, Raderer M, Sedláčková E, et al. Lanreotide in metastatic Enteropancreatic neuroendocrine tumors. NEJM. 2014;371(3):224–33.

79. Rinke A, Wittenberg M, Schade-Brittinger C, Aminossadati B, Ronicke E, Gress TM, et al. Placebo-controlled, double-blind, prospective, randomized study on the effect of Octreotide LAR in the control of tumor growth in Patients with Metastatic Neuroendocrine Midgut Tumors (PROMID): results of long-term survival. Neuroendocrinology. 2017;104(1):26–32.

80. Myrehaug S, Hallet J, Chu W, Yong E, Law C, Assal A, et al. Proof of concept for stereotactic body radiation therapy in the treatment of functional neuroendocrine neoplasms. J Radiosurg SBRT. 2020;6(4):321–4.

81. Chan DL, Thompson R, Lam M, Pavlakis N, Hallet J, Law C, et al. External beam radiotherapy in the treatment of gastroenteropancreatic neuroendocrine tumours: a systematic review. Clin Oncol (R Coll Radiol). 2018;30(7):400–8.

82. Barthet M, Giovannini M, Lesavre N, Boustiere C, Napoleon B, Koch S, et al. Endoscopic ultrasound-guided radiofrequency ablation for pancreatic neuroendocrine tumors and pancreatic cystic neoplasms: a prospective multicenter study. Endoscopy. 2019;51(9):836–42.

83. Larghi A, Rizzatti G, Rimbaş M, Crino SF, Gasbarrini A, Costamagna G. EUS-guided radiofrequency ablation as an alternative to surgery for pancreatic neuroendocrine neoplasms: who should we treat? Endosc Ultrasound. 2019;8(4):220–6.

Jejunoileal Neuroendocrine Tumors

10

Scott K. Sherman and James R. Howe

Introduction

This chapter addresses jejunoileal or small bowel neuroendocrine tumors (SBNETs) arising from enterochromaffin cells between the ligament of Treitz and the ileocecal valve. Neuroendocrine tumors of other sites, as well as management of liver metastases, are covered elsewhere in this volume. While SBNETs share some features with neuroendocrine tumors of the duodenum, pancreas, stomach, and other sites, they are relatively inaccessible to endoscopy, and the primary tumors are frequently small and often elude preoperative identification. Nodal and liver metastases are common at the time of diagnosis. The majority of SBNETs are low grade with slow growth, and with optimal treatment patients can survive for many years, even with metastatic disease. Definitive management includes surgery to remove the primary tumor, associated nodal tissue, and distant metastases, when feasible. For unresectable or recurrent disease, an ever-increasing range of medical therapies including somatostatin analogues (SSAs), peptide receptor radionuclide therapy (PRRT), and targeted molecular inhibitors can delay progression and potentially extend survival.

Epidemiology

Jejunoileal NETs display the much-discussed increase in neuroendocrine tumor incidence reported in population-level databases worldwide over the previous 50 years and have now surpassed adenocarcinoma as the most common primary small intestinal malignancy [1, 2]. A landmark Surveillance, Epidemiology, and End Results (SEER) database study by Yao et al. found that from 1973 to 2004,

S. K. Sherman · J. R. Howe (✉)
Department of Surgery, Division of Surgical Oncology and Endocrine Surgery, University of Iowa Carver College of Medicine, Iowa City, IA, USA
e-mail: scott-sherman@uiowa.edu; james-howe@uiowa.edu

© Springer Nature Switzerland AG 2021
J. M. Cloyd, T. M. Pawlik (eds.), *Neuroendocrine Tumors*,
https://doi.org/10.1007/978-3-030-62241-1_10

overall age-adjusted NET incidence increased by 4.8-fold (1.09 to 5.25/100,000) [1]. More recent follow-up showed these incidences continuing to increase [3]. SBNET incidence increased in line with the overall trend, with incidence up approximately sixfold between 1973 and 2012 [3]. Reasons for this increase surely include more cross-sectional imaging in patients being evaluated for abdominal complaints and improvements in somatostatin receptor-based imaging. A relative increase in locoregional versus metastatic disease over time supports that improved imaging may more often find SBNETs, perhaps due to the increasing recognition that mesenteric lymphadenopathy may suggest the presence of an SBNET [4]. Indeed, a Canadian population-based study reported that even as overall NET incidence increased between 1994 and 2009, the proportion of patients presenting with distant metastatic disease fell from 29% to 13% while locoregional disease increased, suggesting that some incidence trends may reflect earlier diagnoses [5]. Moreover, percent increases in SBNET diagnosis have not risen as sharply as those for gastric and rectal NETs, which closely follow greater use of upper and lower endoscopy (approximately 6-fold increase between 1973 and 2012 for SBNETs vs. 15-fold and 11-fold for gastric and rectal) [3, 6]. Additional factors beyond more or improved imaging contributing to the increasing incidence of SBNETs remain unclear, but could include better recognition of symptoms, changes in the environment, or changing exposure to substances in the gastrointestinal (GI) tract.

Patients with SBNETs are diagnosed at a median age of 66 years and are more often male (54%) [1]. Incidence increases with age, with the maximum occurring in the ninth decade [7]. Low or intermediate grade tumors account for 80–90% of SBNETs [8]. For all NETs, Yao reported that 21% of patients with G1, 30% with G2, and 50% with G3 NETs will have distant metastases at diagnosis [1]. For jejunoileal NETs, 29% present with localized disease, 41% with regional disease, and 30% with distant metastases, and 16% of all NETs arise in the small intestine [1].

Distribution of SBNETs within the small intestine follows a predictable pattern, with most tumors located near the terminal ileum. Multifocal primaries are common in SBNETs and occur in 33–56% of patients [8–11]. A detailed study of tumor location within the small bowel (n = 107 patients) found that <1% of tumors were located within 100 cm of the ligament of Treitz, while 72% were within 100 cm of the ileocecal valve, and 27% fell in between (Fig. 10.1) [10].

Genetics

Unlike in pancreatic NETs, where recurrent mutations in *MEN1, PTEN, DAXX/ATRX,* and *TSC2* lead to malignancy, specific genetic changes involved in the pathogenesis of SBNETs remain poorly understood [12]. While loss and gain of chromosomes often occur, how this causes SBNET tumorigenesis remains unknown. Chromosomal instability is a consistent feature of SBNETs. The most common chromosomal alterations, predicted to represent early events in SBNET formation, are loss of chromosome 18q (40–70% of tumors) and 11q (may occur in 30%) [13–15]. While frequent loss of these regions suggests the presence of a

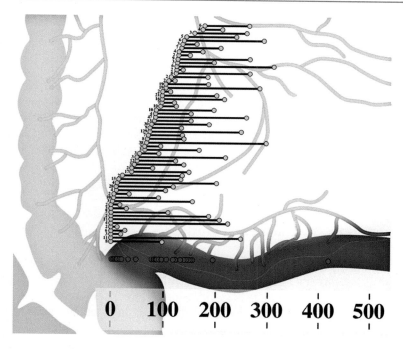

Fig. 10.1 Tumor location along the length of small intestine in 107 primary tumors, reprinted from Keck *et al.* [10]. Bowel length is represented at the bottom as distance from the ileocecal valve. Unifocal tumor locations are shown as blue dots. Multifocal tumors (56% of total patients) are shown by two yellow dots connected with a line, representing the positions of the proximal and distal-most tumors. Tumors were located within 100 cm of the ileocecal valve in 72% of patients, and only one tumor was within 100 cm of the ligament of Treitz

tumor suppressor gene in these locations, extensive investigation has not yet identified it [16]. Candidate genes in these regions include *SMAD4* on chromosome 18 and *SDHD* on chromosome 11, but "second-hit" mutations in the remaining copies of these genes are not commonly observed in these tumors [16]. Amplifications of chromosomes 4, 5, 7, 14, and 20 also occur at lower frequencies [12, 15, 17].

In contrast to their chromosomal instability, SBNETs exhibit a relatively low frequency of somatic gene mutations [18]. The cyclin-dependent kinase inhibitor 1B (*CDKN1B*) represents one of the few recurrent gene mutations observed in SBNETs and is predicted to produce cell-cycle dysregulation and malignancy [12]. Yet while *CDKN1B* represents the most-frequently mutated gene known in SBNETs, this occurs in only 7–9% of patients, implying that additional, as-yet-unknown, mechanisms explain the majority of SBNET cases [12, 19]. Researchers identified another gene involved in SBNETs from studying families with multiple members affected by these tumors. In 181 members of 33 families with SBNETs, genetic linkage identified the inositol polyphosphate multikinase, *IPMK*, as the causative gene in one large family, but mutations were not found in any of the others [20]. While loss of heterozygosity was not seen in resulting tumors, the mutations reduced

IPMK nuclear localization, and this haploinsufficiency decreased *p53* activation and increased cell survival [20]. This finding, along with amplification of *AKT1* and *AKT2* observed in some SBNETs [18], strongly implicates the *PI3K/AKT/mTOR* pathway in SBNET tumorigenesis.

Epigenetic modifications may also play a role in SBNET development. Combining exome sequencing, methylation analysis, copy-number variant analysis, and whole-genome expression profiling, Karpathakis et al. described a high rate of gene methylation and three distinct molecular subgroups of SBNETs [21]. These groups showed differential methylation of *EGFR*, m*TOR*, and *VEGF* signaling pathways, and increased expression of *CDX1*, *CELSR3*, *GIPR*, and other genes which correlated with metastasis and survival outcomes [21].

Presentation, Diagnosis, and Workup

Thorson first described the heart disease, flushing, diarrhea, and bronchospasm typical of the carcinoid syndrome in 1954, which arises from the effects of hormones secreted by these tumors [22]. Occasionally, weakness, arthritis, or pellagra, which occurs as tryptophan is diverted from niacin to serotonin production, can occur [13, 23]. Yet this classic presentation occurs in less than 10% of patients [24]. More commonly, patients with SBNETs present with vague abdominal discomfort, crampy pain, flushing, intermittent obstructive symptoms, or diarrhea [25]. Due to the nonspecific nature of these symptoms, diagnosis frequently takes years [24]. Unlike NETs of the stomach, duodenum, pancreas, and colorectum, jejunoileal NETs are difficult to find endoscopically (unless they are near the ileocecal valve), and preoperative biopsy of the primary site rarely precedes surgical intervention. More often, imaging obtained to investigate abdominal symptoms identifies abnormalities suggestive of an SBNET or metastatic disease. The former would include enlarged nodes in the small bowel mesentery, often with calcification, peritoneal lesions, or an enhancing mass in the wall of the small bowel (Fig. 10.2) [4, 26, 27]. When liver lesions are seen, this often leads to biopsy which will yield the diagnosis of a neuroendocrine tumor, with cells expressing chromogranin A and synaptophysin by immunohistochemistry (IHC) [28]. If the primary site is not clear from imaging, then additional IHC stains may reveal the origin, with CDX2 positivity common in SBNETs, and PAX6 and islet-1 (ISL1) in PNETs [29].

Biochemical Testing – When symptoms raise suspicion for SBNETs, biochemical tests combined with imaging can help make the diagnosis and provide prognostic information. SBNETs, like other neuroendocrine tumors, elaborate a range of hormonal products and bioactive amines [13, 24, 30]. High levels produce the characteristic symptoms of the carcinoid syndrome, which when present, can indicate hepatic or distant metastases or a high tumor burden, as first-pass hepatic inactivation of tumor products often prevents carcinoid symptoms from manifesting when disease is limited to its small bowel primary location [30, 31]. Jejunoileal NETs most often produce high levels of serotonin, chromogranins, 5-hydroxyindoleacetic acid (5-HIAA), pancreastatin, substance P, kallikrein, bradykinins, and others [30,

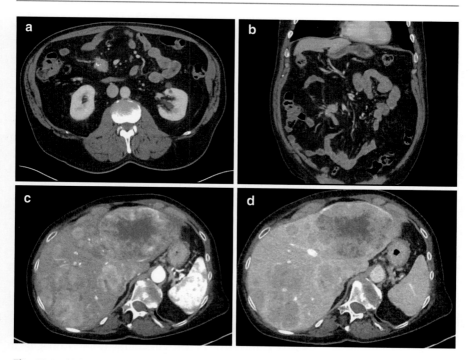

Fig. 10.2 Abdominal CT scans demonstrating findings typical of small bowel neuroendocrine tumor. (**a**) Axial images showing calcified mesenteric mass in the right lower quadrant representing nodal metastasis. (**b**) Coronal view of the same. (**c**) Liver metastases from a different patient demonstrating typical arterial enhancement with tumors appearing brighter than normal liver and (**d**) venous washout with hypoenhancement relative to background liver

32, 33]. Of these, SBNET patients most often have abnormally elevated levels of serotonin, 5-HIAA, and chromogranin A (>75% of metastatic patients) [32].

With many potentially elevated tumor markers, institutional testing practices vary widely, with some centers routinely assessing broad panels, and others pursuing more limited approaches. Current guidelines recommend only assessment of 5-HIAA and chromogranin A [27, 34]. While sensitive for the diagnosis of SBNETs and somewhat correlated to tumor burden and outcomes, both markers can be affected by diet, medications, and the specific assay used, reducing their specificity [23, 27, 31, 32, 35]. In addition to 5-HIAA and chromogranin A, our practice has been to assess levels of pancreastatin and neurokinin A before and after treatment and during follow-up. Although less commonly elevated, high levels of Neurokinin A portend a poorer prognosis [32, 36, 37]. Pancreastatin is a 52 amino acid cleavage product of chromogranin A, commonly elevated in SBNETs, but with levels less affected by diet and medications [32, 38]. Pancreastatin more strongly correlates with recurrence and survival than other NET tumor markers, and may better indicate tumor burden [36, 39–42].

Imaging Evaluation – Once SBNET is suspected, a high-quality arterial and venous contrasted computed tomography (CT) scan of the abdomen and pelvis represents the single most useful imaging study [26]. In addition to providing critical staging information and demonstrating the relationships between key vascular structures and tumors to be resected, CT scan offers the greatest sensitivity for locating the primary tumor site. Optimal SBNET CT imaging includes thin sections with arterial, venous, and delayed venous phases [43]. Jejunoileal NETs often appear hypervascular on arterial phases, but are sometimes hypovascular and better imaged in the venous phase. Triple-phase CT also allows for better definition of potential liver metastases [23, 43]. One tertiary referral center review of preoperative imaging found that CT scan suggested the location of the primary in 150/197 patients with metastatic disease (76%) [4]. CT was most sensitive for pancreatic NETs (32/33) and showed 82% sensitivity for SBNETs (74/90). The primary tumor itself often remained occult by CT imaging, but bowel wall thickening, mesenteric adenopathy, or stellate fibrosis suggested an SBNET primary (Fig. 10.2), which were later confirmed at exploration. CT enteroclysis, in which a water bolus is ingested for oral contrast distension of the bowel, may further increase detection [43, 44]. To supplement CT imaging for treatment of metastases, liver magnetic resonance imaging (MRI) offers better sensitivity to detect metastatic lesions and shows their relationships to hepatic vascular anatomy [45, 46]. For primary SBNETs, contrast-enhanced magnetic resonance (MR)-enterography more often identifies small bowel tumors than non-contrast MR-enterography [47] and has greater reported sensitivity compared to CT [48]. In a prospective comparison of MR-enterography to CT imaging in 150 patients with small bowel disorders, sensitivity for detecting tumors was significantly greater with MR, although only two neuroendocrine tumors were included [48]. Magnetic resonance proves particularly useful in patients with renal dysfunction or contrast allergies and can provide excellent information with optimal technique and equipment, however, variability in radiologists' expertise, capabilities of different MR scanners, complex protocols, and a higher rate of studies with significant motion artifact often renders CT the more practical option [32, 49].

Upon diagnosis of a neuroendocrine tumor, complete staging includes ^{68}Ga-somatostatin receptor-PET imaging (SSTR-PET) [49, 50]. This technique exploits high expression of somatostatin receptors on the surface of lower grade NETs, concentrating the imaging isotope at tumor tissue. A previous SSTR-based technique using ^{111}In-pentetreotide scintigraphy has significant limitations compared to SSTR-PET, including lower sensitivity, two-dimensional images, low resolution, and a 24-hour study acquisition time [32, 51]. Somatostatin receptor-PET fused with CT offers 3-D high-resolution images, high sensitivity, lower radiation dose, and a shorter two-hour acquisition time [32, 50, 52]. In light of these advantages, guidelines now recommend that SSTR-PET replace somatostatin scintigraphy for all of its previous indications [49, 50]. Even in apparently localized disease, the high sensitivity of SSTR-PET to detect occult metastases leads to more accurate staging, and in one single-center prospective study, management decisions changed for 29% of patients based on SSTR-PET results (Fig. 10.3) [52]. Sensitivity to detect metastases in this study was 97% with 100% specificity [52]. A meta-analysis of SSTR-PET studies found sensitivity of 90.9% and specificity of 90.6%, although there was significant heterogeneity for sensitivity across studies [53]. Whether using

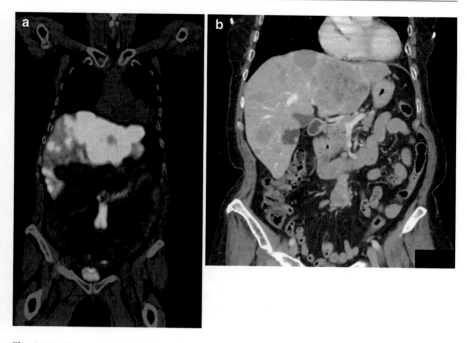

Fig. 10.3 Coronal views of the patient shown in 2C/2D with an ileal primary tumor and liver metastases. (**a**) ^{68}Ga-DOTA-PET/CT showing uptake in nodal metastases at the root of the mesentery and liver metastases. (**b**) Corresponding views on the venous phase CT

additional receptor targets or imaging isotopes can improve receptor-based SBNET imaging performance remains an area of active investigation [54–59], but gallium-PET imaging clearly outperforms somatostatin scintigraphy and is the current standard of care for metastatic staging [49, 50].

Standard 18-fluorodeoxyglucose-PET imaging has a limited role in SBNETs. Most G1-2 SBNETs will not show increased [18]FDG uptake, and it is generally not recommended. For the much less common high-grade SBNETs, which show lower somatostatin receptor expression and greater metabolic activity, [18]FDG-PET can aid staging [32, 49, 50].

Surgical Treatment

Surgical strategies for SBNETs need to take into account their hormonal activity and possibility of obstruction, while balancing the risks of extensive resections against their indolent growth. Whereas resection of extensive or bulky nodal disease (to say nothing of liver metastases) would often not benefit patients with more aggressive malignancies such as small bowel adenocarcinoma, retrospective data support that reducing the volume of disease in low-grade SBNETs can improve quality and length of life [49, 60]. Reducing the volume of SBNET disease contributes to controlling hormonal symptoms and avoiding obstructive and ischemic complications caused by primary tumors blocking the bowel lumen and their nodal metastases encasing and compromising blood vessels [30, 49]. Resecting the primary tumor may also help prevent development of carcinomatosis and obstruction from tumor implants.

Perioperative Considerations – Surgery for SBNET patients presents a risk of precipitating carcinoid crisis, which surgical and anesthesia teams must prepare to treat. Carcinoid crisis manifests as hemodynamic instability, often refractory to vasopressors, and may occur upon induction of anesthesia, during tumor manipulation, or at any point during the procedure [61, 62]. Hypotension in carcinoid crisis may result from tumor secretion of serotonin, histamine, tachykinins, and bradykinin [33]. One study of 46 NET operations, where monitoring included intraoperative echocardiography, pulmonary arterial catheter pressure monitoring, and hormone levels checked at incision, during hypotensive episodes, and at closing, found that the hypothesized massive release of hormones during carcinoid crisis did not happen [33]. While patients with higher serotonin levels were more likely to have carcinoid crises, levels of serotonin, histamine, kallikrein, and bradykinin were not significantly elevated from baseline during hypotensive episodes. Instead, distributive shock from vasodilation seemed responsible for hypotensive symptoms [33].

When hypotension from suspected carcinoid crisis develops, first-line vasopressor treatment includes vasopressin and phenylephrine [63]. Preference for these drugs stands on their efficacy, but also due to concerns that beta-adrenergic drugs might actually stimulate release of carcinoid hormones, thereby worsening the hypotension. A recent retrospective study challenged this dogma, finding no worse hypotension among NET patients who received beta-adrenergic drugs compared to those who did not [63]. The authors concluded that while phenylephrine and vasopressin should be used first, adding norepinephrine, epinephrine, or ephedrine for persistent hypotension may be safe and preferable to prolonged low blood pressure.

To preemptively address potential carcinoid crisis, some NET surgeons provide prophylactic perioperative octreotide. In a study of 97 neuroendocrine operations (including 65 for SBNETs) by Massimino *et al.*, 24% demonstrated evidence of carcinoid crisis after receiving a preoperative octreotide bolus [61]. Carcinoid crisis occurred in both functional and non-functional tumors, but only patients with hepatic metastases showed hemodynamic instability. The authors concluded that prophylactic bolus octreotide is insufficient, and recommended considering additional fluid, vasopressor support, and continuous octreotide infusions to counteract the hormonal effects leading to these symptoms [61]. With the inadequacy of preoperative bolus octreotide, many surgeons provide continuous octreotide infusions at 100–500 ug/hour during surgery [25, 62, 63]. While prospective data supporting intraoperative octreotide are lacking and carcinoid crisis may still occur [33], some authors report low rates (6/179) of clinically meaningful carcinoid crisis symptoms and a favorable risk-benefit profile, supporting its continued use [49, 62].

Carcinoid heart disease, which manifests as fibrosis of the tricuspid and pulmonic valves, should be repaired prior to surgery when significant valvular insufficiency exists [49]. A National Surgical Quality Improvement Database study addressed whether SBNET patients require extended venous thromboembolism (VTE) prophylaxis, as is commonly provided in resections for abdominal adenocarcinomas [64]. In this study, non-pancreatic NETs had significantly lower venous thromboembolism rates than those seen in other malignancies (1.1% vs. 2.4%, p < 0.001), suggesting that extended VTE may not be required.

Indications and Technique – Operative indications for SBNETs include both diagnostic and therapeutic. Not uncommonly, surgeons may discover unsuspected SBNETs during an operation for obstructive symptoms. In this case, a characteristic small, hard, stellate, white primary lesion, possibly accompanied by mesenteric lymphadenopathy should prompt frozen section of the resected lesion (Fig. 10.4a). The characteristic neuroendocrine appearance of the lesion should allow ready diagnosis by the pathologist, permitting the surgeon to perform appropriate inspection of the abdomen and liver for metastatic disease, search the remaining bowel for additional multifocal lesions, and carry out an adequate lymphadenectomy.

When high suspicion for a neuroendocrine tumor exists, such as in a patient with characteristic carcinoid symptoms, mesenteric adenopathy on imaging, positive findings on somatostatin-imaging, or elevated NET markers, careful exploration of the length of the small bowel will identify the primary tumor and permit treatment. Another indication is for a patient with known neuroendocrine liver metastases and an unknown primary site. As gallium-PET/CT imaging, abdominal MRI, and upper and lower endoscopy can locate most lung, gastric, pancreatic, and colon NET primary tumors, primaries sites that remain uncertain after all of these investigations are often found in the small intestine, where their small size and inaccessibility to

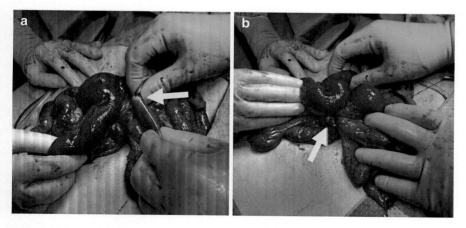

Fig. 10.4 (a) Careful palpation of the small intestine locates a small, hard, white lesion representing the primary tumor, indicated by *arrow*. (b) Large nodal metastases (*arrow*) causing fibrosis and mesenteric foreshortening

endoscopy help them evade preoperative detection [4]. In this situation, careful examination of the small bowel accompanies liver-directed treatment of metastatic disease, and several investigators report a high likelihood of success in locating occult SBNET primaries in this situation [4, 65, 66].

In either case, exploration for a suspected SBNET begins with thorough inspection of the entire length of the bowel. While laparoscopic approaches have been described and can be effective in experienced hands [67], many SBNET primaries are quite small, can be missed by even sensitive imaging techniques, and may only be discovered by careful manual bowel palpation [8, 49]. Importantly, SBNETs are multifocal in >50% of cases [10], and although a larger tumor may be quite evident on laparoscopy, the entire bowel must be carefully palpated in order to not leave additional tumors behind. When surgeons attempt laparoscopic SBNET treatment, manual palpation of extracorporealized bowel is mandatory, and there should be a low threshold for conversion to open to adequately assess for additional multifocal tumors. When bulky nodal disease exists, safe and complete lymphadenectomy most often requires an open technique [49]. Smaller incisions and shorter length of stay should not compromise an optimal oncologic resection.

After identifying all tumor sites, treatment requires resection of affected bowel with associated lymphadenectomy down to the segmental vessels. For solitary lesions, proximal and distal margins of 5–10 cm usually afford adequate regional lymph node resection. For terminal ileum tumors, this may require ileocecectomy or right hemicolectomy. Multifocal primaries often demand multiple segmental resections or longer segmental resections. In this situation, attention to the length of remaining bowel and distance between primary tumors determines which lesions may be resected together with a single anastomosis, and when preservation of bowel length dictates multiple separate anastomoses.

The most technically involved portion of a jejunoileal tumor resection is the lymphadenectomy. Lymphadenopathy associated with SBNETs produces a dense desmoplastic reaction, leading to foreshortening of the mesentery and fibrosis. Large nodal metastases often sit on or surround major vessels in the root of the mesentery (Fig. 10.4b) [49]. Removal of these metastases sometimes risks serious bleeding or devascularization of segments of the intestine; however, bulky nodal disease can produce significant hormonal symptoms, as well as superior mesenteric vein (SMV) thrombosis or intestinal ischemia if left in place. Thorough review of high-quality preoperative cross-sectional imaging allows the surgeon to plan which nodes may be safely approached through meticulous dissection for symptom palliation, and those which must be left in place to avoid an unacceptable surgical risk. Sometimes these nodes are heavily calcified with the major proximal mesenteric vessels running through them. In some cases, resection may not be possible, while other times, nodes can be peeled off these vessels. Some patients with advanced disease also have involved aortocaval, portocaval, and left periaortic nodes seen on preoperative imaging. If these can be removed safely, patients may benefit from this cytoreduction, but this is a judgment call because it is unclear that this improves survival and presents additional risk. A study by Landry *et al.* supports the importance of adequate lymphadenectomy on SBNET outcomes [68]. Among 1143

SBNET patients in SEER who had at least one lymph node removed, improved survival was found among those with more extensive lymphadenectomy (HR 0.66, P = 0.02 for more than eight nodes removed). A caveat regarding mesenteric lymph node counts is that the mesenteric masses in SBNET patients can represent a large conglomeration of many positive nodes, yet be classified as a single mesenteric implant.

Primary Tumor Resection – In jejunoileal NETs, the surgical plan should include resection of the primary tumor and its lymphatic drainage, and when present, removal of as much metastatic disease burden as safely possible, with a goal of at least 70% liver tumor debulking [49, 69, 70]. An important controversy in SBNET surgery concerns the approach to an unresected primary tumor when 70% liver debulking cannot be achieved. When the primary tumor or its nodal metastases cause obstructive or ischemic complications and can be safely removed, operation is clearly indicated. When these symptoms do not exist, some theorize that even if liver or other metastatic disease cannot be adequately resected, surgery to remove the primary tumor prevents future mechanical complications, while removing the source of metastatic spread [49, 71–75]. Others posit that in such advanced disease, unrecognized microscopic metastases are likely already widespread, and surgery to remove the primary is unlikely to extend life, while exposing the patient to unnecessary surgical risk [76].

There are no randomized data addressing this problem, so we only have retrospective series to answer this question. Arguing against primary resection, Daskalakis *et al.* studied asymptomatic SBNET patients in a Swedish registry, comparing those who underwent immediate surgery to those who had surgery only if symptoms developed [76]. In an unmatched analysis, patients undergoing immediate primary resection lived longer than those who underwent medical management with surgery only if needed (HR 0.72 for death, confidence interval [CI] 0.57–0.93, P = 0.009), but in a propensity-matched analysis, there was no difference between the groups (P = 0.9). Notably, among patients in the nonsurgical group who did not have immediate primary resection, 44% ultimately had their primary resected at some point after the study's six-month definition of "immediate" resection, a percentage that was even higher in the propensity-matched group. Such a high rate of crossover to surgery undercuts the paper's conclusion that initial surgery may not benefit SBNET patients [76].

In contrast to these findings, Givi *et al.* argue for resection of asymptomatic primaries, reporting that progression-free and overall survival were significantly better among NET patients who had their primary tumors removed (progression-free survival 56 vs. 25 months; overall survival 159 vs. 47 months) [71]. In the California Cancer Registry, patients undergoing primary tumor resection had significantly lower risk of death regardless of whether liver surgery was performed [77]. Additional support for primary resection comes from the National Cancer Database [78]. Among 4252 patients with metastatic SBNETs who did not undergo surgery for the metastatic site, 59% of patients who underwent primary resection had longer median survival (91.3 vs. 44.2 months, p < 0.001) compared to those whose primary was not resected. On multivariable analysis, primary tumor resection was associated with a hazard ratio (HR) for death of 0.55 [78]. Researchers in the UK and Ireland reached similar conclusions from a multicenter database of midgut NET outcomes. Ahmed *et al.* found on multivariable analysis that among 360 patients followed, age, Ki-67, and resection of the primary tumor independently correlated with better survival [72]. In all of these retrospective and database studies, strong selection biases likely influenced whether patients had surgery, and the impact of primary tumor resection on survival will continue to provoke debate [74].

The ideal treatment for liver metastases is surgical cytoreduction, which will be addressed in a later chapter [49, 79]. Another site of metastatic disease is the peritoneum. As SBNETs grow through the wall of the intestine, cells can spill into the peritoneal cavity, implanting in the pelvis, omentum, mesentery, and under the diaphragms. These lesions can lead to adhesions or grow into loops of bowel, especially the rectosigmoid, and may produce bowel obstructions. Ovarian metastases are frequent, and especially in post-menopausal women, suspicious masses on the ovaries should be removed. There does not appear to be a benefit for hyperthermic intraperitoneal chemotherapy for peritoneal metastases [80, 81], but we suggest an attempt to remove masses >5–10 mm wherever possible, and cauterize or argon-coagulate numerous 1–3 mm lesions.

Medical Treatment

While other chapters in this volume discuss medical treatment of neuroendocrine tumors in detail, this section highlights several points specific to jejunoileal neuroendocrine tumors. As in other gastrointestinal NETs, somatostatin analogues (SSAs) represent first-line medical therapy for those with residual, recurrent, progressive, or unresectable disease [82]. SBNETs markedly overexpress somatostatin receptors, and since 1979, somatostatin analogues have been used to control NET hormonal symptoms [83–86]. In addition to controlling carcinoid syndrome symptoms, the placebo-controlled, double-blind Prospective Randomized study on the effect of Octreotide LAR in the control of tumor growth in patients with metastatic neuroendocrine MIDgut tumors (PROMID) study first provided randomized evidence of SSA's effectiveness in slowing tumor growth [87]. In this study, 85 patients with advanced midgut or unknown primary NETs were randomized to treatment with 30 mg of octreotide long-acting repeatable (LAR) or placebo every 28 days. Median time to progression was longer with octreotide LAR (14.3 vs. 6.0 months; HR 0.34, P < 0.001). Although long-term follow-up showed no overall survival advantage as most placebo patients crossed-over to receiving octreotide, placebo-controlled, double-blind Prospective Randomized study on the effect of Octreotide LAR in the control of tumor growth in patients with metastatic neuroendocrine MIDgut tumors (PROMID) established SSAs as first-line treatment for symptom control and delay of tumor growth in SBNETs [87, 88]. Another randomized SSA trial, Controlled study of Lanreotide Antiproliferative Response In Neuroendocrine Tumors (CLARINET), confirmed that lanreotide also delays tumor growth in advanced, non-functional NETs with progression [89]. Two hundred and four patients were randomized to treatment with 120 mg lanreotide or placebo every 28 days. In this trial, nearly half of the patients had pancreatic NETs;

midgut NETs represented one-third of study subjects. The hazard ratio for progression or death in lanreotide-treated patients was 0.47 (CI 0.30–0.73) and was slightly better in the pre-defined subgroup of midgut NETs (HR 0.35, CI 0.16–0.80) [89]. Thus, for jejunoileal neuroendocrine tumors, high-quality evidence supports SSA use to delay progression in advanced disease [82].

For progressive, unresectable disease, the NETTER-1 trial proved peptide receptor radionuclide therapy's (PRRT) effectiveness in SBNETs [90, 91]. While several European, non-randomized studies had for years reported good PRRT outcomes with both ^{177}Lu and ^{90}Y radiolabeled SSAs, NETTER-1 provided the first phase-III randomized evidence [90]. Patients with low or intermediate grade advanced and unresectable midgut NETs (n = 229) that progressed on octreotide were randomized to treatment with high-dose octreotide (60 mg every 4 weeks) versus 4 cycles of ^{177}Lu-DOTATATE PRRT and 30 mg Octreotide every 4 weeks [90]. The primary endpoint of progression-free survival (PFS) was significantly improved in the treatment group (median not reached versus 8.4 months, p < 0.004), and the objective response rate of 18% was higher than that seen with octreotide alone (3%). Non-significant improvement in the secondary endpoint of overall survival (OS) has been observed, (HR 0.40 vs. control, p = 0.004). Although significant toxicities including renal and bone marrow problems can occur, the treatment was generally well-tolerated, and ^{177}Lu-DOTATATE treatment is currently recommended for patients with unresectable SSTR-positive disease progressing on SSA [91]. The NETTER-1 data are particularly robust in SBNETs considering that of 229 midgut NETs included, 183 were known to arise in the jejunum or ileum, with a further 23 arising in unspecified portions of the small intestine. Only 10% of tumors arose in the colon, appendix, or other midgut sites, making NETTER-1 essentially a jejunoileal NET trial [90].

Patients with carcinoid syndrome can benefit from telotristat, a tryptophan hydroxylase inhibitor that interferes with serotonin production based on recent randomized trials. The Telotristat Etiprate for Somatostatin Analogue Not Adequately Controlled Carcinoid Syndrome (TELESTAR) and Telotristat Etiprate for Carcinoid Syndrome Therapy (TELECAST) trials randomized patients (n = 135 and n = 76, respectively) with well-differentiated NETs not adequately controlled by SSAs to one of two different dose levels of telotristat or placebo [92, 93]. In Telotristat Etiprate for Somatostatin Analogue Not Adequately Controlled Carcinoid Syndrome (TELESTAR), patients with carcinoid syndrome symptoms and diarrhea were included, and drug-treated patients experienced significantly fewer bowel movements (primary endpoint, mean 1.7 and 2.1 fewer per day in low- and high-dose groups, vs. 0.9 fewer per day with placebo, p < 0.001) and reduced urinary 5-HIAA levels compared to placebo [92]. Telotristat Etiprate for Carcinoid Syndrome Therapy (TELECAST) included patients with carcinoid syndrome without diarrhea, and treated patients saw significantly reduced urinary 5-HIAA levels (primary endpoint, 54.0% less for low-dose and 89.7% less for high-dose groups, p < 0.001 for both) [93]. Whether reducing serotonin production impacts other NET outcomes, such as development of carcinoid heart disease, remains to be determined. Importantly, neither trial reported the primary tumor sites of included patients, but carcinoid syndrome with significant diarrhea is most common in patients with SBNETs.

The phase-III randomized RADIANT-2 and RADIANT-4 trials tested everolimus as another option in NETs from multiple primary sites showing progression. However, recent subgroup analyses of these trials suggest that everolimus may have relatively less activity in SBNET tumors compared to lung, stomach, rectal, and pancreatic NETs [94, 95]. In RADIANT-2, 429 patients with progressive low or intermediate grade NETs and carcinoid syndrome were randomized to treatment with everolimus and long-acting octreotide versus placebo plus octreotide [96]. About half of included patients had jejunoileal NETs. The primary endpoint, PFS, was 16.4 months in the treatment group, and 11.3 months in the placebo group. While treatment with everolimus resulted in numerically better PFS, the hazard ratio and p-value of 0.77 and 0.026 fell short of the pre-specified significance bound of 0.0246 [96], and final analysis showed no overall survival benefit [97]. RADIANT-3 included only pancreatic NETs [95], while the subsequent RADIANT-4 trial randomized 302 patients with progressive, advanced non-functional, grade 1–2 gastrointestinal or lung NETs 2:1 to everolimus versus placebo [98]. Median PFS among patients receiving everolimus was 14.0 months versus 5.5 months with placebo (HR 0.39, p < 0.001). Initial analysis of the secondary endpoint of overall survival showed non-significant improvement in the everolimus group (HR 0.64, 95% confidence interval 0.40–1.05). While RADIANT-4 provided evidence for use of everolimus in gastrointestinal NETs, a smaller proportion of tumors were SBNETs compared to RADIANT-2 (30.7% compared to 50%), and more lung NETs were included (30% compared to 10%) [96, 98]. Post-hoc analysis revealed that hazard ratio confidence intervals crossed 1.00 for jejunal and ileal primary tumors, and the efficacy shown in RADIANT-4 may have been driven more by results in lung, stomach, and rectal NETs [94]. Whether this was due to lack of efficacy or insufficient power to detect an effect in smaller subgroups could not be determined.

Finally, chemotherapy with capecitabine/temozolomide or other regimens remains an option for unresectable or higher-grade well-differentiated SBNETs [99]. Although no randomized studies exist, institutional series report partial response rates of around 20–40%, with stable disease in up to 50% of SBNETs [100–102]. Such studies may include multiple types of NETs, with generally lower response rates in SBNETs compared to other primary sites. Grade 3 well-differentiated NETs (with Ki-67 > 20%) and poorly differentiated neuroendocrine carcinomas are very uncommon in jejunoileal primaries [23]. When they do occur, poorly differentiated, high Ki-67 small or large cell neuroendocrine carcinomas typically respond better to platinum-based chemotherapies (such as cisplatin/etoposide) [100, 103, 104]. Unfortunately, randomized trials comparing the several medical options for progressive SBNETs against one another are lacking, as is sequencing of treatments, and guidance in choosing one therapy versus another remains mainly in the domain of expert opinion.

Outcomes and Survival

Despite the high incidence of nodal and liver metastases, patients with SBNETs generally enjoy long survival. Between 1973 and 2004, NET patients of all primary sites identified in SEER had median OS of 75 months [1]. Tumor grade represents the single most important prognostic factor, with patients with G1 tumors enjoying median OS of 124 months, compared to 10 months in patients with high-grade tumors [1]. Tumor stage also strongly influences survival. Among patients in SEER presenting with metastatic disease, even low-grade NETs have significantly shortened survival at 33 months [1]. Patients with jejunoileal NETs lived longer both with localized (median 111 months) and metastatic disease (median 56 months) [1]. Survival in gastrointestinal NETs has increased over time. Earlier studies found improved survival for metastatic NETs in the post-octreotide era (1987–2004) compared to before [1], and more recent studies confirmed that this trend has continued, with an HR for death of 0.71 in advanced tumors diagnosed in 2009–2012 compared to 2000–2004 [3].

While these results paint a general picture, and NETs clearly have better survival than many malignant tumors, SBNET patients receiving treatment at experienced centers may live longer still than these figures suggest, although significant selection and referral biases in non-population-based or institutional databases complicate comparisons. A French series of 107 SBNETs, 70% of whom had metastatic disease reported median overall survival of 128 months [8]. In our own series of 218 surgically treated SBNETs, 73% of whom had distant metastases, median survival was 119 months [36].

It remains under investigation whether multifocal SBNETs have different outcomes from unifocal primaries. A small series of 68 patients, 18 with multifocal SBNETs reported worse survival among those with multifocal tumors [105]. Another study by Gangi *et al.* reported that while multifocal tumors more commonly presented with metastatic disease and more involved lymph nodes, multifocality did not correlate with increased risk of recurrence or death on multivariable analysis [9]. Still another study found no difference in rates of metastases, grade, *SSTR2* expression, or survival between unifocal and multifocal SBNETs [11].

Surveillance

Even in apparently completely resected SBNETs, as many as 50% will recur, and guidelines recommend long-term imaging surveillance and follow-up for at least ten years [82]. Although no prospective studies establish superiority of one regimen over another, expert opinion supports initial CT imaging every six months, moving later to annual imaging if no recurrence is identified [82].

Tumor hormonal markers also may inform prognosis and therapy during follow-up, but false positive and negative results historically have limited their utility, and institutional practices regarding use of blood markers during follow-up vary widely [82]. In addition to current guidelines which discuss monitoring chromogranin A (CgA) levels [34, 82, 106], emerging data support pancreastatin as a more specific SBNET biomarker [36, 39]. In surgically treated SBNET patients, those with normal postoperative pancreastatin had median PFS of 7.3 years, compared to 1.5 years among those with elevated postoperative levels [39]. Woltering *et al.* found that among SBNET patients undergoing surgical cytoreduction, those with postoperative pancreastatin levels within the normal range had >90% five-year survival whether or not their preoperative levels were elevated (n = 155), compared to 58% five-year survival among the 145 patients whose postoperative pancreastatin levels remained elevated (p < 0.001) [40]. Serial determination of pancreastatin levels during follow-up may also provide superior information relative to other tumor markers. In 218 resected SBNETs, pancreastatin showed overall accuracy in detecting progression of 78.9%, compared to 63.3% for CgA (p < 0.001) [36]. Serotonin and neurokinin A performed more poorly. Thus, pancreastatin identifies patients at higher risk of progression who might benefit from additional treatment and shows utility in detecting progression during long-term follow-up.

Conclusions

Jejunoileal neuroendocrine tumors present with symptoms of carcinoid syndrome, bowel obstruction, or can be discovered incidentally on imaging studies. Tumors are most often low-grade and indolent, although nodal or distant metastases commonly exist at diagnosis. Imaging with contrasted CT and ^{68}Ga-PET/CT can identify distant metastases and often primary tumors, but in many cases, small primary tumors are not detected, and their presence is inferred by indirect signs such as mesenteric thickening. Biochemical markers, including chromogranin A and pancreastatin assist in preoperative evaluation, and correlate with risk of recurrence and long-term outcomes. Surgical management seeks to remove both primary and metastatic disease. Small bowel NETs are often small and multifocal, making careful manual palpation of the entire bowel length of critical importance. Along with segmental bowel resection, careful removal of often large and calcified lymph nodes to the level of segmental mesenteric blood vessels completes operative treatment of the primary tumor. Following resection, somatostatin analogues control hormonal symptoms and delay progression for those with residual or recurrent disease. For unresectable progressive disease, peptide receptor radionuclide therapy offers an encouraging response rate, and early data suggest a possible overall survival benefit. With such multimodal treatment, long-term survival for patients with low-grade disease is excellent, even among patients with metastases.

Acknowledgments This work was supported by NIH Grants No. T32CA078586 (SKS) and P50 CA1724521-01 (JRH).

Disclosures None

References

1. Yao JC, Hassan M, Phan A, et al. One hundred years after "carcinoid": epidemiology of and prognostic factors for neuroendocrine tumors in 35,825 cases in the United States. J Clin Oncol. Jun 2008;26(18):3063–72.

2. Bilimoria KY, Bentrem DJ, Wayne JD, Ko CY, Bennett CL, Talamonti MS. Small bowel cancer in the United States: changes in epidemiology, treatment and survival over the last 20 years. Ann Surg. Jan 2009;249(1):63–71.
3. Dasari A, Shen C, Halperin D, et al. Trends in the incidence, prevalence, and survival outcomes in patients with neuroendocrine tumors in the United States. JAMA Oncol. 2017;3(10):1335–42.
4. Keck KJ, Maxwell JE, Menda Y, et al. Identification of primary tumors in patients presenting with metastatic gastroenteropancreatic neuroendocrine tumors. Surgery. 2017;161(1):272–9.
5. Hallet J, Law CH, Cukier M, Saskin R, Liu N, Singh S. Exploring the rising incidence of neuroendocrine tumors: a population-based analysis of epidemiology, metastatic presentation, and outcomes. Cancer. 2015;121(4):589–97.
6. Fraenkel M, Kim M, Faggiano A, de Herder WW, Valk GD, Knowledge N. Incidence of gastroenteropancreatic neuroendocrine tumours: a systematic review of the literature. Endocr Relat Cancer. 2014;21(3):R153–63.
7. Hemminki K, Li X. Incidence trends and risk factors of carcinoid tumors: a nationwide epidemiologic study from Sweden. Cancer. 2001;92(8):2204–10.
8. Pasquer A, Walter T, Hervieu V, et al. Surgical management of small bowel neuroendocrine tumors: specific requirements and their impact on staging and prognosis. Ann Surg Oncol. 2015;22(Suppl 3):S742–9.
9. Gangi A, Siegel E, Barmparas G, et al. Multifocality in small bowel neuroendocrine tumors. J Gastrointest Surg. 2018;22(2):303–9.
10. Keck KJ, Maxwell JE, Utria AF, et al. The distal predilection of small bowel neuroendocrine tumors. Ann Surg Oncol. 2018;25(11):3207–13.
11. Choi AB, Maxwell JE, Keck KJ, et al. Is multifocality an indicator of aggressive behavior in small bowel neuroendocrine tumors? Pancreas. 2017;46(9):1115–20.
12. Francis JM, Kiezun A, Ramos AH, et al. Somatic mutation of CDKN1B in small intestine neuroendocrine tumors. Nat Genet. 2013;45(12):1483–6.
13. Modlin IM, Kidd M, Latich I, Zikusoka MN, Shapiro MD. Current status of gastrointestinal carcinoids. Gastroenterology. 2005;128(6):1717–51.
14. Kytola S, Hoog A, Nord B, et al. Comparative genomic hybridization identifies loss of 18q22-qter as an early and specific event in tumorigenesis of midgut carcinoids. Am J Pathol. 2001;158(5):1803–8.
15. Hashemi J, Fotouhi O, Sulaiman L, et al. Copy number alterations in small intestinal neuroendocrine tumors determined by array comparative genomic hybridization. BMC Cancer. 2013;13:505.
16. Stålberg P, Westin G, Thirlwell C. Genetics and epigenetics in small intestinal neuroendocrine tumours. J Intern Med. 2016;280(6):584–94.
17. Kulke MH, Freed E, Chiang DY, et al. High-resolution analysis of genetic alterations in small bowel carcinoid tumors reveals areas of recurrent amplification and loss. Genes Chromosomes Cancer. 2008;47(7):591–603.
18. Banck MS, Kanwar R, Kulkarni AA, et al. The genomic landscape of small intestine neuroendocrine tumors. J Clin Invest. 2013;123(6):2502–8.
19. Maxwell JE, Sherman SK, Li G, et al. Somatic alterations of CDKN1B are associated with small bowel neuroendocrine tumors. Cancer Genet. Sep 15 2015.
20. Sei Y, Zhao X, Forbes J, et al. A hereditary form of small intestinal carcinoid associated with a Germline mutation in inositol polyphosphate multikinase. Gastroenterology. 2015;149(1):67–78.
21. Karpathakis A, Dibra H, Pipinikas C, et al. Prognostic impact of novel molecular subtypes of small intestinal neuroendocrine tumor. Clin Cancer Res. 2016;22(1):250–8.
22. Thorson A, Biorck G, Bjorkman G, Waldenstrom J. Malignant carcinoid of the small intestine with metastases to the liver, valvular disease of the right side of the heart (pulmonary stenosis and tricuspid regurgitation without septal defects), peripheral vasomotor symptoms, bronchoconstriction, and an unusual type of cyanosis; a clinical and pathologic syndrome. Am Heart J. 1954;47(5):795–817.

23. Scott AT, Howe JR. Management of small bowel neuroendocrine tumors. J Oncol Pract. 2018;14(8):471–82.
24. Vinik AI, Silva MP, Woltering EA, Go VL, Warner R, Caplin M. Biochemical testing for neuroendocrine tumors. Pancreas. 2009;38(8):876–89.
25. Scott AT, Howe JR. Management of small bowel neuroendocrine tumors. Surg Oncol Clin N Am. 2020;29(2):223–41.
26. Dahdaleh FS, Lorenzen A, Rajput M, et al. The value of preoperative imaging in small bowel neuroendocrine tumors. Ann Surg Oncol. 2013;20(6):1912–7.
27. Pape UF, Perren A, Niederle B, et al. ENETS consensus guidelines for the management of patients with neuroendocrine neoplasms from the jejuno-ileum and the appendix including goblet cell carcinomas. Neuroendocrinology. 2012;95(2):135–56.
28. Klimstra DS, Modlin IR, Adsay NV, et al. Pathology reporting of neuroendocrine tumors: application of the Delphic consensus process to the development of a minimum pathology data set. Am J Surg Pathol. 2010;34(3):300–13.
29. Maxwell JE, Sherman SK, Stashek KM, O'Dorisio TM, Bellizzi AM, Howe JR. A practical method to determine the site of unknown primary in metastatic neuroendocrine tumors. Surgery. 2014;156(6):1359–65; discussion 1365–1356
30. Vinik AI, Chaya C. Clinical presentation and diagnosis of neuroendocrine Tumors. Hematol Oncol Clin North Am. 2016;30(1):21–48.
31. Tran CG, Sherman SK, Howe JR. Small bowel neuroendocrine tumors. Curr Probl Surg. 2020.
32. Maxwell JE, O'Dorisio TM, Howe JR. Biochemical diagnosis and preoperative imaging of Gastroenteropancreatic neuroendocrine tumors. Surg Oncol Clin N Am. 2016;25(1):171–94.
33. Condron ME, Jameson NE, Limbach KE, et al. A prospective study of the pathophysiology of carcinoid crisis. Surgery. 2019;165(1):158–65.
34. Shah MH, Goldner WS, Halfdanarson TR, et al. NCCN guidelines insights: neuroendocrine and adrenal tumors, version 2.2018. J Natl Compr Cancer Netw. 2018;16(6):693–702.
35. Arnold R, Wilke A, Rinke A, et al. Plasma chromogranin a as marker for survival in patients with metastatic endocrine gastroenteropancreatic tumors. Clin Gastroenterol Hepatol. 2008;6(7):820–7.
36. Tran CG, Sherman SK, Scott AT, et al. It's time to rethink biomarkers for surveillance of small bowel neuroendocrine tumors. Ann Surg Oncol. 2020.
37. Woltering EA, Voros BA, Thiagarajan R, et al. Plasma Neurokinin A levels predict survival in well-differentiated neuroendocrine Tumors of the small bowel. Pancreas. 2018;47(7):843–8.
38. O'Dorisio TM, Krutzik SR, Woltering EA, et al. Development of a highly sensitive and specific carboxy-terminal human pancreastatin assay to monitor neuroendocrine tumor behavior. Pancreas. 2010;39(5):611–6.
39. Sherman SK, Maxwell JE, O'Dorisio MS, O'Dorisio TM, Howe JR. Pancreastatin predicts survival in neuroendocrine tumors. Ann Surg Oncol. 2014;21(9):2971–80.
40. Woltering EA, Voros BA, Beyer DT, et al. Plasma Pancreastatin predicts the outcome of surgical Cytoreduction in neuroendocrine tumors of the small bowel. Pancreas. 2019;48(3):356–62.
41. Strosberg D, Schneider EB, Onesti J, et al. Prognostic impact of serum Pancreastatin following chemoembolization for neuroendocrine tumors. Ann Surg Oncol. 2018;25(12):3613–20.
42. Khan TM, Garg M, Warner RR, Uhr JH, Divino CM. Elevated serum Pancreastatin is an indicator of hepatic metastasis in patients with small bowel neuroendocrine tumors. Pancreas. 2016;45(7):1032–5.
43. Sundin A, Arnold R, Baudin E, et al. ENETS consensus guidelines for the standards of care in neuroendocrine tumors: radiological, nuclear medicine & hybrid imaging. Neuroendocrinology. 2017;105(3):212–44.
44. Pilleul F, Penigaud M, Milot L, Saurin JC, Chayvialle JA, Valette PJ. Possible small-bowel neoplasms: contrast-enhanced and water-enhanced multidetector CT enteroclysis. Radiology. 2006;241(3):796–801.
45. Dromain C, de Baere T, Lumbroso J, et al. Detection of liver metastases from endocrine tumors: a prospective comparison of somatostatin receptor scintigraphy, computed tomography, and magnetic resonance imaging. J Clin Oncol. 2005;23(1):70–8.

46. Kunz PL, Reidy-Lagunes D, Anthony LB, et al. Consensus guidelines for the management and treatment of neuroendocrine tumors. Pancreas. 2013;42(4):557–77.
47. Amzallag-Bellenger E, Soyer P, Barbe C, Diebold MD, Cadiot G, Hoeffel C. Prospective evaluation of magnetic resonance enterography for the detection of mesenteric small bowel tumours. Eur Radiol. 2013;23(7):1901–10.
48. Masselli G, Di Tola M, Casciani E, et al. Diagnosis of small-bowel diseases: prospective comparison of multi-detector row CT enterography with MR enterography. Radiology. 2016;279(2):420–31.
49. Howe JR, Cardona K, Fraker DL, et al. The surgical management of small bowel neuroendocrine tumors: Consensus guidelines of the North American Neuroendocrine Tumor Society. Pancreas. 2017;46(6):715–31.
50. Hope TA, Bergsland EK, Bozkurt MF, et al. Appropriate use criteria for somatostatin receptor PET imaging in neuroendocrine tumors. J Nucl Med. 2018;59(1):66–74.
51. Maxwell JE, Sherman SK, Menda Y, Wang D, O'Dorisio TM, Howe JR. Limitations of somatostatin scintigraphy in primary small bowel neuroendocrine tumors. J Surg Res. 2014;190(2):548–53.
52. Naswa N, Sharma P, Kumar A, et al. Gallium-68-DOTA-NOC PET/CT of patients with gastroenteropancreatic neuroendocrine tumors: a prospective single-center study. AJR Am J Roentgenol. 2011;197(5):1221–8.
53. Deppen SA, Blume J, Bobbey AJ, et al. 68Ga-DOTATATE compared with 111In-DTPA-Octreotide and conventional imaging for pulmonary and Gastroenteropancreatic neuroendocrine tumors: a systematic review and meta-analysis. J Nucl Med. 2016;57(6):872–8.
54. Waser B, Rehmann R, Sanchez C, Fourmy D, Reubi JC. Glucose-dependent insulinotropic polypeptide receptors in most gastroenteropancreatic and bronchial neuroendocrine tumors. J Clin Endocrinol Metab. 2012;97(2):482–8.
55. Sherman SK, Carr JC, Wang D, O'Dorisio MS, O'Dorisio TM, Howe JR. Gastric inhibitory polypeptide receptor (GIPR) is a promising target for imaging and therapy in neuroendocrine tumors. Surgery. 2013;154(6):1206–13; discussion 1214
56. Gourni E, Waser B, Clerc P, Fourmy D, Reubi JC, Maecke HR. The glucose-dependent insulinotropic polypeptide receptor: a novel target for neuroendocrine tumor imaging-first preclinical studies. J Nucl Med. 2014;55(6):976–82.
57. Reubi JC, Maecke HR. Approaches to multireceptor targeting: hybrid radioligands, Radioligand cocktails, and sequential radioligand applications. J Nucl Med. 2017;58(Suppl 2):10S–6S.
58. Nicolas GP, Morgenstern A, Schottelius M, Fani M. New Developments in Peptide Receptor Radionuclide Therapy. J Nucl Med. Dec 20 2018.
59. Navalkissoor S, Grossman A. Targeted alpha particle therapy for neuroendocrine tumours: the next generation of peptide receptor radionuclide therapy. Neuroendocrinology. 2019;108(3):256–64.
60. Norlen O, Stalberg P, Oberg K, et al. Long-term results of surgery for small intestinal neuroendocrine tumors at a tertiary referral center. World J Surg. 2012;36(6):1419–31.
61. Massimino K, Harrskog O, Pommier S, Pommier R. Octreotide LAR and bolus octreotide are insufficient for preventing intraoperative complications in carcinoid patients. J Surg Oncol. 2013;107(8):842–6.
62. Woltering EA, Wright AE, Stevens MA, et al. Development of effective prophylaxis against intraoperative carcinoid crisis. J Clin Anesth. 2016;32:189–93.
63. Limbach KE, Condron ME, Bingham AE, Pommier SJ, Pommier RF. Beta-adrenergic agonist administration is not associated with secondary carcinoid crisis in patients with carcinoid tumor. Am J Surg. 2019;217(5):932–6.
64. Skertich NJ, Gerard J, Poirier J, et al. Do all abdominal neuroendocrine tumors require extended postoperative VTE prophylaxis? A NSQIP Analysis. J Gastrointest Surg. 2019;23(4):788–93.
65. Bartlett EK, Roses RE, Gupta M, et al. Surgery for metastatic neuroendocrine tumors with occult primaries. J Surg Res. 2013;184(1):221–7.

66. Wang SC, Parekh JR, Zuraek MB, et al. Identification of unknown primary tumors in patients with neuroendocrine liver metastases. Arch Surg (Chicago, Ill. 1960). 2010;145(3):276–80.

67. Massimino KP, Han E, Pommier SJ, Pommier RF. Laparoscopic surgical exploration is an effective strategy for locating occult primary neuroendocrine tumors. Am J Surg. 2012;203(5):628–31.

68. Landry CS, Lin HY, Phan A, et al. Resection of at-risk mesenteric lymph nodes is associated with improved survival in patients with small bowel neuroendocrine tumors. World J Surg. 2013;37(7):1695–700.

69. Scott AT, Breheny PJ, Keck KJ, et al. Effective cytoreduction can be achieved in patients with numerous neuroendocrine tumor liver metastases (NETLMs). Surgery. 2019;165(1):166–75.

70. Wonn SM, Limbach KE, Pommier SJ, et al. Outcomes of cytoreductive operations for peritoneal carcinomatosis with or without liver cytoreduction in patients with small bowel neuroendocrine tumors. Surgery. May 27 2020.

71. Givi B, Pommier SJ, Thompson AK, Diggs BS, Pommier RF. Operative resection of primary carcinoid neoplasms in patients with liver metastases yields significantly better survival. Surgery. 2006;140(6):891–7; discussion 897–898

72. Ahmed A, Turner G, King B, et al. Midgut neuroendocrine tumours with liver metastases: results of the UKINETS study. Endocr Relat Cancer. 2009;16(3):885–94.

73. Citterio D, Pusceddu S, Facciorusso A, et al. Primary tumour resection may improve survival in functional well-differentiated neuroendocrine tumours metastatic to the liver. Eur J Surg Oncol. 2017;43(2):380–7.

74. Howe JR. It may not be too little or too late: resecting primary small bowel neuroendocrine tumors in the presence of metastatic disease. Ann Surg Oncol. Jun 4 2020.

75. Pommier RF. Re-evaluating resection of primary pancreatic neuroendocrine tumors. Surgery. 2019;165(3):557–8.

76. Daskalakis K, Karakatsanis A, Hessman O, et al. Association of a prophylactic surgical approach to stage IV small intestinal neuroendocrine tumors with survival. JAMA Oncol. 2018;4(2):183–9.

77. Lewis A, Raoof M, Ituarte PHG, et al. Resection of the primary gastrointestinal neuroendocrine tumor improves survival with or without liver treatment. Ann Surg. 2019;270(6):1131–7.

78. Tierney JF, Chivukula SV, Wang X, et al. Resection of primary tumor may prolong survival in metastatic gastroenteropancreatic neuroendocrine tumors. Surgery. 2019;165(3):644–51.

79. Keutgen XM, Schadde E, Pommier RF, Halfdanarson TR, Howe JR, Kebebew E. Metastatic neuroendocrine tumors of the gastrointestinal tract and pancreas: a surgeon's plea to centering attention on the liver. Semin Oncol. 2018;45(4):232–5.

80. Elias D, David A, Sourrouille I, et al. Neuroendocrine carcinomas: optimal surgery of peritoneal metastases (and associated intra-abdominal metastases). Surgery. 2014;155(1):5–12.

81. Chicago Consensus WG. The Chicago Consensus on peritoneal surface malignancies: management of neuroendocrine tumors. Ann Surg Oncol. 2020;27(6):1788–92.

82. Strosberg JR, Halfdanarson TR, Bellizzi AM, et al. The North American Neuroendocrine Tumor Society consensus guidelines for surveillance and medical management of midgut neuroendocrine tumors. Pancreas. 2017;46(6):707–14.

83. Long RG, Barnes AJ, Adrian TE, et al. Suppression of pancreatic endocrine tumour secretion by long-acting somatostatin analogue. Lancet. 1979;2(8146):764–7.

84. Reubi JC, Hacki WH, Lamberts SW. Hormone-producing gastrointestinal tumors contain a high density of somatostatin receptors. J Clin Endocrinol Metab. 1987;65(6):1127–34.

85. Reubi JC, Maurer R, von Werder K, Torhorst J, Klijn JG, Lamberts SW. Somatostatin receptors in human endocrine tumors. Cancer Res. 1987;47(2):551–8.

86. Carr JC, Sherman SK, Wang D, et al. Overexpression of membrane proteins in primary and metastatic gastrointestinal neuroendocrine tumors. Ann Surg Oncol. 2013;20(Suppl 3):S739–46.

87. Rinke A, Muller HH, Schade-Brittinger C, et al. Placebo-controlled, double-blind, prospective, randomized study on the effect of octreotide LAR in the control of tumor growth in

patients with metastatic neuroendocrine midgut tumors: a report from the PROMID Study Group. J Clin Oncol. 2009;27(28):4656–63.

88. Rinke A, Wittenberg M, Schade-Brittinger C, et al. Placebo-controlled, double-blind, prospective, randomized study on the effect of octreotide LAR in the control of tumor growth in Patients with Metastatic Neuroendocrine Midgut Tumors (PROMID): results of long-term survival. Neuroendocrinology. 2017;104(1):26–32.

89. Caplin ME, Pavel M, Cwikla JB, et al. Lanreotide in metastatic enteropancreatic neuroendocrine tumors. N Engl J Med. 2014;371(3):224–33.

90. Strosberg J, El-Haddad G, Wolin E, et al. Phase 3 Trial of (177)Lu-Dotatate for Midgut Neuroendocrine Tumors. N Engl J Med. 2017;376(2):125–35.

91. Hope TA, Bodei L, Chan JA, et al. NANETS/SNMMI consensus statement on patient selection and appropriate use of (177)Lu-DOTATATE peptide receptor radionuclide therapy. J Nucl Med. 2020;61(2):222–7.

92. Kulke MH, Horsch D, Caplin ME, et al. Telotristat ethyl, a tryptophan hydroxylase inhibitor for the treatment of carcinoid syndrome. J Clin Oncol. 2017;35(1):14–23.

93. Pavel M, Gross DJ, Benavent M, et al. Telotristat ethyl in carcinoid syndrome: safety and efficacy in the TELECAST phase 3 trial. Endocr Relat Cancer. 2018;25(3):309–22.

94. Singh S, Carnaghi C, Buzzoni R, et al. Everolimus in neuroendocrine tumors of the gastrointestinal tract and unknown primary. Neuroendocrinology. 2018;106(3):211–20.

95. Yao JC, Shah MH, Ito T, et al. Everolimus for advanced pancreatic neuroendocrine tumors. N Engl J Med. 2011;364(6):514–23.

96. Pavel ME, Hainsworth JD, Baudin E, et al. Everolimus plus octreotide long-acting repeatable for the treatment of advanced neuroendocrine tumours associated with carcinoid syndrome (RADIANT-2): a randomised, placebo-controlled, phase 3 study. Lancet. 2011;378(9808):2005–12.

97. Pavel ME, Baudin E, Oberg KE, et al. Efficacy of everolimus plus octreotide LAR in patients with advanced neuroendocrine tumor and carcinoid syndrome: final overall survival from the randomized, placebo-controlled phase 3 RADIANT-2 study. Ann Oncol. 2017;28(7):1569–75.

98. Yao JC, Fazio N, Singh S, et al. Everolimus for the treatment of advanced, non-functional neuroendocrine tumours of the lung or gastrointestinal tract (RADIANT-4): a randomised, placebo-controlled, phase 3 study. The Lancet. 2016;387(10022):968–77.

99. Garcia-Carbonero R, Rinke A, Valle JW, et al. ENETS consensus guidelines for the standards of care in neuroendocrine neoplasms. systemic therapy 2: chemotherapy. Neuroendocrinology. 2017;105(3):281–94.

100. Ramirez RA, Beyer DT, Chauhan A, Boudreaux JP, Wang YZ, Woltering EA. The role of capecitabine/temozolomide in metastatic neuroendocrine tumors. Oncologist. 2016;21(6):671–5.

101. Fine RL, Gulati AP, Tsushima D, et al. Prospective phase II study of capecitabine and temozolomide (CAPTEM) for progressive, moderately, and well-differentiated metastatic neuroendocrine tumors. J Clin Oncol. 2014;32(3):179.

102. de Mestier L, Walter T, Brixi H, et al. Comparison of temozolomide-capecitabine to 5-fluorouracile-dacarbazine in 247 patients with advanced digestive neuroendocrine tumors using propensity score analyses. Neuroendocrinology. 2019;108(4):343–53.

103. Mitry E, Baudin E, Ducreux M, et al. Treatment of poorly differentiated neuroendocrine tumours with etoposide and cisplatin. Br J Cancer. 1999;81(8):1351–5.

104. Heetfeld M, Chougnet CN, Olsen IH, et al. Characteristics and treatment of patients with G3 gastroenteropancreatic neuroendocrine neoplasms. Endocr Relat Cancer. 2015;22(4):657–64.

105. Yantiss RK, Odze RD, Farraye FA, Rosenberg AE. Solitary versus multiple carcinoid tumors of the ileum: a clinical and pathologic review of 68 cases. Am J Surg Pathol. 2003;27(6):811–7.

106. Oberg K, Couvelard A, Delle Fave G, et al. ENETS consensus guidelines for standard of care in neuroendocrine tumours: biochemical markers. Neuroendocrinology. 2017;105(3):201–11.

Colon and Rectal Neuroendocrine Tumors

Adam C. Fields, Pamela W. Lu, and Nelya Melnitchouk

Colon

Introduction Neuroendocrine tumors (NETs) of the colon are a rare entity, accounting for only 10–17% of NETs arising from the gastrointestinal tract and comprise only 1% of colonic malignancies [1–3]. However, despite its rarity, the incidence of these tumors is increasing, and high grade NETs of the colon carry a particularly poor prognosis when compared to that seen with other primary gastro-intestinal sites [1, 4, 5]. Given this, it is critical for clinicians to be able to appropriately identify these tumors and recognize important management steps in treating this disease.

Incidence In the United States, the estimated incidence of NETs arising from the colon is approximately 0.3 per 100,000 [6]. Unlike rectal NETs, the majority of patients diagnosed with this malignancy are white, and there is a slight female predominance seen [3, 6]. The mean age of diagnosis of colonic NETs is 63.3 years [6].

Terminology and Pathology Similar to the case of all NETs, the terminology used to describe the malignancies has changed considerably since its first description in 1867 [7]. Gastroenteropancreatic neuroendocrine tumors had previously been described by the embryologic origin of the primary site and were divided into fore-gut, midgut, and hindgut tumors [8]. This nomenclature divided colonic neuroendo-crine tumors into midgut (cecum, ascending, and two-thirds of the transverse colon) and hindgut (remaining transverse, descending colon) tumors [8]. However, more recent studies have instead taken to viewing small bowel, colonic, and rectal NETs

A. C. Fields · P. W. Lu · N. Melnitchouk (✉)
Department of Surgery, Division of Gastrointestinal Surgery, Brigham and Women's Hospital, Harvard Medical School, Boston, MA, USA
e-mail: Acfields@partners.org; pwlu@partners.org; nmelnitchouk@bwh.harvard.edu

© Springer Nature Switzerland AG 2021
J. M. Cloyd, T. M. Pawlik (eds.), *Neuroendocrine Tumors*,
https://doi.org/10.1007/978-3-030-62241-1_11

as separate entities, with differential survival, prognosis, and recommended treatment guidelines for each primary site [9]. Critical components to describing NETs include the grade and differentiation. The most recent World Health Organization (WHO) classification for NETs of gastrointestinal primary sites is defined by grade and differentiation. Well-differentiated tumors are called NETs and are divided into three grades based on mitoses/mm^2 and Ki-67 proliferation index. G1 or low grade tumors have <2 mitoses/mm^2 and Ki-67 < 3%. G2 or intermediate grade tumors have 2–20 mitoses/mm^2 and Ki-67 from 3–20%. G3 or high grade tumors have >20 mitoses/mm^2 and Ki-67 > 20%. Poorly differentiated tumors, also called neuroendocrine carcinomas (NECs), are divided into small cell type or large cell type. NECs are all high grade based on the above criteria [10]. The pathologic descriptions of these tumors are critical, as they have significantly different natural histories and prognostic implications [11].

Presentation The majority of colonic NETs are non-functioning, thus are often asymptomatic at the time of diagnosis [12]. While the diagnosis of smaller, superficial NETs of the colon is increasing over time, hypothesized to be related to incidentally identified lesions seen on screening colonoscopies, more than half of colonic NETs are of advanced stage, or metastatic at time of diagnosis [3, 7, 13]. If symptomatic at diagnosis, reported symptoms are often vague and can be abdominal pain, bleeding, change in bowel habits, or weight loss; rarely are symptoms consistent with carcinoid syndrome reported [7]. Patients with gastrointestinal tract NETs who do present with these symptoms (e.g., flushing, diarrhea, bronchoconstriction, cardiac valvular fibrosis) tend to have extensive metastases [9].

Workup, Diagnosis, and Staging The staging of colonic NETs follow the T, N, and M staging system as defined by the National Comprehensive Cancer Network (NCCN). The definitions for T, N, and M staging for colonic and rectal primary sites are described in Table 11.1 [9]. T staging is defined by the size of the primary tumor and depth of invasion. Although nodal status is dichotomous based on this TNM staging system, it has been previously suggested that the number of positive nodes is an important predictor of overall survival in this patient population [14]. Also recommended as part of the workup for colonic NETs is abdominal and pelvic imaging, either with CT or with MRI. Additionally, colonoscopy can be considered to evaluate the remainder of the colon for additional lesions, along with small bowel imaging (CT enterography or capsule endoscopy) [9]. Somatostatin receptor-based imaging can also be considered to better define the location of NETs. Biochemical testing, such as urine 5-HIAA or serum serotonin, is not routinely recommended as only a very small proportion of colonic neuroendocrine tumors are hormone producing [6]. According to NCCN guidelines, it is generally recommended only when symptoms of hormone secretion are present [9]. In a study of over 35,000 patients diagnosed with NETs in the Surveillence, Epidemiology, and End Results Program (SEER) database, it was found that approximately 45% of colonic NETs are diagnosed with localized disease, 23% with regional disease, and 32% with distant metastases [15].

Table 11.1 American Joint Cancer Commission TNM staging classification of colorectal NETs

Tx	Primary tumor cannot be assessed
T0	No evidence of primary tumor
T1	Tumor invades lamina propria or submucosa and size ≤2 cm
T1a	Tumor size <1 cm in greatest dimension
T1b	Tumor size 1–2 cm in greatest dimension
T2	Tumor invades muscularis propria or size >2 cm with invasion of lamina propria or submucosa
T3	Tumor invades through muscularis propria into subserosa or into nonperitonealized pericolic or perirectal tissue
T4	Tumor invades peritoneum or other organs
Nx	Regional lymph nodes cannot be assessed
N0	No regional lymph node metastases
N1	Regional lymph node metastases
M0	No distant metastases
M1	Distant metastases
Stage I	T1, N0, M0
Stage IIa	T2, N0, M0
Stage IIb	T3, N0, M0
Stage IIIa	T4, N0, M0
Stage IIIB	Any T, N1, M0
Stage IV	Any T, any N, M1

Management The utility of systemic medical treatments in managing NETs of the colon depends on the histology of the tumor and the patient's symptoms. Low grade well-differentiated tumors tend to have indolent courses and thus are refractory to standard chemotherapy agents [16, 17]. Patients who have metastatic disease, local disease with somatostatin receptor-positive imaging, or patients with symptoms related to carcinoid syndrome can benefit from somatostatin analogues (SSAs) either in its original or long acting formulations [9, 18]. With respect to cytotoxic chemotherapy use, some studies have shown that patients with high grade NECs of colorectal origin may benefit from such aggressive treatment [5, 13]. However, the data on this topic is sparse, and debate remains on the most appropriate use and regimens of cytotoxic agents in treating this disease [17, 19].

For primary tumors arising from the colon, resection of the bowel with regional lymphadenectomy is the recommended surgical treatment for NETs [9] (Fig. 11.1). It is important to note that during surgery, careful examination of the remainder of the bowel should be performed to rule out synchronous lesions [9]. For NECs, the European Neuroendocrine Tumor Society (ENETS) recommends surgery for localized or locoregional disease and no debulking for metastatic disease [20]. Unfortunately, in cases of advanced high grade disease, some prior studies have

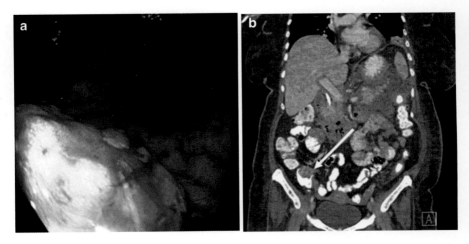

Fig. 11.1 70–year-old woman who was found to have a nonobstructing submucosal mass in the cecum on screening colonoscopy with biopsies demonstrating well-differentiated NET. (**a**). Abdominal CT showed a cecal mass near the appendiceal orifice without metastatic disease. (**b**). She underwent right hemicolectomy with pathology findings revealing a 2.8 cm G1 Ki67 < 2% NET with 2/22 lymph nodes involved

shown that surgical resection does not improve survival – especially in patients with metastatic disease [16, 21]. Unlike NETs of rectal origin, endoscopic resection is not currently recommended, though it has been suggested that intramucosal tumors of the colon that are <1 cm in size may be appropriate for endoscopic resection based on low rates of lymph node metastases [3, 9].

Survival Unfortunately, survival associated with NETs of the colon is worse than many other primary sites [6, 11, 20]. For patients diagnosed with grade 1 or 2 tumors, the median survival is as follows: 261 months for localized disease, 36 months for regionally invasive disease, and only 5 months for disease with distant metastases [15]. Patients with high grade NECs fare worse: reported median survival for all-comers with high grade colorectal NECs range from 7.1 to 9.0 months [5, 22].

Surveillance Current recommendations set forth by the NCCN include serial follow-ups every 3–4 months for one year after resection, with biochemical markers and abdominal/pelvic imaging. Following one year post-resection, follow-up every 12–24 months is recommended until ten years post-resection with the same testing procedures [9]. With respect to biochemical markers, Chromogranin A levels have been previously suggested as a surveillance tool in patients with known metastatic disease or in patients who have undergone resection of locally advanced disease; however, this biochemical test can be easily affected by the use of proton pump inhibitors, is often elevated in cases of other primary malignancies, and concerns have been raised about its utility in NETs of colorectal sites [6, 9, 23].

Conclusion NETs arising from the colon are rare and the prognosis depends on traditional TNM staging as well as histologic grading using Ki67 and mitotic rate. While the mainstay of treatment for localized disease remains segmental resection with regional lymphadenectomy, the optimal use of various systemic cytotoxic agents in treating this disease requires further study.

Rectum

Introduction The incidence of rectal neuroendocrine tumors (NETs) is estimated to be 1 in 100,000 and this rate is increasing [1, 24]. Rectal NETs represent 27% of gastrointestinal NETs and approximately 2% of rectal neoplasms [25]. The mean age of diagnosis is 56, higher rates are reported in Asian and Black patients, and there are more males affected [26, 27]. Well-differentiated rectal NETs are associated with five-year survival exceeding 85% [1, 26, 28] while poorly differentiated rectal NETs are associated with low overall survival [5]. The North American Neuroendocrine Tumor Society (NANETS) and ENETS both provide guidelines for the management of rectal NETs [29, 30].

Terminology and Pathology The WHO grading for rectal NETs and NECs is the same as for colon NETs and NECs [31]. As previously discussed, well-differentiated tumors are comprised of low and intermediate grade tumors (grades 1–2) while poorly differentiated rectal NETs are considered high grade (grade 3) and are divided into small and large cell neuroendocrine carcinomas. It is important to differentiate between well-differentiated and poorly differentiated rectal NETs because their tumor behavior is distinctive; well-differentiated tumors are typically indolent while poorly differentiated tumors are aggressive. Management for each type of tumor also differs.

Presentation Rectal NETs are often found incidentally during surveillance endoscopy [32]. The majority of rectal NETs are submucosal and located in the mid-rectum [33, 34]. Over 50% of patients are asymptomatic at the time of diagnosis [33, 35]. Symptoms that can be associated with rectal NETs include rectal bleeding, pain, bowel habit changes, bowel obstruction, and weight loss [30, 33, 36]. If widespread metastasis is present, symptoms of carcinoid syndrome could occur such as flushing, diarrhea, cardiac valvular disease, and bronchoconstriction [30].

Workup, Diagnosis, and Staging The majority of rectal NETs are localized to the rectum at the time of diagnosis [26, 37]. The median tumor size at the time of diagnosis is 0.6 cm [38]. Although metastases are rare at the time of diagnosis, 2% of patients with rectal NETs with tumors less than 1.0 cm, 10–15% of patients with rectal NETs with tumors 1–2 cm, and 60–80% of patients with tumors greater than 2 cm will have metastases [39].

In 2010, the American Joint Cancer Commission published the first TNM classification for rectal NETs [40] (Table 11.1). This staging matches staging guidelines put forth by NANETS and ENETS [29, 30]. Other staging systems have been proposed to better account for survival differences based on the number of lymph node metastases [41]. Patients with a new rectal NET diagnosis should have a complete colonoscopy to rule out synchronous lesions [42]. Rectal NETs with ulceration or mucosal depression have been shown to have higher metastatic potential [19].

Patients with rectal NETs that measure less than about 1 cm do not require cross-sectional imaging, although some guidelines recommend imaging for all new diagnoses of rectal NETs [42]. Patients who have larger or invasive tumors require computed tomography or magnetic resonance imaging (MRI) to rule out distant metastases. High grade rectal NETs are often negative for octreotide uptake on somatostatin receptor scintigraphy and thus it has not been suggested as a first-line imaging modality [30]. Endoscopic ultrasonography (EUS) or MRI can be used to further characterize localized tumors measuring greater than 1 cm to accurately determine tumor size, depth of invasion, and lymph node involvement [43, 44]. EUS should be performed in patients that have tumors >0.5 cm, atypical features such as ulceration or hyperpigmentation, or local lymph node invasion [37].

Less than 1% of rectal NETs produce serotonin and thus testing for serotonin or 5-hydroxyindoleacetic acid is not recommended [29]. Serum chromogranin A is a tumor marker that can be used to monitor patients over time, monitor patients with metastatic disease, or act as a surveillance marker for patients with resected tumors [45].

Management There are no large multicenter investigations or controlled trials focused on the treatment of rectal NETs. Treatment algorithms are derived from consensus guidelines and retrospective cohort studies.

For well-differentiated NETs, the NCCN recommends local excision for rectal NETs less than 1 cm and radical resection for rectal NETs larger than 2 cm and for tumors that have metastasized to lymph nodes [42]. Endoscopic resection is typically reserved for small (<1 cm) tumors that do not invade beyond the submucosa and when there is no locoregional lymph node metastasis [44]. Prior work has demonstrated low rates of recurrence (0%) [46] and low rates of positive margins (17%) following endoscopic resection [44, 47]. Endoscopic polypectomy can be performed for small tumors (Fig. 11.2). Other endoscopic techniques including band snares, submucosal dissection, and ligation have been described [46, 48, 49]. Endoscopic submucosal dissection and endoscopic mucosal resection are similar in efficacy in establishing negative margins for small tumors (0.5 cm) [50, 51]. For larger lesions >0.5 cm, endoscopic submucosal dissection has been shown to have higher rates of negative margins compared to endoscopic mucosal resection [52]. Tattooing of the rectal NET is recommended in the event that a secondary therapy is required or for surveillance.

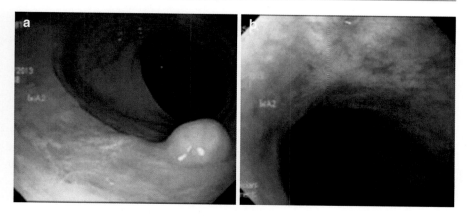

Fig. 11.2 52-year-old man who underwent routine colonoscopy for history of colonic polyps was found to have a small polyp in the upper rectum. Snare polypectomy was performed. Pathology showed 0.4 cm well-differentiated NET Ki67 < 1% (**a**). Repeat sigmoidoscopy one year later showed only a polypectomy scar (**b**)

A transanal excision is often utilized for rectal NETs that are intermediate in size (1–2 cm) that are confined to the submucosa/muscularis propria and located distally in the rectum. Rectal NETs within 5 cm of the anal verge can be resected with conventional transanal excision techniques [53]. Rectal NETs in the middle and upper portions of the rectum can be resected with transanal endoscopic microsurgery [54]. Transanal excision allows for a full-thickness excision of the tumor. If lymphovascular invasion is present in the specimen, further resection with low anterior resection or abdominoperineal resection should be considered.

Oncologic resection, consisting of low anterior resection or abdominoperineal resection with total mesorectal excision, depending on the tumor location within the rectum should take place for larger rectal NETs (> 2 cm), tumors invading the muscularis propria, or tumors with locoregional lymph node involvement. The optimal surgical strategy for patients with rectal NETs measuring 1–2 cm has not been well defined. The risk of metastasis has been reported at 10–15%. Some studies have shown no difference in survival with local excision versus radical excision for these intermediate sized tumors [55, 56].

Metastatic NETs have been treated with SSAs, interferon alpha, chemotherapy, and cytoreductive surgery [57–59]. To date, no trials have evaluated these treatment options for rectal NETs.

Little is known about the optimal treatment for patients with poorly differentiated NETs. Few studies with small patient populations have focused on treatment for these NETs. Unlike for the treatment of well-differentiated NETs, surgery alone is likely not curative for poorly differentiated NETs. A combination of an oncologic resection with low anterior resection and abdominoperineal resection and systemic chemotherapy is often utilized [5, 60, 61]. NANETS recommends surgical resection followed by adjuvant chemotherapy for early stage high grade extrapulmonary neuroendocrine carcinomas [62].

Survival Patients with well-differentiated rectal NETs have excellent five-year survival with rates exceeding 85% [1, 26, 28]. If the rectal NET has metastasized to lymph nodes five-year survival decreases to 54–70% and if there is distant metastasis, five-year survival drops considerably to 15–32% [1, 26, 63]. Tumor size, grade, mitotic count, and lymphovascular invasion are associated with survival [28, 63, 64]. For patients with poorly differentiated rectal NETs, survival is significantly lower. In assessing patients with poorly differentiated colorectal NETs, five-year survival was approximately 13–33% [5, 65].

Surveillance It is possible for rectal NETs to recur years after diagnosis and treatment. For patients with rectal NETs <1 cm, long-term surveillance with endoscopy or imaging is not recommended [30, 42]. For patients with tumors between 1 and 2 cm or who undergo local excision, EUS or MRI is recommended at 6 and 12 months, although studies have not evaluated the efficacy of surveillance [42]. Patients with tumors >2 cm or who have formal resections should be followed closely for up to ten years [30, 42].

Conclusions Rectal NETs are rare tumors that are often diagnosed incidentally on endoscopy. Although well-differentiated tumors are known to be indolent, the first-line treatment for all locoregional tumors is resection, either endoscopic or surgical depending on risks of lymphatic metastasis. Five-year survival is high for well-differentiated locoregional tumors that are resected. Further investigation is needed to better risk stratify patients with well-differentiated rectal NETs who may benefit from less invasive resection and to evaluate treatment options for patients with poorly differentiated rectal NETs.

References

1. Maggard MA, O'Connell JB, Ko CY. Updated population-based review of carcinoid tumors. Ann Surg. 2004;240(1):117–22.
2. Frilling A, Akerström G, Falconi M, Pavel M, Ramos J, Kidd M, et al. Neuroendocrine tumor disease: an evolving landscape. Endocr Relat Cancer. 2012;19(5):R163–85.
3. Al Natour RH, Saund MS, Sanchez VM, Whang EE, Sharma AM, Huang Q, et al. Tumor size and depth predict rate of lymph node metastasis in colon carcinoids and can be used to select patients for endoscopic resection. J Gastrointest Surg. 2012;16(3):595–602.
4. Dasari A, Shen C, Halperin D, Zhao B, Zhou S, Xu Y, et al. Trends in the incidence, prevalence, and survival outcomes in patients with neuroendocrine tumors in the United States. JAMA Oncol. 2017;3(10):1335–42.
5. Fields AC, Lu P, Vierra BM, Hu F, Irani J, Bleday R, et al. Survival in patients with high-grade colorectal neuroendocrine carcinomas: the role of surgery and chemotherapy. Ann Surg Oncol. 2019;26(4):1127–33.

6. Ford MM. Neuroendocrine tumors of the colon and rectum. Dis Colon Rectum. 2017;60(10):1018–20.
7. Eggenberger JC. Carcinoid and other neuroendocrine tumors of the colon and rectum. Clin Colon Rectal Surg. 2011;24(3):129–34.
8. Díez M, Teulé A, Salazar R. Gastroenteropancreatic neuroendocrine tumors: diagnosis and treatment. Ann Gastroenterol. 2013;26(1):29–36.
9. NCCN. National Comprehensive Cancer Network clinical practice guidelines in oncology: neuroendocrine and adrenal tumors. Version 1.2019 2019. Available from: https://www.nccn.org/professionals/physician_gls/pdf/neuroendocrine.pdf
10. Nagtegaal ID, Odze RD, Klimstra D, Paradis V, Rugge M, Schirmacher P, et al. The 2019 WHO classification of tumours of the digestive system. Histopathology. 2020;76(2):182–8.
11. Hrabe J. Neuroendocrine Tumors of the appendix, Colon, and rectum. Surg Oncol Clin N Am. 2020;29(2):267–79.
12. Chung TP, Hunt SR. Carcinoid and neuroendocrine tumors of the colon and rectum. Clin Colon Rectal Surg. 2006;19(2):45–8.
13. Wang R, Zheng-Pywell R, Chen HA, Bibb JA, Chen H, Rose JB. Management of Gastrointestinal Neuroendocrine Tumors. Clin Med Insights Endocrinol Diabetes. 2019;12:1179551419884058.
14. Fields AC, McCarty JC, Lu P, Vierra BM, Pak LM, Irani J, et al. Colon neuroendocrine Tumors: a new lymph node staging classification. Ann Surg Oncol. 2019;26(7):2028–36.
15. Yao JC, Hassan M, Phan A, Dagohoy C, Leary C, Mares JE, et al. One hundred years after "carcinoid": epidemiology of and prognostic factors for neuroendocrine tumors in 35,825 cases in the United States. J Clin Oncol. 2008;26(18):3063–72.
16. Smith JD, Reidy DL, Goodman KA, Shia J, Nash GM. A retrospective review of 126 high-grade neuroendocrine carcinomas of the colon and rectum. Ann Surg Oncol. 2014;21(9):2956–62.
17. Vilar E, Salazar R, Pérez-García J, Cortes J, Oberg K, Tabernero J. Chemotherapy and role of the proliferation marker Ki-67 in digestive neuroendocrine tumors. Endocr Relat Cancer. 2007;14(2):221–32.
18. Costa F, Gumz B. Octreotide – a review of its use in treating neuroendocrine tumours. Eur Endocrinol. 2014;10(1):70–4.
19. Ramage JK, De Herder WW, Delle Fave G, Ferolla P, Ferone D, Ito T, et al. ENETS consensus guidelines update for colorectal neuroendocrine neoplasms. Neuroendocrinology. 2016;103(2):139–43.
20. Garcia-Carbonero R, Sorbye H, Baudin E, et al. ENETS consensus guidelines for high-grade gastroenteropancreatic neuroendocrine tumors and neuroendocrine carcinomas. Neuroendocrinology. 2016;103:186–94.
21. Aytac E, Ozdemir Y, Ozuner G. Long term outcomes of neuroendocrine carcinomas (high-grade neuroendocrine tumors) of the colon, rectum, and anal canal. J Visc Surg. 2014;151(1):3–7.
22. Shafqat H, Ali S, Salhab M, Olszewski AJ. Survival of patients with neuroendocrine carcinoma of the colon and rectum: a population-based analysis. Dis Colon Rectum. 2015;58(3):294–303.
23. Koenig A, Krug S, Mueller D, Barth PJ, Koenig U, Scharf M, et al. Clinicopathological hallmarks and biomarkers of colorectal neuroendocrine neoplasms. PLoS One. 2017;12(12):e0188876.
24. Yao JC, Phan AT, Chang DZ, et al. Efficacy of RAD001 (everolimus) and octreotide LAR in advanced low- to intermediate-grade neuroendocrine tumors: results of a phase II study. J Clin Oncol. 2008;1926:4311–8.
25. Godwin JD. Carcinoid tumors. An analysis of 2,837 cases. Cancer. 1975;36(2):560–9.
26. Modlin IM, Lye KD, Kidd M. A 5-decade analysis of 13,715 carcinoid tumors. Cancer. 2003;97(4):934–59.
27. Taghavi S, Jayarajan SN, Powers BD, Davey A, Willis AI. Examining rectal carcinoids in the era of screening colonoscopy: a surveillance, epidemiology, and end results analysis. Dis Colon Rectum. 2013;56(8):952–9.
28. Tsang ES, McConnell YJ, Schaeffer DF, et al. Prognostic factors for locoregional recurrence in neuroendocrine tumors of the rectum. Dis Colon Rectum. 2018;61:187–92.

29. Anthony LB, Strosberg JR, Klimstra DS, et al. The NANETS consensus guidelines for the diagnosis and management of gastrointestinal neuroendocrine tumors (NETs): well differentiated NETs of the distal colon and rectum. Pancreas. 2010;39:767–74.
30. Ramage JK, Goretzki PE, Manfredi R, et al. Consensus guidelines for the management of patients with digestive neuroendocrine tumors: well-differentiated colon and rectum tumour/carcinoma. Neuroendocrinology. 2008;87:31–9.
31. Rindi G, Arnold R, Bosman FT, et al. Nomenclature and classification of neuroendocrine neoplasms of the digestive system. WHO classification of tumors in the digestive system. 4th ed. Lyon: International Agency for Research on Cancer (IARC); 2010. p. 13–4.
32. Yoon SN, Yu CS, Shin US, Kim CW, Lim SB, Kim JC. Clinicopathological characteristics of rectal carcinoids. Int J Color Dis. 2010;25:1087–92.
33. Wang AY, Ahmad NA. Rectal carcinoids. Curr Opin Gastroenterol. 2006;22(5):529–35.
34. Shim KN, Yang SK, Myung SJ, et al. Atypical endoscopic features of rectal carcinoids. Endoscopy. 2004;36(4):313–6.
35. Jetmore AB, Ray JE, Gathright JB Jr, McMullen KM, Hicks TC, Timmcke AE. Rectal carcinoids: the most frequent carcinoid tumor. Dis Colon Rectum. 1992;35:717–25.
36. Merg A, Wirtzfeld D, Wang J, et al. Viability of endoscopic and excisional treatment of early rectal carcinoids. J Gastrointest Surg. 2007;11(7):893–7.
37. Basuroy R, Haji A, Ramage JK, Quaglia A, Srirajaskanthan R. Review article: the investigation and management of rectal neuroendocrine tumours. Aliment Phamacol Ther. 2016;44:332–45.
38. Landry CS, Brock G, Scoggins CR, et al. A proposed staging system for rectal carcinoid tumors based on an analysis of 4701 patients. Surgery. 2008;144(3):460–6.
39. Mani S, Modlin IM, Ballantyne G, et al. Carcinoids of the rectum. J Am Coll Surg. 1994;179(2):231–48.
40. Edge SB, Byrd DR, Compton CC. AJCC cancer staging manual. 7th ed. New York: Springer; 2010.
41. Fields AC, McCarty JC, Ma-Pak L, et al. New lymph node staging for rectal neuroendocrine tumors. J Surg Oncol. 2019;119(1):156–62.
42. Kulke MH, Shah MH, Benson AB 3rd, et al. Neuroendocrine tumors, version 1.2015. J Natl Compr Cancer Netw. 2015;13:78–108.
43. Ishii N, Horiki N, Itoh T, et al. Endoscopic submucosal dissection and preoperative assessment with endoscopic ultrasonography for the treatment of rectal carcinoid tumors. Surg Endosc. 2010;24:1413–9.
44. Kobayashi K, Katsumata T, Yoshizawa S, et al. Indications of endoscopic polypectomy for rectal carcinoid tumors and clinical usefulness of endoscopic ultrasonography. Dis Colon Rectum. 2005;48(2):285–91.
45. Eriksson B, Oberg K, Stridsberg M, et al. Tumor markers in neuroendocrine tumors. Digestion. 2000;62:33–8.
46. Berkelhammer C, Jasper I, Kirvaitis E, et al. "Band-snare" resection of small rectal carcinoid tumors. Gastrointest Endosc. 1999;50(4):582–5.
47. Higaki S, Nishiaki M, Mitani N, et al. Effectiveness of local endoscopic resection of rectal carcinoid tumors. Endoscopy. 1997;29(3):171–5.
48. Fujishiro M, Yahagi N, Nakamura M, et al. Successful outcomes of a novel endoscopic treatment for GI tumors: endoscopic submucosal dissection with a mixture of high-molecular-weight hyaluronic acid, glycerin, and sugar. Gastrointest Endosc. 2006;63(2):243–9.
49. Okamoto Y, Fujii M, Tateiwa S, et al. Treatment of multiple rectal carcinoids by endoscopic mucosal resection using a device for esophageal variceal ligation. Endoscopy. 2004;36(5):469–70.
50. Niimi K, Goto O, Fujishiro M, et al. Endoscopic mucosal resection with a ligation device or endoscopic submucosal dissection for rectal carcinoid tumors: an analysis of 24 consecutive cases. Dig Endosc. 2012;24:443–7.
51. Choi CW, Kang DH, Kim HW, et al. Comparison of endoscopic resection therapies for rectal carcinoid tumor: endoscopic submucosal dissection versus endoscopic mucosal resection using band ligation. J Clin Gastroenterol. 2013;47:432–6.

52. Wang X, Xiang L, Li A, et al. Endoscopic submucosal dissection for the treatment of rectal carcinoid tumors 7–16 mm in diameter. Int J Color Dis. 2015;30:375–80.
53. Ishikawa K, Arita T, Shimoda K, Hagino Y, Shiraishi N, Kitano S. Usefulness of transanal endoscopic surgery for carcinoid tumor in the upper and middle rectum. Surg Endosc Other Interv Tech. 2005;19:1151–4.
54. Kinoshita T, Kanehira E, Omura K, Tomori T, Yamada H. Transanal endoscopic microsurgery in the treatment of rectal carcinoid tumor. Surg Endosc. 2007;21:970–4.
55. Fields AC, Saadat LV, Scully R, et al. Local excision versus radical resection for 1- to 2-cm neuroendocrine tumors of the rectum: a national cancer database analysis. Dis Colon Rectum. 2019;62(4):417–21.
56. Koura AN, Giacco GG, Curley SA, Skibber JM, Feig BW, Ellis LM. Carcinoid tumors of the rectum: effect of size, histopathology, and surgical treatment on metastasis-free survival. Cancer. 1997;79:1294–8.
57. Arnold R, Trautmann ME, Creutzfeldt W, et al. Somatostatin analogue octreotide and inhibition of tumour growth in metastatic endocrine gastroenteropancreatic tumours. Gut. 1996;38(3):430–8.
58. Arnold R, Rinke A, Klose KJ, et al. Octreotide versus octreotide plus interferon-alpha in endocrine gastroenteropancreatic tumors: a randomized trial. Clin Gastroenterol Hepatol. 2005;3(8):761–71.
59. Norton JA, Warren RS, Kelly MG, et al. Aggressive surgery for metastatic liver neuroendocrine tumors. Surgery. 2003;134(6):1057–63.
60. Sorbye H, Welin S, Langer SW, et al. Predictive and prognostic factors for treatment and survival in 305 patients with advanced gastrointestinal neuroendocrine carcinoma (WHO G3): the NORDIC NEC study. Ann Oncol. 2013;24(1):152–60.
61. Brenner B, Shah MA, Gonen M, Klimstra DS, Shia J, Kelsen DP. Small-cell carcinoma of the gastrointestinal tract: a retrospective study of 64 cases. Br J Cancer. 2004;90(9):1720–6.
62. Kunz PL, Reidy-Lagunes D, Anthony LB, et al. Consensus guidelines for the management and treatment of neuroendocrine tumors. Pancreas. 2013;42(4):557–77.
63. Shields CJ, Tiret E, Winter DC. Carcinoid tumors of the rectum: a multi-institutional international collaboration. Ann Surg. 2010;252:750–5.
64. Fahy BN, Tang LH, Klimstra D, et al. CARCINOID of the rectum risk stratification (CaRRS): a strategy for preoperative outcome assessment. Ann Surg Oncol. 2007;14:396–404.
65. Weinstock B, Ward SC, Harpaz N, Warner RRP, Itzkowitz S, Kim MK. Clinical and prognostic features of rectal neuroendocrine tumors. Neuroendocrinology. 2013;98(3):180–7.

Surgical Evaluation of Appendiceal Neuroendocrine Tumors

12

Xavier M. Keutgen and Tanaz M. Vaghaiwalla

Introduction

Neuroendocrine tumors (NETs) are a heterogeneous group of tumors which originate from specialized cells that secrete neuro-hormonal peptides. They are characterized as neuroendocrine cells because of their similar features to both neuronal cells which have dense core granules and endocrine cells which produce and secrete various hormones [1]. Neuroendocrine cells are located throughout the body including the bronchial and gastroenteropancreatic tracts and therefore NETs may arise from various organ systems. Appendiceal NETs arise from neuroendocrine cells located within the appendix [2]. In 1907 Siegfried Oberndorfer first described neuroendocrine tumors as "carcinoid" or little carcinomas which he believed to be benign tumors at that time; however, their potential for aggressive behavior was later identified [3, 4]. Today the term carcinoid is rarely used anymore and generally reserved for neuroendocrine tumors of the gastrointestinal tract. Appendiceal NETs are also described as midgut NETs along with NETs of the jejunum, ileum, and cecum given their common embryologic origin [1, 2, 4].

The appendix is the most common site for gastrointestinal NETs [5]. Appendiceal NETs comprise 38% of all gastrointestinal NETs and represent up to 88% of all appendiceal tumors [6]. The incidence rate of appendiceal NET ranges from 0.15 to 0.6 cases per 100,000 each year [7]. Appendiceal NETs are typically diagnosed in the third through fifth decades of life and appear to have no racial predilection [4, 8]. There appears to be no gender predominance; however, some studies have identified a slight incidence increase in women [7, 9, 10]. The majority of appendiceal NETs are diagnosed incidentally upon pathological examination of specimens removed during appendectomy for appendicitis or other reasons [5, 7, 9, 10].

X. M. Keutgen · T. M. Vaghaiwalla (✉)
Department of Surgery, Endocrine Research Program, University of Chicago Medical Center, Chicago, IL, USA
e-mail: xkeutgen@surgery.bsd.uchicago.edu; Tanaz.vaghaiwalla@uchospitals.edu

© Springer Nature Switzerland AG 2021
J. M. Cloyd, T. M. Pawlik (eds.), *Neuroendocrine Tumors*,
https://doi.org/10.1007/978-3-030-62241-1_12

Surgical treatment is the mainstay for management of localized appendiceal NETs and offers the chance for curative resection. While the majority of patients are diagnosed with early stage tumors, both lymph node and distant metastases can occur and portend a worse prognosis [10, 11]. There are many non-surgical treatment modalities for patients with advanced or distant metastases, and a multidisciplinary approach is necessary to establish the optimal management and timing of intervention. The purpose of this text is to review the diagnosis and surgical management of well-differentiated appendiceal NETs. Appendiceal tumors may also include adenocarcinoma, goblet cell carcinoma, adenocarcinoid tumors, and a variety of benign tumors, which will not be the focus of this chapter.

Diagnosis and Workup

Clinical Presentation

Neuroendocrine tumors may be classified as functioning tumors which produce a hormonal syndrome and non-functioning tumors which do not produce clinical symptoms. While 55% of midgut and hindgut NETs are diagnosed with functional tumors producing primarily serotonin, only 2% of appendiceal NETs are found to be functioning [12]. Appendiceal NETs are most often located at the tip of the appendix and less likely to cause locoregional symptoms. These tumors are more often diagnosed incidentally upon pathology review after appendectomy is performed for other reasons, such as acute appendicitis. Studies have shown that <1.5% of appendectomies demonstrated an appendiceal NET [5, 9]. Non-functioning asymptomatic tumors can be identified at later stages and therefore represent a diagnostic challenge. Rarely, patients with metastatic disease may present with symptoms related to the location of their tumor metastases or symptoms of carcinoid syndrome [7, 9–11].

Biochemical Evaluation

Several key biochemical markers are used in the diagnosis and surveillance of neuroendocrine tumors, including appendiceal NETs. However, it is worth noting that asymptomatic patients with early stage appendiceal tumors who have undergone complete resection do not require measurement of biochemical markers [7, 11].

Appendiceal neuroendocrine tumor cells may release chromogranin A, an acidic glycoprotein present in the dense-core granules of endocrine and neuroendocrine cells [13]. Serum chromogranin A is a sensitive and specific marker for NETs and may serve as a diagnostic marker in asymptomatic patients; however, its role in diagnosing appendiceal NETs specifically is unknown [14]. Guidelines generally support measurement of chromogranin A in patients in the surveillance of patients with advanced or metastatic disease, including appendiceal NETs [7, 11, 15–17].

5-Hydroxyindoleacetic acid (5-HIAA) is a breakdown product in serotonin metabolism that can be measured in the blood, serum, or urine [13]. Screening with

5-HIAA or plasma serotonin is not recommended for appendiceal NETs, unless in the rare case of suspected carcinoid syndrome [7, 10, 11, 17, 18].

Preoperative Imaging

Since most appendiceal tumors are diagnosed after an operation has been performed for another reason, determining what type of imaging modality is to be performed is often part of the follow-up rather than the preoperative planning (see section "Pathologic Classification"). If an incidental appendiceal tumor is discovered on imaging the authors recommend assessment of other sites of disease, such as mesenteric lymph nodes and the liver since this can change operative management (i.e., performing a right hemicolectomy for gross mesenteric lymphadenopathy vs. appendectomy alone). If a completion right hemicolectomy is to be performed after an appendectomy for appendiceal NET, it is the authors' recommendation to also carefully evaluate the liver with dedicated triple phase computerized tomography (CT) or an magnetic resonance imaging (MRI) abdomen with gadoxetic acid-enhanced (marketed as EOVIST in the United States and PRIMOVIST in Europe) as liver metastases may influence surgical therapy. There is no consensus among guidelines for the selection and timing of imaging in the diagnosis, staging, and follow-up of neuroendocrine tumors [7, 11, 18, 19]. The imaging modality selected is often a result of a combination of factors including surgeon or clinician preference, institutional availability, expense, and risk of irradiation exposure.

Pathological Classification

Gross Features and Histopathology

The location of the tumor within the appendix has an important role in surgical decision-making. While >70% of appendiceal NETs are located at the tip of the appendix, the tumor may also be located at the mid-portion in 15–20% or the base of the appendix in 5–10% [20–22]. On gross examination, appendiceal NETs have a yellow appearance with well-defined borders. Microscopically, tumors are made up of uniform polygonal cells in large nests with peripheral palisading and glandular patterns [20]. There are no studies at present that confirm whether tumor location has a survival impact, but guidelines do recommend oncologic resection, which includes right hemicolectomy and mesenteric lymphadenectomy, for tumors located at the base of the appendix due to concerns of positive margins and lymph node involvement metastases [7, 10, 18, 21–23].

Appendiceal NETs like other neuroendocrine neoplasms are classified according to the World Health Organization (WHO) classification [24]. The WHO defines the grade of NETs according to their morphology, mitotic index, and Ki-67 index. Neuroendocrine neoplasms of the appendix may also have mixed histologies including goblet cell and adenocarcinoid types which have mutations similar to neuroendocrine carcinomas or adenocarcinomas (Fig. 12.1) [25, 26].

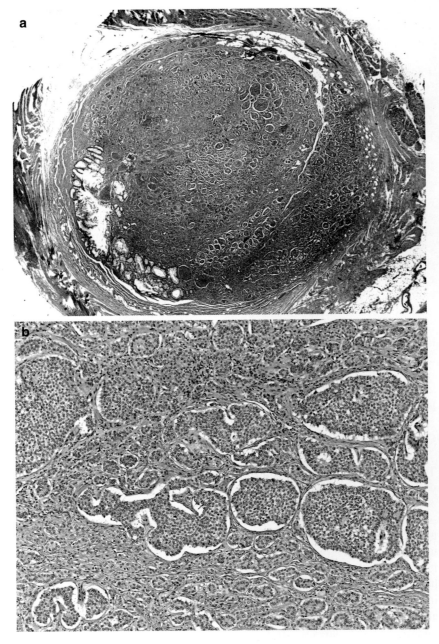

Fig. 12.1 Microscopic and Gross Images of Appendiceal Neuroendocrine Tumor. (**a**) Cross-section of an appendix with infiltration of the wall by nests of well-differentiated neuroendocrine tumor [H&E, 12.5×]. (**b**) Higher magnification shows solid nests of small-medium cells with amphophilic cytoplasm and uniform round nuclei with "salt and pepper" (finely stippled) chromatin [H&E, 100×]. (**c**) Ki-67 immunostain in a well-differentiated neuroendocrine tumor showing a proliferation index of less than 3% [immunostain, 200×]. (**d**) Hemicolectomy specimen with appendiceal neuroendocrine tumor (black arrow) involving the appendiceal stump

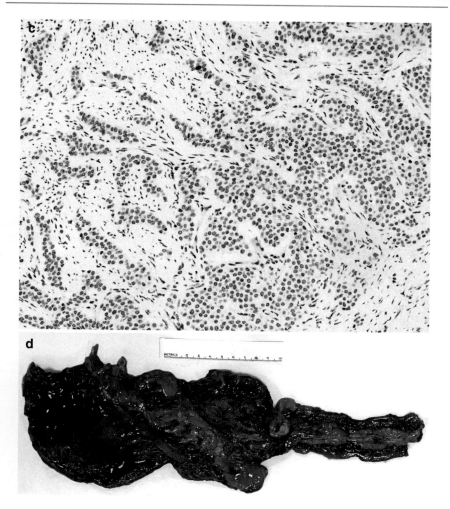

Fig. 12.1 (continued)

High Risk Features

Certain high risk features described in pathology reports influence the recommendation on surgical management of appendiceal NETs.

Tumor Location at Appendiceal Base

Tumor location at the base may confer a higher risk of recurrence and subsequent metastases due to positive resection margins after incomplete resection with appendectomy alone. Positive margins have been associated with shortened survival [27]. Guidelines do recognize that incomplete resection is more likely with an appendectomy for a tumor located at the base and this may increase the risk of local recurrence or metastases; however, the association between tumor location and risk of tumor recurrence remains unclear [28, 29].

Tumor Invasion of the Mesoappendix

Tumor invasion of the mesoappendix >3 mm is often cited as a high risk feature of appendiceal NETs, although this finding is controversial. Invasion of the mesoappendix may be found in as high as 35% of patients with appendiceal NETs [30]. Early studies had identified a possible correlation between tumor invasion of the mesoappendix with nodal metastases and tumor size; however, more recent studies have not found a significant correlation with lymph node involvement [21, 30–34]. A systematic review found no significant difference in the rate of lymph node metastases in patients with invasion of the mesoappendix (30%) compared to patients without (26%) [33]. Another study found that patients who underwent appendectomy for tumors <2 cm had an excellent prognosis despite the presence of tumor invasion into the mesoappendix [30]. Although the presence of this feature on outcomes remains unproven, both North American Neuroendocrine Tumor Society (NANETS) and European Neuroendocrine Tumor Society (ENETS) guidelines recommend consideration of right hemicolectomy when invasion of the mesoappendix is present, and ENETS guidelines include depth of invasion in their Tumor–node–metastasis (TNM) staging (Table 12.1) [28].

Table 12.1 TNM staging of appendiceal NETs

TNM stage	ENETS guidelines[a]	AJCC classification system[b]
Primary tumor (T)		
Tx	Primary tumor not evaluated	
T0	No evidence of primary tumor	
T1	Tumor ≤1 cm in size with submucosa and muscularis propria infiltration	
T1a		Tumor ≤1 cm
T1b		Tumor >1 cm and ≤ 2 cm
T2	Tumor ≤2 cm and infiltration of submucosa, muscularis propria and/or ≤ 3 mm infiltration of subserosa or mesoappendix	Tumor >2 cm and ≤ 4 cm; tumor extension to cecum
T3	Tumor >2 cm and/or > 3 mm infiltration of subserosa or mesoappendix	Tumor >4 cm; tumor extension to ileum
T4	Tumor infiltration of peritoneum and/or adjacent structures	
Lymph node metastases (N)		
Nx	Regional lymph nodes not evaluated	
N0	No regional lymph nodes	
N1	Locoregional lymph node metastases	
Distant metastases (M)		
Mx	Distant metastases not evaluated	
M0	No distant metastases	
M1	Distant metastases	

[a]Pape et al. [17]
[b]Edge and Edge [39]
Abbreviations: *T* tumor; *N* nodal; *M* metastases; *ENETS* European Neuroendocrine Tumor Society; *AJCC* American Joint Commission on Cancer

Lymphovascular Invasion

Lymphovascular invasion is a histopathologic finding of tumor cell invasion into adjacent lymphatic channels and vasculature. Lymphovascular invasion is considered an indicator of aggressive tumor biology for patients with appendiceal NETs between 1 and 2 cm in size. An estimated 18% of all appendiceal NETs and 27% of tumors 1–2 cm in size were found to have lymphovascular invasion on histopathology review [35]. Multiple studies have shown that lymphovascular invasion and angioinvasion to be independently associated with lymph node metastases [33–36]. Guidelines recognize that lymph node metastases, however, have an unclear impact on the development of distant metastases and survival. One study showed ten-year overall survival rates of patients with tumor size ≤1.0 cm, 1–2 cm, and > 2.0 cm were high regardless of lymph node metastases at 100%, 92%, and 91%, respectively, and several studies found similar good prognosis despite the presence of lymph node metastases [37, 38]. Despite these conflicting results, at this time guidelines suggest consideration of completion right hemicolectomy for patients with appendiceal NETs between 1 and 2 cm in size with presence of lymphovascular invasion on histopathologic review.

Grade 2

As mentioned previously, histopathology is the gold standard for diagnosis of appendiceal NETs, and increasing grade is considered a marker of aggressive tumor behavior. Grade 2 tumors were independently associated with lymph node involvement [33, 36]. The rate of lymph node metastases in patients with G1 appendiceal NETs was 22% compared to 55% for G2 tumors [33]. When tumors > G1 are identified on pathology after appendectomy, guidelines recommend consideration of completion right hemicolectomy [7, 10, 28].

Tumor Staging

Two staging systems, the European Neuroendocrine Tumor Society (ENETS) and the American Joint Committee on Cancer (AJCC) classify appendiceal NETs but with slight variations in their definitions. Both systems use the Tumor–node–metastasis (TNM) cancer staging system. Multiple studies have demonstrated the prognostic significance of tumor size on presence of lymph node involvement, distant metastasis, and survival [27, 33, 36–39].

Appendiceal NETs <1 cm in size (ENETS and AJCC classification T1) are the earliest stage and cured by complete tumor resection with appendectomy. Despite conflicting reports of the presence of lymph node involvement (2.7–11.6%), T1 appendiceal NETs have excellent prognosis with five-year survival estimates of 95–100% [4, 7, 27, 37–40]. While still low stage, tumors >1 cm and < 2 cm in size (ENETS guidelines T2; AJCC classification T1b) have shown to have lymph node metastases in 18–56.8% of cases [7, 21, 27, 37–39]. Some studies have suggested a cutoff value of >1.5 cm as tumor size to determine whether a patient needs a completion right hemicolectomy, since that size threshold appeared to be a better predictor of lymph node metastasis [36]. Appendiceal NETs >2 cm in size (ENETS guidelines T3; AJCC classification T2) have a higher risk of metastases and guidelines recommend oncological resection of tumors this size. Studies have reported rates of lymph node metastases of 64–86% in patients with appendiceal NETs >2 cm in size [27, 38]. Distant metastases are more frequently encountered for tumors >2 cm in size (4.1%) [41].

Both ENETS guidelines and AJCC classification similarly characterize tumors which invade the peritoneal surface or adjacent organs (T4), invade regional ileocolic lymph nodes (N1), and metastases to distant sites (M1) [7, 39]. Appendiceal NETs with these characteristics are recommended to undergo evaluation for systemic treatments and long-term surveillance given their worse prognosis [7, 10, 11, 18, 39].

Surgical Management

Perioperative Considerations

Carcinoid syndrome is a clinical syndrome resulting from the release of serotonin and other peptide hormones such as histamine, bradykinins, and prostaglandins in patients with metastatic NET [42–44]. For patients with appendiceal NETs, carcinoid syndrome is a rare occurrence in approximately 2% of patients. In these very rare cases of functioning appendiceal NETs symptom control should be achieved prior to surgery with octreotide analogues in order to minimize the risk of carcinoid crisis which can occur during period of stress such as operative resection [43–45].

Locoregional Disease

While surgical management may need to be individualized for each patient, there are general guidelines for the treatment of appendiceal NETs based on tumor size and high risk pathological features. Most patients may be cured with appendectomy alone, but oncologic resection which includes a right-sided hemicolectomy and mesenteric lymphadenectomy is recommended in certain situations. More often, oncologic resection is performed at a second operation following pathologic review of the tumor specimen.

Appendectomy Alone

Appendiceal NETs are often diagnosed incidentally after appendectomy for presumed appendicitis or for other indications. Appendiceal NETs <1 cm in size are treated with curative appendectomy in which the tumor is completely resected along with the appendix. Oncologic resection is recommended for tumors <1 cm in size in the event of an incomplete tumor resection or tumor location at the base of the appendix [7, 10, 18]. ENETS guidelines highlight concerning features that place individuals with small appendiceal NETs at higher risk of lymph node metastases (Table 12.2) [7].

Table 12.2 Surgical management of appendiceal NETs

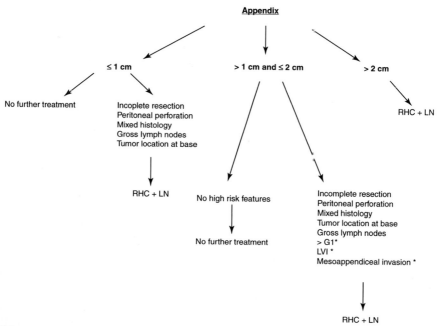

Abbreviations: RHC right hemicolectomy; *LN* lymph nodes; *G1* Grade 1; *LVI* lymphovascular invasion

*High risk feature, ≥ 1 consideration of right hemicolectomy and lymphadenectomy

*Mesoappendiceal invasion ≥3 mm only, ENETS; depth not specified, NANETS

For appendiceal NETs between 1 and 2 cm in size, the recommendations for surgery are less clear. Reports of the presence of lymph node involvement and risk of recurrence are conflicting. While some studies have reported lymph node involvement in 18–56.8% of appendiceal NETs between 1 and 2 cm in size, studies have also shown there may not be a survival difference compared to appendiceal NETs <1 cm in size [21, 27, 37, 38, 46]. The oncologic value of resection should be weighed against the morbidity of further surgical intervention.

Completion Right Hemicolectomy and Mesenteric Lymphadenectomy

According to NANETS guidelines, an oncologic resection is recommended for appendiceal NETs between 1 and 2 cm in size or in the presence of high risk features [10]. National Comprehensive Cancer Network (NCCN) guidelines also advocate for oncologic resection for appendiceal NETs <2 cm in the presence of high risk features such as lymphatic or vascular invasion or tumor invasion of the mesoappendix [18]. ENETS guidelines highlight concerning features that place individuals with small appendiceal NETs at higher risk of lymph node metastases. These features include grade 2 histology, vascular or lymphatic invasion, and invasion of the mesoappendix >3 mm. When ≥1 of these features exist, an oncologic resection should be considered [7, 28].

Guidelines recommend that low-grade appendiceal NETs >2 cm in size be treated by oncologic resection because of a higher risk of lymphatic metastases, recurrence, and distant metastases [7, 10, 18]. During oncologic resection, an ideal cut-point of 12 lymph nodes during lymphadenectomy has been identified. Patients who underwent resection of ≤12 lymph nodes had significantly worse overall survival than the patients with >12 lymph nodes resected (five-year survival, 88% vs. 96%) [27]. The morbidity and 30-day mortality after hemicolectomy remain low at were 2% and 0%, respectively [9].

Surgical Management of Hepatic Metastases

Perioperative Considerations

While majority of appendiceal NETs have an indolent course, cases of liver metastases can occur, though typically in <10% of patients [7, 10, 38, 47–49]. Liver failure secondary to tumor replacement is the leading cause of death among patients with neuroendocrine hepatic metastases; therefore, strategies to manage hepatic metastases are paramount to improving survival [10, 50–51]. Diagnostic evaluation of suspected hepatic metastases should begin with a fine needle or core needle pathologic specimen or a ^{68}-Ga-DOTATATE (dodecanetetraacetic acid tyrosine-3-octreotate) PET/CT (positron emisson tomography) if a biopsy is to be avoided. Histopathologic characteristics such as tumor differentiation and grade, including, mitotic rate and Ki-67 proliferative index, are often helpful to assist in the timing and selection of treatment modality in addition to providing prognostic information and can only be obtained preoperatively with a biopsy [11]. While many treatment modalities are available, surgery remains the only potentially curative option. Surgical candidates are recommended to undergo cross-sectional imaging with CT or MRI to evaluate for resectability [7]. Functional imaging such as ^{68}-Gallium-DOTATATE positron emission tomography PET/CT (^{68}Ga-PET/CT) is also recommended in the staging workup of metastatic NETs and may change management, including surgical planning, in a majority of patients [52]. Patients with elevated serotonin or 5-HIAA levels are recommended to undergo screening for carcinoid heart disease with echocardiography to evaluate for tricuspid and pulmonic valve abnormalities [11, 45].

Hepatic Debulking

Surgical management includes anatomical resections, hepatic debulking, and a variety of ablative techniques. Complete curative resection is recommended when possible, but this is often not the case, as neuroendocrine hepatic metastases may present with multiple and bilobar tumors [53]. Hepatic debulking has emerged as an important treatment option for surgical candidates as it offers survival benefit and symptom palliation. Neuroendocrine metastases seldom invade or envelop critical structures such as the biliary ducts or hepatic vasculature; therefore, surgical debulking with parenchyma-sparing techniques, such as enucleations and wedge resections are feasible [54]. Historically, hepatic resection was only recommended when resection ≥90% of liver tumor burden was possible; however, in the past decade multiple studies demonstrated that this criterion may be too restrictive [51, 54–59]. Lower debulking thresholds may allow for similar symptom improvement, functional quality of life, and survival benefit [45, 48, 51, 53, 60]. Intraoperative ultrasound is highly recommended to identify additional metastases and character-ize tumors in proximity to critical structures. Ultrasound also allows for ablative procedures to be performed concurrently [54]. Ablative techniques including radio-frequency ablation and microwave ablation of hepatic metastases have been per-formed concurrently with hepatic resection, hepatic debulking, and primary tumor resections [10]. Open and laparoscopic approaches to surgical management are pos-sible; however, selection depends on anatomical considerations, ability to perform a thorough exploration, and surgeon preference or expertise.

Guidelines currently recommend complete resection with curative intent when possible and hepatic debulking operations in select patients even if curative resec-tion cannot be achieved [45, 53]. Given the high rate of recurrence rates that also occur with curative resection, hepatic debulking has emerged as a treatment option as it still offers similar benefits. By allowing both a lower threshold for debulking operations and including patients with extrahepatic disease, more patients are eli-gible for surgical treatment while benefiting from increased survival and symptom palliation [17]. Hepatic resection and debulking operations have low morbidity and mortality rates ranging 13–24% and 0–2.7%, respectively [57, 58, 61].

Follow-up and Surveillance

The follow-up recommendations vary according to the patient's risk for tumor recurrence and the development of distant metastases. No follow-up or surveillance strategy is necessary for low-grade well-differentiated appendiceal NETs ≤1 cm in size which were completely resected with appendectomy [10, 18, 28]. Individuals with appendiceal NET who underwent oncologic resection for >1 cm size without high risk features do not require surveillance. Individuals with tumors >2 cm in size or between 1 and 2 cm in size with high risk features should be evaluated for resid-ual, locoregional, and metastatic disease [7, 11, 18, 19]. There are no prospective validated studies on type of imaging or frequency of surveillance of appendiceal NETs. Guidelines generally suggest surveillance with CT or MRI at intervals of 6 and 12 months after complete resection and annually for 5–10 years. Individuals with tumors of any size with lymph node involvement or distant metastatic disease require long-term surveillance [28].

For patients who underwent resection of hepatic metastases, increased frequency in surveillance is recommended at 3–6 months for the first 1–2 years and every 6–12 months for life [7, 11, 18, 19]. The selection of imaging modality may vary by institutional availability or physician preference, but generally multiphasic CT or MRI and recommended for evaluating local tumor recurrence or vascular invasion. The sensitivities of MRI and CT scan to identify neuroendocrine hepatic metastases are 95% and 78% respectively [62]. Consideration should be given for performing surveillance with MRI given the risk of repetitive exposure to irradiation from CT scanning [63]. Gadoxetic acid-enhanced MRI (EOVIST) has excellent capability of detecting hepatic metastases [62, 64, 65]. Some studies have reported the superiority of gadoxetic acid-enhanced MRI (EOVIST), a hepatocyte specific contrast, compared to other imaging modalities including CT scan with respect to tumor characterization [62, 65]. Functional imaging modalities, including somatostatin receptor imaging such as octreotide scan or ^{68}Ga-PET/CT, take advantage of somatostatin receptor expression on well-differentiated NETs. ^{68}Ga-PET/CT has largely replaced the octreotide scan because of its higher sensitivity, improved image quality, and lower radiation exposure [19, 66]. Studies report ^{68}Ga-PET/CT is able to detect NETs with a reported sensitivity of 88–99% compared to 60–80% for octreotide scan [19, 66–69].

For patients who are undergoing routine surveillance, the visit should include a complete history and physical examination of the patient. Biochemical markers, such as chromogranin A level may be obtained at intervals particularly if levels were elevated pre-operatively. Patients who exhibited symptoms of carcinoid syndrome or who had elevated levels of 5-HIAA pre-operatively may be surveilled after surgery, as well.

Prognosis

Most patients with appendiceal NETs are diagnosed at lower stages and have excellent prognosis. Patients with localized or regional disease have an estimated five-year survival of 95–100% and 78–100%, respectively [4, 38]. Tumor size is considered the major predictor of prognosis, as cases <1 cm almost invariably have favorable outcome, whereas those with a diameter exceeding 2 cm are associated with a five-year survival of 70% [6, 46]. High risk factors have been identified to help further stratify patients most at risk of recurrence or distant metastases. These factors include tumor location at the base of the appendix, tumor invasion of the mesoappendix, and lymph node or vascular invasion [7, 11, 38]. Increase in tumor stage correlates with a statistically worse prognosis, particularly for patients with hepatic metastases; however, optimal strategies to manage the liver remain an intense area of investigation [69].

References

1. Klöppel G, Perren A, Heitz PU. The gastroenteropancreatic neuroendocrine cell system and its tumors: the WHO classification. Ann N Y Acad Sci. 2004;1014(1):13–27.
2. Oronsky B, Ma PC, Morgensztern D, Carter CA. Nothing but NET: a review of neuroendocrine tumors and carcinomas. Neoplasia. 2017;19(12):991–1002.
3. Oberndorfer S. Karzinoide tumoren des dünndarms. Frankf Z Pathol. 1907;1:426–32.
4. Yao JC, Hassan M, Phan A, Dagohoy C, Leary C, Mares JE, Abdalla EK, Fleming JB, Vauthey JN, Rashid A, Evans DB. One hundred years after "carcinoid": epidemiology of and prog-

nostic factors for neuroendocrine tumors in 35,825 cases in the United States. J Clin Oncol. 2008;26(18):3063–72.

5. Amr B, Froghi F, Edmond M, Haq K, Kochupapy RT. Management and outcomes of appendicular neuroendocrine tumours: retrospective review with 5-year follow-up. Eur J Surg Oncol (EJSO). 2015;41(9):1243–6.

6. Ellis L, Shale MJ, Coleman MP. Carcinoid tumors of the gastrointestinal tract: trends in incidence in England since 1971. Am J Gastroenterol. 2010;105(12):2563–9.

7. Pape UF, Niederle B, Costa F, Gross D, Kelestimur F, Kianmanesh R, Knigge U, Öberg K, Pavel M, Perren A, Toumpanakis C. ENETS consensus guidelines for neuroendocrine neoplasms of the appendix (excluding goblet cell carcinomas). Neuroendocrinology. 2016;103(2):144–52.

8. Modlin IM, Lye KD, Kidd M. A 5-decade analysis of 13,715 carcinoid tumors. Cancer: Interdiscip Inter J American Cancer Soc. 2003;97(4):934–59.

9. Pawa N, Clift AK, Osmani H, Drymousis P, Cichocki A, Flora R, Goldin R, Patsouras D, Baird A, Malczewsk A, Kinross J. Surgical management of patients with neuroendocrine neoplasms of the appendix: appendectomy or more. Neuroendocrinology. 2018;106(3):242–51.

10. Boudreaux JP, Klimstra DS, Hassan MM, Woltering EA, Jensen RT, Goldsmith SJ, Nutting C, Bushnell DL, Caplin ME, Yao JC. The NANETS consensus guideline for the diagnosis and management of neuroendocrine tumors: well-differentiated neuroendocrine tumors of the jejunum, ileum, appendix, and cecum. Pancreas. 2010;39(6):753–66.

11. Strosberg JR, Halfdanarson TR, Bellizzi AM, Chan JA, Dillon J, Heaney AP, Kunz PL, O'Dorisio TM, Salem R, Segelov E, Howe J. The North American Neuroendocrine Society (NANETS) consensus guidelines for surveillance and medical management of midgut neuroendocrine tumors. Pancreas. 2017;46(6):707.

12. Halperin DM, Shen C, Dasari A, Xu Y, Chu Y, Zhou S, Shih YCT, Yao JC. Frequency of carcinoid syndrome at neuroendocrine tumour diagnosis: a population-based study. Lancet Oncol. 2017;18(4):525–34.

13. Taupenot L, Harper KL, O'Connor DT. The chromogranin–secretogranin family. N Engl J Med. 2003;348(12):1134–49.

14. Yang X, Yang Y, Li Z, Cheng C, Yang T, Wang C, Liu L, Liu S. Diagnostic value of circulating chromogranin A for neuroendocrine tumors: a systematic review and meta-analysis. PLoS One. 2015;10(4):e0124884.

15. Yao JC, Hainsworth JD, Wolin EM, Pavel ME, Baudin E, Gross D, Ruszniewski P, Tomassetti P, Panneerselvam A, Saletan S, Klimovsky J. Multivariate analysis including biomarkers in the phase III RADIANT-2 study of octreotide LAR plus everolimus (E+ O) or placebo (P+ O) among patients with advanced neuroendocrine tumors (NET). J Clin Oncol. 2012;30:157.

16. Nobels FR, Kwekkeboom DJ, Coopmans W, Schoenmakers CH, Lindemans J, De Herder WW, Krenning EP, Bouillon R, Lamberts SW. Chromogranin A as serum marker for neuroendocrine neoplasia: comparison with neuron-specific enolase and the α-subunit of glycoprotein hormones. J Clin Endocrinol Metab. 1997;82(8):2622–8.

17. O'Toole D, Grossman A, Gross D, Delle Fave G, Barkmanova J, O'Connor J, Pape UF, Plöckinger U. ENETS consensus guidelines for the standards of care in neuroendocrine tumors: biochemical markers. Neuroendocrinology. 2009;90(2):194–202.

18. National Comprehensive Cancer Network. NCCN clinical practice guidelines in oncology: neuroendocrine tumors. Ver. 1.2019. Fort Washington: NCCN; 2017.

19. Sundin A, Arnold R, Baudin E, Cwikla JB, Eriksson B, Fanti S, Fazio N, Giammarile F, Hicks RJ, Kjaer A, Krenning E. ENETS consensus guidelines for the standards of care in neuroendocrine tumors: radiological, nuclear medicine and hybrid imaging. Neuroendocrinology. 2017;105(3):212–44.

20. Assarzadegan N, Montgomery E. What is new in 2019 World Health Organization (WHO) classification of tumors of the digestive system: review of selected updates on neuroendocrine neoplasms, appendiceal tumors, and molecular testing. Arch Pathol Lab Med. 2020;

21. Rault-Petit B, Do Cao C, Guyétant S, Guimbaud R, Rohmer V, Julié C, Baudin E, Goichot B, Coriat R, Tabarin A, Ramos J. Current management and predictive factors of lymph node

metasasis of appendix neuroendocrine tumors: a national study from the french group of endocrine tumors (GTE). Ann Surg. 2019;270(1):165–71.

22. Debnath D, Rees J, Myint F. Are we missing diagnostic opportunities in cases of carcinoid tumours of the appendix? Surgeon. 2008;6(5):266–72.

23. Safioleas MC, Moulakakis KG, Kontzoglou K, Stamoulis J, Nikou GC, Toubanakis C, Lygidakis NJ. Carcinoid tumors of the appendix. Prognostic factors and evaluation of indications for right hemicolectomy. Hepato-Gastroenterology. 2005;52(61):123–7.

24. Lloyd RV, Osamura RY, Klöppel G, et al., editors. WHO classification of tumours of endocrine organs, vol. 10. 4th ed. Lyon: International Agency for Research on Cancer; 2017.

25. Nagtegaal ID, Odze RD, Klimstra D, Paradis V, Rugge M, Schirmacher P, Washington KM, Carneiro F, Cree IA, WHO Classification of Tumours Editorial Board. The 2019 WHO classification of tumours of the digestive system. Histopathology. 2020;76(2):182–8.

26. Rindi G, Klimstra DS, Abedi-Ardekani B, Asa SL, Bosman FT, Brambilla E, Busam KJ, de Krijger RR, Dietel M, El-Naggar AK, Fernandez-Cuesta L. A common classification framework for neuroendocrine neoplasms: an International Agency for Research on Cancer (IARC) and World Health Organization (WHO) expert consensus proposal. Mod Pathol. 2018;31(12):1770–86.

27. Raoof M, Dumitra S, O'Leary MP, Singh G, Fong Y, Lee B. Mesenteric lymphadenectomy in well-differentiated appendiceal neuroendocrine tumors. Dis Colon Rectum. 2017;60(7):674–81.

28. Pape UF, Perren A, Niederle B, Gross D, Gress T, Costa F, Arnold R, Denecke T, Plöckinger U, Salazar R, Grossman A. ENETS consensus guidelines for the management of patients with neuroendocrine neoplasms from the jejuno-ileum and the appendix including goblet cell carcinomas. Neuroendocrinology. 2012;95(2):135–56.

29. Grozinsky-Glasberg S, Alexandraki KI, Barak D, Doviner V, Reissman P, Kaltsas GA, Gross DJ. Current size criteria for the management of neuroendocrine tumors of the appendix: are they valid? Clinical experience and review of the literature. Neuroendocrinology. 2013;98(1):31–7.

30. Rossi G, Valli R, Bertolini F, Sighinolfi P, Losi L, Cavazza A, Rivasi F, Luppi G. Does mesoappendix infiltration predict a worse prognosis in incidental neuroendocrine tumors of the appendix? A clinicopathologic and immunohistochemical study of 15 cases. Am J Clin Pathol. 2003;120(5):706–11.

31. Syracuse DC, Perzin KH, Price JB, Wiedel PD, Mesa-Tejada R. Carcinoid tumors of the appendix. Mesoappendiceal extension and nodal metastases. Ann Surg. 1979;190:58–63.

32. Moertel CG, Weiland LH, Nagorney DM, Dockerty MB. Carcinoid tumor of the appendix: treatment and prognosis. N Engl J Med. 1987;317(27):1699–701.

33. Daskalakis K, Alexandraki K, Kassi E, Tsoli M, Angelousi A, Ragkousi A, Kaltsas G. The risk of lymph node metastases and their impact on survival in patients with appendiceal neuroendocrine neoplasms: a systematic review and meta-analysis of adult and paediatric patients. Endocrine. 2019;67:20–34.

34. Galanopoulos M, McFadyen R, Drami I, Naik R, Evans N, Luong TV, Watkins J, Caplin M, Toumpanakis C. Challenging the current risk factors of appendiceal neuroendocrine neoplasms: can they accurately predict local lymph nodal invasion? Results from a large case series. Neuroendocrinology. 2019;109(2):179–86.

35. Blakely AM, Raoof M, Ituarte PH, Fong Y, Singh G, Lee B. Lymphovascular invasion is associated with lymph node involvement in small appendiceal neuroendocrine tumors. Ann Surg Oncol. 2019;26(12):4008–15.

36. Brighi N, La Rosa S, Rossi G, Grillo F, Pusceddu S, Rinzivillo M, Spada F, Tafuto S, Massironi S, Faggiano A, Antonuzzo L. Morphological factors related to nodal metastases in neuroendocrine tumors of the appendix: a multicentric retrospective study. Ann Surg. 2020;271(3):527–33.

37. Sarshekeh AM, Advani S, Halperin DM, Conrad C, Shen C, Yao JC, Dasari A. Regional lymph node involvement and outcomes in appendiceal neuroendocrine tumors: a SEER database analysis. Oncotarget. 2017;8(59):99541.

38. Mullen JT, Savarese DM. Carcinoid tumors of the appendix: a population-based study. J Surg Oncol. 2011;104(1):41–4.
39. Edge SB, Edge SB. AJCC Cancer staging manual. 8th ed. New York: Springer; 2017.
40. Goede AC, Caplin ME, Winslet MC. Carcinoid tumour of the appendix. Br J Surg. 2003;90(11):1317–22.
41. Hsu C, Rashid A, Xing Y, Chiang YJ, Chagpar RB, Fournier KF, Chang GJ, You YN, Feig BW, Cormier JN. Varying malignant potential of appendiceal neuroendocrine tumors: importance of histologic subtype. J Surg Oncol. 2013;107(2):136–43.
42. Fanciulli G, Ruggeri RM, Grossrubatscher E, Calzo FL, Wood TD, Faggiano A, Isidori A, Colao A. Serotonin pathway in carcinoid syndrome: clinical, diagnostic, prognostic and therapeutic implications. Rev Endocr Metab Disord. 2020;21:1–14.
43. Clement D, Ramage J, Srirajaskanthan R. Update on pathophysiology, treatment, and complications of carcinoid syndrome. J Oncol. 2020;2020:1–11.
44. Loughrey PB, Zhang D, Heaney AP. New treatments for the carcinoid syndrome. Endocrinol Metab Clin. 2018;47(3):557–76.
45. Howe JR, Cardona K, Fraker DL, Kebebew E, Untch BR, Wang YZ, Law CH, Liu EH, Kim MK, Menda Y, Morse BG. The surgical management of small bowel neuroendocrine tumors: consensus guidelines of the North American Neuroendocrine Tumor Society (NANETS). Pancreas. 2017;46(6):715.
46. Landry CS, Woodall C, Scoggins CR, McMasters KM, Martin RC. Analysis of 900 appendiceal carcinoid tumors for a proposed predictive staging system. Arch Surg. 2008;143(7):664–70.
47. Hallet J, Law CHL, Cukier M, Saskin R, Liu N, Singh S. Exploring the rising incidence of neuroendocrine tumors: a population-based analysis of epidemiology, metastatic presentation, and outcomes. Cancer. 2015;121(4):589–97.
48. Chambers AJ, Pasieka JL, Dixon E, Rorstad O. The palliative benefit of aggressive surgical intervention for both hepatic and mesenteric metastases from neuroendocrine tumors. Surgery. 2008;144(4):645–53.
49. Cai B, Broder MS, Chang E, Yan T, Metz DC. Predictive factors associated with carcinoid syndrome in patients with gastrointestinal neuroendocrine tumors. World J Gastroenterol. 2017 Oct 28;23(40):7283.
50. Givi B, Pommier SJ, Thompson AK, Diggs BS, Pommier RF. Operative resection of primary carcinoid neoplasms in patients with liver metastases yields significantly better survival. Surgery. 2006;140(6):891–8.
51. Graff-Baker AN, Sauer DA, Pommier SJ, Pommier RF. Expanded criteria for carcinoid liver debulking: maintaining survival and increasing the number of eligible patients. Surgery. 2014;156(6):1369–77.
52. Tierney JF, Kosche C, Schadde E, Ali A, Virmani S, Pappas SG, Poirier J, Keutgen XM. 68Gallium-DOTATATE positron emission tomography–computed tomography (PET CT) changes management in a majority of patients with neuroendocrine tumors. Surgery. 2019;165(1):178–85.
53. Pavel M, Costa F, Capdevila J, Gross D, Kianmanesh R, Krenning E, Knigge U, Salazar R, Pape UF, Öberg K. ENETS consensus guidelines update for the management of distant metastatic disease of intestinal, pancreatic, bronchial neuroendocrine neoplasms (NEN) and NEN of unknown primary site. Neuroendocrinology. 2016;103(2):172–85.
54. Wright BE, Lee CC, Bilchik AJ. Hepatic cytoreductive surgery for neuroendocrine cancer. Surg Oncol Clin N Am. 2007;16(3):627–37.
55. Anthony LB, Strosberg JR, Klimstra DS, Maples WJ, O'Dorisio TM, Warner RR, Wiseman GA, Benson AB III, Pommier RF. The NANETS consensus guidelines for the diagnosis and management of gastrointestinal neuroendocrine tumors (nets): well-differentiated nets of the distal colon and rectum. Pancreas. 2010;39(6):767–74.
56. Mayo SC, De Jong MC, Pulitano C, Clary BM, Reddy SK, Gamblin TC, Celinksi SA, Kooby DA, Staley CA, Stokes JB, Chu CK. Surgical management of hepatic neuroendocrine tumor metastasis: results from an international multi-institutional analysis. Ann Surg Oncol. 2010;17(12):3129–36.

57. Que FG, Nagorney DM, Batts KP, Linz LJ, Kvols LK. Hepatic resection for metastatic neuroendocrine carcinomas. Am J Surg. 1995;169(1):36–43.
58. Sarmiento JM, Heywood G, Rubin J, Ilstrup DM, Nagorney DM, Que FG. Surgical treatment of neuroendocrine metastases to the liver: a plea for resection to increase survival. J Am Coll Surg. 2003;197(1):29–37.
59. Knox CD, Feurer ID, Wise PE, Lamps LW, Wright JK, Chari RS, Gorden DL, Pinson CW. Survival and functional quality of life after resection for hepatic carcinoid metastasis. J Gastrointest Surg. 2004;8(6):653–9.
60. Scott AT, Breheny PJ, Keck KJ, Bellizzi AM, Dillon JS, O'Dorisio TM, Howe JR. Effective cytoreduction can be achieved in patients with numerous neuroendocrine tumor liver metastases (NETLMs). Surgery. 2019;165(1):166–75.
61. Maxwell JE, Sherman SK, O'Dorisio TM, Bellizzi AM, Howe JR. Liver-directed surgery of neuroendocrine metastases: what is the optimal strategy? Surgery. 2016;159(1):320–35.
62. Dromain C, de Baere T, Lumbroso J, Caillet H, Laplanche A, Boige V, Ducreux M, Duvillard P, Elias D, Schlumberger M, Sigal R. Detection of liver metastases from endocrine tumors: a prospective comparison of somatostatin receptor scintigraphy, computed tomography, and magnetic resonance imaging. J Clin Oncol. 2004;23(1):70–8.
63. Maxwell JE, Howe JR. Imaging in neuroendocrine tumors: an update for the clinician. Int J Endocr Oncol. 2015;2(2):159–68.
64. Morin C, Drolet S, Cousineau J, Daigle C, Deshaies I, Ouellet JF, Ball CG, Dixon E, Marceau J, Ouellet JFB. Additional value of gadoxetic acid-enhanced MRI to gadolinium-enhanced MRI for the surgical management of colorectal and neuroendocrine liver metastases. HPB. 2017;19:S69.
65. Giesel FL, Kratochwil C, Mehndiratta A, Wulfert S, Moltz JH, Zechmann CM, Kauczor HU, Haberkorn U, Ley S. Comparison of neuroendocrine tumor detection and characterization using DOTATOC-PET in correlation with contrast enhanced CT and delayed contrast enhanced MRI. Eur J Radiol. 2012;81(10):2820–5.
66. Deppen SA, Blume J, Bobbey AJ, Shah C, Graham MM, Lee P, Delbeke D, Walker RC. 68Ga-DOTATATE compared with 111In-DTPA-octreotide and conventional imaging for pulmonary and gastroenteropancreatic neuroendocrine tumors: a systematic review and meta-analysis. J Nucl Med. 2016;57(6):872–8.
67. Deppen SA, Liu E, Blume JD, Clanton J, Shi C, Jones-Jackson LB, Lakhani V, Baum RP, Berlin J, Smith GT, Graham M. Safety and efficacy of 68Ga-DOTATATE PET/CT for diagnosis, staging, and treatment management of neuroendocrine tumors. J Nucl Med. 2016;57(5):708–14.
68. Skoura E, Michopoulou S, Mohmaduvesh M, Panagiotidis E, Al Harbi M, Toumpanakis C, Almukhailed O, Kayani I, Syed R, Navalkissoor S, Ell PJ. The impact of 68Ga-DOTATATE PET/CT imaging on management of patients with neuroendocrine tumors: experience from a national referral center in the United Kingdom. J Nucl Med. 2016;57(1):34–40.
69. Quaedvlieg PF, Visser O, Lamers CB, Janssen-Heijen MLG, Taal BG. Epidemiology and survival in patients with carcinoid disease in the Netherlands: an epidemiological study with 2391 patients. Ann Oncol. 2001;12(9):1295–300.

Part III

Other Primary NETs

Primary Neuroendocrine Tumors of the Lung

13

Pier Luigi Filosso, Elisa Carla Fontana,
and Matteo Roffinella

Abbreviations

AC:	Atypical carcinoid
ACTH:	Adrenocorticotropic hormone
ADH:	Antidiuretic hormone
BC:	Bronchial carcinoid
CS:	Cushing's syndrome
CT:	Chemotherapy
DIPNECH:	Diffuse idiopathic pulmonary neuroendocrine cell hyperplasia
EBUS:	Endobronchial ultrasound biopsy
G:	Tumor grading
GEP:	Gastroenteropancreatic
GH:	Growth hormone
IASLC:	International Association for the Study of Lung Cancer
LCNC:	Large-cell neuroendocrine carcinoma
MEN 1:	Multiple endocrine neoplasia type 1
NET:	Neuroendocrine tumor
NSCLC:	Non-small-cell lung cancer
OS:	Overall survival
PET:	Positron emission tomography
PTH:	Parathyroid hormone
SCLC:	Small-cell lung carcinoma
SUV:	Standardized uptake value

P. L. Filosso (✉) · E. C. Fontana · M. Roffinella
University of Torino, Department of Surgical Sciences, Unit of General Thoracic Surgery,
Torino, Italy
e-mail: pierluigi.filosso@unito.it

© Springer Nature Switzerland AG 2021
J. M. Cloyd, T. M. Pawlik (eds.), *Neuroendocrine Tumors*,
https://doi.org/10.1007/978-3-030-62241-1_13

TC: Typical carcinoid
UICC/AJCC: Union Internationale Contre le Cancer/American Joint Committee
                   on Cancer
WHO: World Health Organization

Introduction: Neuroendocrine Tumors of the Lung – Definition and Classification

Lung neuroendocrine tumors (NETs) are a group of primary lung cancers with shared neuroendocrine differentiation though with distinct molecular, morphological, and immunohistochemical features and biological behavior. They account for approximately 20–30% of NETs and 1–2% of all primary lung cancers in adults.

The recent (2015) World Health Organization (WHO) classification system groups those neoplasms into four major histological subtypes, ranging from low-grade typical carcinoid (TC), intermediate-grade atypical carcinoid (AC) to high-grade poorly differentiated large-cell neuroendocrine carcinoma (LCNC) and small-cell lung carcinoma (SCLC), according to the absence/presence of necrosis and the number of mitoses [1]. NET classification is shown in Table 13.1.

Diffuse idiopathic pulmonary neuroendocrine cell hyperplasia (DIPNECH) is regarded as a preneoplastic lesion. It consists in a generalized proliferation of pulmonary neuroendocrine cells, usually observed as the final evolution of chronic obstructive complaints. A minority of patients with DIPNECH may develop TC and very rarely AC [2–4].

The Ki67 proliferative index (the product of *MKI67* gene mapping to *10q26.2* gene involved in the cell proliferation) has emerged as a new promising prognostic marker in pulmonary NETs [5–6] and also to evaluate their grading (G).

With the aim to standardize lung and gastroenteropancreatic (GEP) NET classification, a recent consensus conference suggested to similarly classify neuroendocrine neoplasms at all anatomical locations. Well-differentiated neoplasms, which include lung TCs and ACs, are defined neuroendocrine tumors (NETs), while poorly differentiated neuroendocrine neoplasms are defined neuroendocrine carcinomas (NECs) [7]. TC corresponds to NET G1 and AC to NET G2. However, this approach is not currently officially integrated in the WHO classification of lung neuroendocrine neoplasms, and more data are needed to confirm Ki67 utility in lung NETs, as

Table 13.1 Lung NET histological classification

	Mitotic count (per 2 mm²)	Necrosis	Ki67 (%)	Cell size
Typical carcinoid (TC)	<2	No	<5	
Atypical carcinoid (AC)	2–10	Focal	<20	
Large-cell neuroendocrine carcinoma (LCNC)	>10	Extensive	40–80	Large
Small-cell neuroendocrine carcinoma (SCLC)	>10	Extensive	50–100	<3 lymphocytes

opposed to GEP NETs, where it is an integral part of the actual grading system. Preliminary reports suggest an overlapping in the Ki67 index between TCs and ACs but also its potential role to improve prognostication [6, 8].

Lung NETs are currently staged according to the 2017 revision of the Union Internationale Contre le Cancer/American Joint Committee on Cancer (UICC/ AJCC) TNM classification [9]. However, the possible role of some tumor descriptors should be refined: nodal status has been extensively studied, but T denominator, pleural invasion, and multicentricity must be better outlined.

The aim of the remainder of this chapter is to focus on diagnosis and surgical management of those neuroendocrine tumors more commonly observed in the General Thoracic Surgery common clinical practice.

Bronchial Carcinoid (BC) Tumors

Epidemiology

BCs are rare primary malignant tumors of the lung, with an age-adjusted incidence which ranges from 0.2 to 2/100,000 person/year in Europe and the United States [10–11]. An increased prevalence in the past 30 years was observed, probably due to the improved awareness [12] and the augmented use of special immunohistochemistry stains [10, 13]. An increased prevalence was also observed as a consequence of lung cancer screening programs worldwide, with a greater prevalence of TC over AC.

BCs' highest incidence is around the sixth decade of age, with a younger mean time (45 years) for TCs and an older one (55 years) for ACs [14–15]. Moreover, BCs are the most common primary lung neoplasm in childhood, with TCs more prevalent [16–17]. The chance to have an AC is about 25% in patients older than 50 years and less than 10% in younger than 30 [18].

Smoking habits have been sometimes evaluated in BCs: the majority of patients (especially young ones) are never or very light smokers, albeit some AC patients are current or former smokers [19].

BCs are very often sporadic lesions; nevertheless rare cases of familiarity have been described [20]. In about 5% of multiple endocrine neoplasia type 1 (MEN 1) patients, a BC is observed, usually a TC and very rarely an AC [21–22].

Clinical Presentation and Diagnosis

In general, BC's location may vary between central and peripheral, according to its origin in respect to the bronchial tree. Using Detterbeck's classification, central ones are those visible at bronchoscopy [15] (Fig. 13.1).

Clinical symptoms are also influenced by the tumor's location. The most frequent respiratory symptoms in central forms are recurrent chest infections, cough, chest pain, hemoptysis, dyspnea and wheezing. Peripheral forms are usually

Fig. 13.1 Endobronchial centrally located typical carcinoid (TC) observed during bronchoscopy. The presence of tumor-rich vascular network puts the maneuver at high risk of bleeding

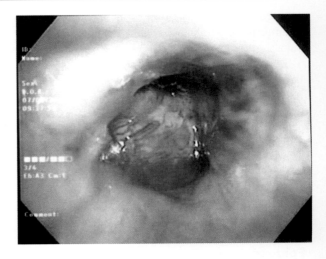

asymptomatic. Asthma that does not improve with medical therapy or prolonged pneumonia is sometimes observed in central forms, and often this precedes tumor diagnosis [23].

In about 40% of cases, BC is incidentally discovered by performing a chest X-ray for other reasons [24–25]. Unlike GEP NETs, functional BCs are relatively infrequent, accounting for no more than 10–15% of cases. The most common associated endocrine syndrome is the ectopic adrenocorticotropic hormone (ACTH) secretion (Cushing's syndrome, CS). In approximately 1% of all CS cases, ACTH ectopic secretion is caused by a BC [26]. Other less common paraneoplastic endocrine syndromes include growth hormone (GH), antidiuretic hormone (ADH), and parathyroid hormone (PTH) ectopic secretions.

For diagnostic purposes, contrast thoracic CT scan represents the gold standard. CT features of BC may be non-specific (Fig. 13.2a), and the tumor can be round or lobular with occasional spicular margins [25]. Approximately 1/3 of peripheral BCs are ACs. On CT scan, BC central form is frequently associated with indirect signs of bronchial obstruction (atelectasis, obstructive pneumonia, bronchiectasis, or sometimes lung abscess) (Fig. 13.2b). Central BCs are commonly TCs; lymph node enlargement (hilar and/or mediastinal) (Fig. 13.2c) is sometimes evident, but it is generally difficult to distinguish an adjacent lymph node from a central mass. Furthermore, atelectasis or obstructive pneumonia can cause a reactive (and not neoplastic) lymph node enlargement. Finally, for DIPNECH diagnosis, high-resolution CT scan with expiratory study is the gold standard and shows air trapping with/without multiple nodules (Fig. 13.2d).

Hilar and mediastinal lymph nodal involvement detected by thoracic CT scan has a false-positive rate of 20–40%, whereas the false-negative rate is only 6–8% [15–27].

[18]F positron emission tomography (PET) uptake in BCs is usually low, especially in TCs [28]. For this reason, a different SUV_{max} (standardized uptake value) cutoff

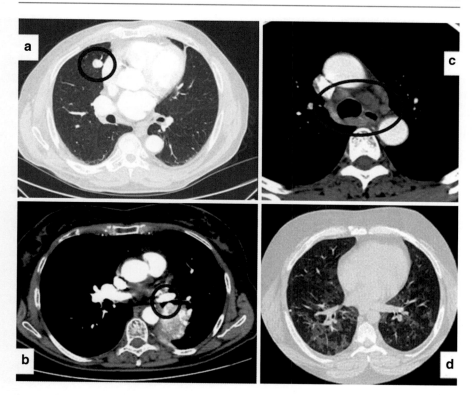

Fig. 13.2 (**a**) Peripheral bronchial carcinoid, as a right round solitary pulmonary nodule; (**b**) left central endobronchial carcinoid; direct signs of bronchial obstruction (atelectasis) are also evident; (**c**) mediastinal bilateral lymph nodal involvement (red circle); (**d**) high-resolution CT scan in diffuse idiopathic pulmonary neuroendocrine cell hyperplasia (DIPNECH): air trapping with some small nodules is evident

should be used for less ^{18}F-avid neoplasms. ACs usually present with a significantly higher ^{18}F uptake, as result of their more aggressive biological behavior and high proliferative rate [29–30]. ^{68}Ga-tetraazacyclododecane-tetraacetic acid (DOTA) somatostatin analog PET scan is more sensitive and preferable to somatostatin receptor scintigraphy (Octreoscan®) [31–33]. The problem is its low availability in many countries and institutions.

Bronchoscopy is indicated in BC's central forms [14, 34–35] and also for the possibility to perform a biopsy. Flexible bronchoscopy is always used; rigid bronchoscopy may be preferable in case of high risk of bleeding during biopsy for highly vascularized endobronchial lesions. Bronchoscopy is usually negative in peripheral forms of BCs, and biopsies may be obtained through transthoracic CT-guided method. However, an accurate differentiation between TC and AC is not always achievable through this technique [36]. If clinically needed, to rule out mediastinal lymph nodal metastasis, mediastinoscopy or endobronchial ultrasound biopsy (EBUS) is indicated.

Treatment

Currently, complete BC surgical resection represents the mainstay of treatment. The aim of surgery is to completely resect the lesion, preserving as much functional lung tissue as possible. Surgical approach generally depends on (1) tumor size and location and (2) tumor histology.

Despite BCs' moderate malignant behavior (compared to other primary lung cancers), resections should be anatomical in principle [37–39].

For *peripheral BCs*, the best surgical approach is an anatomic resection (segmentectomy/lobectomy); this procedure must be always accompanied by lymph node exeresis, according to the current IASLC guidelines [40], which recommend the sampling/resection of a minimum of six nodes/stations (three hilar, three mediastinal), always including the subcarinal one. Systematic lymphadenectomy is strongly recommended since lymph nodal metastases are not rare and may be observed in up to 25% of TCs and in more than 50% of ACs [41]. A wide wedge resection can be proposed for patients with poor and limited respiratory functional reserve though lymphadenectomy should still be performed in such cases. Finally, an increased probability to develop local recurrence is sometimes observed when an AC is treated with a wedge resection [39].

For *centrally located tumors* (very often TCs), the use of parenchymal-sparing resections (sleeve bronchial resection – no lung tissue is removed – or sleeve lobectomy) has recently become increasingly familiar among thoracic surgeons. These surgical procedures facilitate the avoidance of a pneumonectomy and therefore a greater sacrifice of lung parenchyma, but with consolidated results in terms of overall survival [42–44]. An intraoperative bronchial margin frozen section is needed, to rule out the presence of neoplastic cell on bronchial suture's edge. Furthermore, the need to avoid pneumonectomy is prioritized when we consider that central TC affects preferentially young people. When distant pneumonitis and/or destroyed lung parenchyma is present, an initial local endobronchial resection to disobliterate the airway may be performed before reassessment for lung parenchymal-sparing surgery [15].

Currently, the indications to perform a pneumonectomy in BC are very few, apart from vascular accidents or other intraoperative surgical complications: (1) central tumors with distant severe pneumonitis or destroyed lung, where endobronchial approach has not been able to reconvert for a parenchymal-sparing approach; (2) central or (3) very large tumors in whom bronchoplastic procedure is not deemed feasible; and (4) tumor recurrence after bronchial sleeve resection/lobectomy (completion pneumonectomy).

While surgical resection is traditionally the preferred approach for patients with BCs, in very selected cases, laser endobronchial treatment (EBT) has shown promising results [45–46].

With the intent to bring order to EBT indications, a systematic literature review was recently reported [47]. Results showed that (1) tumor histology, (2) the presence of lymph nodal involvement, (3) tumor location, and (4) tumor size were identified as negative prognostic factors for this technique. For patients with a more favorable prognosis, tumor location and its diameter may influence the optimal treatment strategy, in the sense that small central tumors with an exclusive intraluminal growth and without signs of lymph node involvement can benefit positively from a minimally invasive approach (EBT or pure bronchoplastic sleeve resection).

Table 13.2 shows BCs' clinical characteristics and overall survival in recent and large series. According to the literature, the most significant factors influencing

Table 13.2 Bronchial carcinoid tumors: clinical characteristics and survival in recent large clinical series

Authors	[a]Filosso	[b]Rea	[c]Cardillo	[d]Garcia Yuste (multicentric)	[e]Filosso	[f]Lee
Year	2002	2007	2004	2007	2013	2016
Sample size	126	252	163	661	126	142
Histology						
TC	82	174	121	569	83	108
AC	44	78	42	92	43	34
Location						
Central	103	195	98	439	57	93
Peripheral	23	57	65	222	69	49
Nodal mets						
N1	9 (7 AC)	19	32 (18 AC)	46 (32 TC)	14	10
N2	11 (7 AC)	10	9 (all AC)	39 (20 TC)	12	10
Surgical procedures						
Wedge	16	13	9	66 (+ segm)		20
Segmental	3	10	1		14 (+wedge)	10
Lobectomy	64	139 (+bilob)	112	374 (+bilob)	94	99
Bilobectomy	17		21		11	3
Pneumonectomy	15	14	12	63	3	2
Bronchoplastic	7	76	8	66	4	8
Survival						
5-y OS	97% TC 77% AC		98.6% TC 70% AC	97% TC 78% AC	91% TC 68% AC	92% TC 72% AC
10-y OS	93% TC 52% AC	93% TC 64% AC			86% TC 43% AC	85% TC 32% AC
15-y OS	84% TC 52% AC					
Recurrences						
TC	4/72	6/174			3/83	1/108
AC	8/44	14/78			5/43	6/34

References: [a]Filosso PL et al.: J Thorac Cardiovasc Surg. 2002;123:303–309
[b]Rea F et al.: Eur J Cardiothorac Surg. 2007;31:186–191
[c]Cardillo G et al.: Ann Thorac Surg. 2004;77:1781–1785
[d]Garcia-Yuste M et al.: Eur J Cardiothorac Surg. 2007;31:192–197
[e]Filosso PL et al.: J Thorac Oncol. 2013;8:1282–1288
[f]Lee PC et al.: Thorac Cardiovasc Surg. 2016;64:159–165

outcome are (1) tumor histology, (2) tumor stage, (3) the presence of lymph node involvement, and (4) the presence of local recurrence/distant metastases. Less significant factors are (1) the type of surgical resection (especially in early-stage tumors), (2) tumor size, and (3) the Ki67 proliferating index.

Diagnosis of synchronous bilateral multiple BCs is extremely rare, though probably underestimated, since a thorough systematic pathological examination of the resected lobe in a patient with BC shows neuroendocrine cell hyperplasia in three-quarters of cases [48]. This might indicate that genetic factors may be involved, but their exact role still remains unclear. Few articles describe this rare condition: in general, when bilateral BCs take the form of solitary pulmonary nodules, surgical resection is performed [49–50]. When two or more endobronchial lesions are detected, surgical approach seems questionable and depends on several factors: (1) patient's age and presence of other important comorbidities; (2) ability to perform lung-sparing procedure(s); and (3) feasibility to perform an oncologically radical intervention. Questions still remain about the type of surgical resections in synchronous bilateral multiple BCs: anatomical or wedge resections? This choice depends on (1) number and location of multiple/bilateral lesions; (2) their size; (3) tumor histology; (4) presence/absence of lymph node involvement; and (5) patient's respiratory/cardiac reserve and possible associated comorbidities. A radical resection of the lesion usually results in long survival, especially in case of TCs without lymph node metastases. As a case example, the authors had a young patient alive and disease-free 12 years after the resection of seven TCs (three on the left, four on the right lung), followed by adjuvant treatment with octreotide for 4 years.

Endobronchial palliative treatment plus chemotherapy and a close follow-up are offered for patients with multiple BCs, unfit for surgery [51].

Thoracic recurrent disease is an uncommon occurrence after surgical resection of BC: anecdotal cases diagnosed 10–30 years after surgery have been reported [51–55]. Very often, a new surgical resection may be offered so far as (1) it is deemed oncologically radical and (2) the respiratory/cardiac functional reserve of the patient allows it.

Large-Cell Neuroendocrine Carcinoma (LCNC) of the Lung

Epidemiology and Clinical Characteristics

Large-cell neuroendocrine carcinoma (LCNC) of the lung is a relatively rare and very aggressive subset of lung primary NETs, belonging to the group of poorly differentiated NECs (see above). LCNC was first described by Travis et al. in 1991, recognizing a separate category of lung NETs, distinct from TC, AC, and SCLC [56]. LCNC was described as a tumor composed of large cells, with neuroendocrine characteristics (detected by electron microscopy and immunohistochemistry), with a low nuclear-to-cytoplasmic ratio, frequent nucleoli, a very high mitotic rate, and abundant necrosis. In the last WHO tumor classification, LCNC is definitively included in the NETs group, after which, for a long time, it was regarded as a part of large-cell carcinoma group.

LCNC's incidence is low among resected primary lung cancers: it is reported ranging between 2.1% and 3.5% according to the different clinical series [57–59]. LCNC shows a significant prevalence in men [58, 60] and smokers [58, 61–62].

LCNC mostly presents as a peripheral tumor/mass, as opposed to central lesions, which are more typical in TC and SCLC; clinical symptoms are therefore infrequently present. Similar to SCLC, LCNC commonly occurs with lymph node metastases at time of diagnosis. Moreover, LCNC is significantly more ^{18}F-FDG-avid than low/intermediate-grade NETs, with a mean SUV_{max} of 13 [63], very similar to SCLC.

Despite presenting as a peripheral neoplasm, and therefore susceptible to transthoracic needle biopsy, a preoperative correct cytohistologic diagnosis is extremely difficult, and therefore LCNC is frequently diagnosed postoperatively.

Treatment and Survival

Surgical approach still represents the best option for LCNC treatment, especially in early stage. Adjuvant chemotherapy should be offered when lymph nodal involvement is demonstrated. Due to the high risk of distant metastasis, a correct preoperative clinical staging must be performed, with the use of thoracic, brain, and abdomen CT scan and ^{18}F-FDG PET scan. Surgical options closely follow those offered for non-small cell lung cancer (NSCLC): in general, an anatomical resection with systematic lymphadenectomy should be performed.

The reported 5-year overall survival (OS) in patients with resected LCNC may range between 13% and 57%. Table 13.3 reports clinical characteristics and outcome in the most recent LCNC clinical series. If compared to TC and AC, even stage I and II survival rates appear significantly low, confirming LCNC's extremely aggressive biological behavior. Tumor recurrences (both local and distant) are frequent and often appear very shortly even after a complete tumor surgical resection; percentages of 70% after 1 year and 85% after 3 years have been recently reported [57–58]. Brain, liver, and bone are the most common sites of LCNC distant metastases.

Surgical resection alone is therefore not enough, even in LCNC early stage: adjuvant chemotherapy should be offered, and it may improve survival [64–67]. Rossi and colleagues. [68] for the first time observed a significant improved outcome when LCNC was treated with adjuvant SCLC-based chemotherapy (*cisplatin/etoposide*), compared to those who received platin combined with other agents. Similar results were obtained by Iyoda et al. [69] who reported 89% 5-year survival rate in patients treated with SCLC-based chemotherapy, compared to 47% in those who did not. Finally, the role of induction chemotherapy has not yet been well demonstrated, despite some recent clinical experiences, based however on limited number of patients [62].

Table 13.3 Large-cell neuroendocrine carcinomas: clinical characteristics and survival in recent large clinical series

Authors						
	Takei[a]	Battafarano[b]	Asamura[c]	Veronesi[d] *(multicentric)*	Filosso[e] *(multicentric)*	Filosso[f] *(multicentric)*
Year	2002	2005	2006	2006	2014	2017
Numb of patients	87	20	141	144	135	400
Survival						
5-y OS (%)	57%	30.2%	40.3%	43%	28%	54%
Stage I	67%	67%	58%	52%		56%
Stage II	75%	24%	32%	59%		42%
Stage III	45%	7%		20%		24%
Recurrences						
Number	35 (40%)		68 (48%)	58 (40%)	26 (20%)	201 (50%)

References: [a]Takei H et al.: J Thorac Cardiovasc Surg. 2002;124:285–292
[b]Battafarano RJ et al.: J Thorac Cardiovasc Surg. 2005;130:166–172
[c]Asamura H et al.: J Clin Oncol. 2006;24:70–76
[d]Veronesi G et al.: Lung Cancer. 2006;53:111–115
[e]Filosso PL et al.: Eur J Cardiothorac Surg. 2015;48:55–64
[f]Filosso PL et al.: Eur J Cardiothorac Surg. 2017;52:339–345

References

1. Travis WD, Brambilla E, Burke AP, et al. WHO classification of tumours of the lung, pleura, thymus and heart. World Health Organization Classification Tumours. 4th ed. Lyon: IARC Press; 2015.
2. Rossi G, Cavazza A, Spagnolo P, Sverzellati N, Longo L, Jukna A, Montanari G, Carbonelli C, Vincenzi G, Bogina G, Franco R, Tiseo M, Cottin V, Colby TV. Diffuse idiopathic pulmonary neuroendocrine cell hyperplasia syndrome. Eur Respir J. 2016;47:1829–41.
3. Wirtschafter E, Walts AE, Liu ST, Marchevsky AM. Diffuse Idiopathic Pulmonary Neuroendocrine Cell Hyperplasia of the Lung (DIPNECH): current best evidence. Lung. 2015;193:659–67.
4. Myint ZW, McCormick J, Chauhan A, Behrens E, Anthony LB. Management of diffuse idiopathic pulmonary neuroendocrine cell hyperplasia: review and a single center experience. Lung. 2018 Oct;196(5):577–81.
5. Rindi G, Klersy C, Inzani F, Fellegara G, Ampollini L, Ardizzoni A, Campanini N, Carbognani P, De Pas TM, Galetta D, Granone PL, Righi L, Rusca M, Spaggiari L, Tiseo M, Viale G, Volante M, Papotti M, Pelosi G. Grading the neuroendocrine tumors of the lung: an evidence-based proposal. Endocr Relat Cancer. 2013;21:1–16.
6. Pelosi G, Rindi G, Travis WD, Papotti M. Ki-67 antigen in lung neuroendocrine tumors: unraveling a role in clinical practice. J Thorac Oncol. 2014;9:273–84.
7. Rindi G, Klimstra DS, Abedi-Ardekani B, Asa SL, Bosman FT, Brambilla E, Busam KJ, de Krijger RR, Dietel M, El-Naggar AK, Fernandez-Cuesta L, Klöppel G, WG MC, Moch H, Ohgaki H, Rakha EA, Reed NS, Rous BA, Sasano H, Scarpa A, Scoazec JY, Travis WD, Tallini G, Trouillas J, van Krieken JH, Cree IA. A common classification framework for neuroendocrine neoplasms: an International Agency for Research on Cancer (IARC) and World Health Organization (WHO) expert consensus proposal. Mod Pathol. 2018;31:1770–86.

8. Walts AE, Ines D, Marchevsky AM. Limited role of Ki-67 proliferative index in predicting overall short-term survival in patients with typical and atypical pulmonary carcinoid tumors. Mod Pathol. 2012;25:1258–64.

9. Travis WD, Giroux DJ, Chansky K, Crowley J, Asamura H, Brambilla E, Jett J, Kennedy C, Rami-Porta R, Rusch VW, Goldstraw P. International staging committee and participating institutions: the IASLC lung cancer staging project: proposals for the inclusion of broncho-pulmonary carcinoid tumors in the forthcoming (seventh) edition of the TNM classification for lung cancer. J Thorac Oncol. 2008;3:1213–23.

10. Yao JC, Hassan M, Phan A, et al. One hundred years after "carcinoid": epidemiology of and prognostic factors for neuroendocrine tumors in 35,825 cases in the United States. J Clin Oncol. 2008;26:3063–72.

11. Hallet J, Law CH, Cukier M, Saskin R, Liu N, Singh S. Exploring the rising incidence of neuroendocrine tumors: a population-based analysis of epidemiology metastatic presentation, and outcomes. Cancer. 2015;121:589–97.

12. Carter D, Vazquez M, Flieder DB, Brambilla E, Gazdar A, Noguchi M, Travis WD, Kramer A, Yip R, Yankelevitz DF, Henschke CI, ELCAP, NY-ELCAP Comparison of pathologic findings of baseline and annual repeat cancers diagnosed on CT screening. Lung Cancer. 2007;56:193–9.

13. Gustafsson BI, Kidd M, Chan A, Malfertheiner MV, Modlin IM. Bronchopulmonary neuroendocrine tumors. Cancer. 2008;113:5–21.

14. Filosso PL, Rena O, Donati G, Casadio C, Ruffini E, Papalia E, Cliaro A, Maggi G. Bronchial carcinoid tumors: surgical management and long-term outcome J Thorac Cardiovasc Surg. 2002;123:303–9.

15. Detterbeck FC. Clinical presentation and evaluation of neuroendocrine tumors of the lung. Thorac Surg Clin. 2014;24(3):267–76.

16. Broaddus RR, Herzog CE, Hicks MJ. Neuroendocrine tumors (carcinoid and neuroendocrine carcinoma) presenting at extra-appendiceal sites in childhood and adolescence. Arch Pathol Lab Med. 2003;127:1200–3.

17. Dishop MK, Kuruvilla S. Primary and metastatic lung tumors in the pediatric population: a review and 25-year experience at a large children's hospital. Arch Pathol Lab Med. 2008;132:1079–103.

18. Paladugu RR, Benfield JR, Pak HY, Ross RK, Teplitz RL. Bronchopulmonary Kulchitzky cell carcinomas. A new classification scheme for typical and atypical carcinoids. Cancer. 1985;55:1303–11.

19. Beasley MB, Thunnissen FB, Brambilla E, Hasleton P, Steele R, Hammar SP, Colby TV, Sheppard M, Shimosato Y, Koss MN, Falk R, Travis WD. Pulmonary atypical carcinoid: predictors of survival in 106 cases. Hum Pathol. 2000;31:1255–65.

20. Oliveira AM, Tazelaar HD, Wentzlaff KA, Kosugi NS, Hai N, Benson A, Miller DL, Yang P. Familial pulmonary carcinoid tumors. Cancer. 2001;1(91):2104–9.

21. Leotlela PD, Jauch A, Holtgreve-Grez H, Thakker RV. Genetics of neuroendocrine and carcinoid tumours. Endocr Relat Cancer. 2003;10:437–50.

22. Sachithanandan N, Harle RA, Burgess JR. Bronchopulmonary carcinoid in multiple endocrine neoplasia type 1. Cancer. 2005;103:509–15.

23. Godwin JD 2nd. Carcinoid tumors. An analysis of 2,837 cases. Cancer. 1975;36:560–9.

24. Jeung MY, Gasser B, Gangi A, Charneau D, Ducroq X, Kessler R, Quoix E, Roy C. Bronchial carcinoid tumors of the thorax: spectrum of radiologic findings. Radiographics. 2002;22:351–65.

25. Meisinger QC, Klein JS, Butnor KJ, Gentchos G, Leavitt BJ. CT features of peripheral pulmonary carcinoid tumors. AJR Am J Roentgenol. 2011;197:1073–80.

26. Isidori AM, Kaltsas GA, Grossman AB. Ectopic ACTH syndrome. Front Horm Res. 2006;35:143–56.

27. Chughtai T, Morin J, Sheiner N, Wilson J, et al. Bronchial carcinoid: twenty years' experience defines a selective surgical approach. Surgery. 1997;122:801–8.

28. Higashi K, Ueda Y, Ayabe K, Sakurai A, Seki H, Nambu Y, Oguchi M, Shikata H, Taki S, Tonami H, Katsuda S. Yamamoto: FDG PET in the evaluation of the aggressiveness of pulmonary adenocarcinoma: correlation with histopathological features. Nucl Med Commun. 2000;21:707–14.

29. Wartski M, Alberini JL, Leroy-Ladurie F, De Montpreville V, Nguyen C, Corone C, Dartevelle P, Pecking AP. Typical and atypical bronchopulmonary carcinoid tumors on FDG PET/CT imaging. Clin Nucl Med. 2004;29:752–3.

30. Daniels CE, Lowe VJ, Aubry MC, Allen MS, Jett JR. The utility of fluorodeoxyglucose positron emission tomography in the evaluation of carcinoid tumors presenting as pulmonary nodules. Chest. 2007;131:255–60.

31. Kayani I, Bomanji JB, Groves A, Conway G, Gacinovic S, Win T, Dickson J, Caplin M, Ell PJ. Functional imaging of neuroendocrine tumors with combined PET/CT using 68Ga-DOTATATE (DOTA-DPhe1,Tyr3-octreotate) and 18F-FDG. Cancer. 2008;112:2447–55.

32. Kayani I, Conry BG, Groves AM, Win T, Dickson J, Caplin M, Bomanji JB. A comparison of 68Ga-DOTATATE and 18F-FDG PET/CT in pulmonary neuroendocrine tumors. J Nucl Med. 2009;50:1927–32.

33. Santhanam P, Chandramahanti S, Kroiss A, Yu R, Ruszniewski P, Kumar R, Taïeb D. Nuclear imaging of neuroendocrine tumors with unknown primary: why, when and how? Eur J Nucl Med Mol Imaging. 2015;42:1144–55.

34. Daddi N, Ferolla P, Urbani M, Semeraro A, Avenia N, Ribacchi R, Puma F, Daddi G. Surgical treatment of neuroendocrine tumors of the lung. Eur J Cardiothorac Surg. 2004;26:813–7.

35. Marty-Ané C, Alauzen M, Costes V, Serres-Cousiné O, Mary H. Heterogeneity of bronchial carcinoid tumors. Place of atypical forms. Ann Chir. 1994;48:253–8.

36. Steinfort DP, Finlay M, Irving LB. Diagnosis of peripheral pulmonary carcinoid tumor using endobronchial ultrasound. Ann Thorac Med. 2008;3:146–8.

37. Filosso PL, Guerrera F, Falco NR, Thomas P, Garcia Yuste M, Rocco G, Welter S, Moreno Casado P, Rendina EA, Venuta F, Ampollini L, Nosotti M, Raveglia F, Rena O, Stella F, Larocca V, Ardissone F, Brunelli A, Margaritora S, Travis WD, Sagan D, Sarkaria I. Evangelista A; ESTS NETs-WG steering committee: anatomical resections are superior to wedge resections for overall survival in patients with stage 1 typical carcinoids. Eur J Cardiothorac Surg. 2019;55:273–9.

38. Filosso PL, Guerrera F, Evangelista A, Welter S, Thomas P, Casado PM, Rendina EA, Venuta F, Ampollini L, Brunelli A, Stella F, Nosotti M, Raveglia F, Larocca V, Rena O, Margaritora S, Ardissone F, Travis WD, Sarkaria I, Sagan D. ESTS NETs-WG steering committee: prognostic model of survival for typical bronchial carcinoid tumours: analysis of 1109 patients on behalf of the European Association of Thoracic Surgeons (ESTS) Neuroendocrine Tumours Working Group. Eur J Cardiothorac Surg. 2015;48:441–7.

39. Filosso PL, Rena O, Guerrera F, Moreno Casado P, Sagan D, Raveglia F, Brunelli A, Welter S, Gust L, Pompili C, Casadio C, Bora G, Alvarez A, Zaluska W, Baisi A, Roesel C, Thomas PA. ESTS NETs-WG steering committee: clinical management of atypical carcinoid and large-cell neuroendocrine carcinoma: a multicentre study on behalf of the European Association of Thoracic Surgeons (ESTS) neuroendocrine tumours of the lung working group. Eur J Cardiothorac Surg. 2015;48:55–64.

40. Goldstraw P. International Association for the Study of Lung Cancer (IASLC) staging manual in thoracic oncology. Florida: Editorial Rx Press; 2009.

41. Lim E, Yap YK, De Stavola BL, Nicholson AG, Goldstraw P. The impact of stage and cell type on the prognosis of pulmonary neuroendocrine tumors. J Thorac Cardiovasc Surg. 2005;130:969–72.

42. Okada M, Tsubota N, Yoshimura M, Miyamoto Y, Matsuoka H, Satake S, Yamagishi H. Extended sleeve lobectomy for lung cancer: the avoidance of pneumonectomy. J Thorac Cardiovasc Surg. 1999;118:710–3.

43. Takeda S, Maeda H, Koma M, Matsubara Y, Sawabata N, Inoue M, Tokunaga T, Ohta M. Comparison of surgical results after pneumonectomy and sleeve lobectomy for non-small

cell lung cancer: trends over time and 20-year institutional experience. Eur J Cardiothorac Surg. 2006;29:276–80.

44. Berthet JP, Paradela M, Jimenez MJ, Molins L, Gómez-Caro A. Extended sleeve lobectomy: one more step toward avoiding pneumonectomy in centrally located lung cancer. Ann Thorac Surg. 2013;96:1988–97.

45. Dalar L, Ozdemir C, Abul Y, et al. Endobronchial treatment of carcinoid tumors of the lung. Thorac Cardiovasc Surg. 2016;64:166–71.

46. Reuling EMBP, Dickhoff C, Plaisier PW, et al. Endobronchial treatment for bronchial carcinoid: patient selection and predictors of outcome. Respiration. 2018;95:220–7.

47. Reuling EMBP, Dickhoff C, Plaisier PW, et al. Endobronchial and surgical treatment of pulmonary carcinoid tumors: a systematic literature review. Lung Cancer. 2019;134:85–95.

48. Miller RR, Müller NL. Neuroendocrine cell hyperplasia and obliterative bronchiolitis in patients with peripheral carcinoid tumors. Am J Surg Pathol. 1995;19:653–8.

49. Beshay M, Roth T, Stein R, Schmid RA. Synchronous bilateral typical pulmonary carcinoid tumors. Eur J Cardiothorac Surg. 2003;23:251–3.

50. Camargo SM, Machuca TN, Moreira AL, Schio SM, Moreira JS, Camargo JJ. Multiple synchronous bronchial carcinoid tumors: report of a case. Thorac Cardiovasc Surg. 2009;57:58–60.

51. Erelel M, Toker SA, Yakar F, Yakar AA, Yildiz R, Kaya ZB. Multifocal endobronchial carcinoid tumors: a rare case. J Bronchology Interv Pulmonol. 2010;17:158–61.

52. Okike N, Bernatz PE, Woolner LB. Carcinoid tumors of the lung. Ann Thorac Surg. 1976;22:270–7.

53. Vadasz P, Palffy G, Egervary M, Schaff Z. Diagnosis and treatment of bronchial carcinoid tumors: clinical and pathological review of 120 operated patients. Eur J Cardiothorac Surg. 1993;7:8–11.

54. Hurt R, Bates M. Carcinoid tumours of the bronchus: a 33 year experience. Thorax. 1984;39:617–23.

55. Francioni F, Rendina EA, Venuta F, Pescarmona E, De Giacomo T, Ricci C. Low grade neuroendocrine tumors of the lung (bronchial carcinoids) – 25 years experience. Eur J Cardiothorac Surg. 1990;4:472–6.

56. Travis WD, Linnoila RI, Tsokos MG, Hitchcock CL, Cutler GB Jr, Nieman L, Chrousos G, Pass H, Doppman J. Neuroendocrine tumors of the lung with proposed criteria for large-cell neuroendocrine carcinoma. An ultrastructural, immunohistochemical, and flow cytometric study of 35 cases. Am J Surg Pathol. 1991;15:529–53.

57. Iyoda A, Hiroshima K, Toyozaki T, Haga Y, Fujisawa T, Ohwada H. Clinical characterization of pulmonary large cell neuroendocrine carcinoma and large cell carcinoma with neuroendocrine morphology. Cancer. 2001;91:1992–2000.

58. Takei H, Asamura H, Maeshima A, Suzuki K, Kondo H, Niki T, Yamada T, Tsuchiya R, Matsuno Y. Large cell neuroendocrine carcinoma of the lung: a clinicopathologic study of eighty-seven cases. J Thorac Cardiovasc Surg. 2002;124:285–92.

59. Battafarano RJ, Fernandez FG, Ritter J, Meyers BF, Guthrie TJ, Cooper JD, Patterson GA. Large cell neuroendocrine carcinoma: an aggressive form of non-small cell lung cancer. J Thorac Cardiovasc Surg. 2005;130:166–72.

60. Asamura H, Kameya T, Matsuno Y, Noguchi M, Tada H, Ishikawa Y, Yokose T, Jiang SX, Inoue T, Nakagawa K, Tajima K, Nagai K. Neuroendocrine neoplasms of the lung: a prognostic spectrum. J Clin Oncol. 2006;24:70–6.

61. Hage R, Seldenrijk K, de Bruin P, van Swieten H, van den Bosch J. Pulmonary large-cell neuroendocrine carcinoma (LCNEC). Eur J Cardiothorac Surg. 2003 23:457–60.

62. Sarkaria IS, Iyoda A, Roh MS, Sica G, Kuk D, Sima CS, Pietanza MC, Park BJ, Travis WD, Rusch VW. Neoadjuvant and adjuvant chemotherapy in resected pulmonary large cell neuroendocrine carcinomas: a single institution experience. Ann Thorac Surg. 2011;92:1180–6.

63. Kaira K, Murakami H, Endo M, Ohde Y, Naito T, Kondo H, Nakajima T, Yamamoto N, Takahashi T. Biological correlation of ^{18}F-FDG uptake on PET in pulmonary neuroendocrine tumors. Anticancer Res. 2013;33:4219–28.

64. Iyoda A, Travis WD, Sarkaria IS, Jiang SX, Amano H, Sato Y, Saegusa M, Rusch VW, Satoh Y. Expression profiling and identification of potential molecular targets for therapy in pulmonary large-cell neuroendocrine carcinoma. Exp Ther Med. 2011;2:1041–5.
65. Makino T, Mikami T, Hata Y, Otsuka H, Koezuka S, Isobe K, Tochigi N, Shibuya K, Homma S, Iyoda A. Comprehensive biomarkers for personalized treatment in pulmonary large cell neuroendocrine carcinoma: a comparative analysis with adenocarcinoma. Ann Thorac Surg. 2016;102:1694–701.
66. Filosso PL, Guerrera F, Evangelista A, Galassi C, Welter S, Rendina EA, Travis W, Lim E, Sarkaria I, Thomas PA. ESTS lung neuroendocrine working group contributors: adjuvant chemotherapy for large-cell neuroendocrine lung carcinoma: results from the European Society for Thoracic Surgeons Lung Neuroendocrine Tumours retrospective database. Eur J Cardiothorac Surg. 2017;52:339–45.
67. Raman V, Jawitz OK, Yang CJ, Tong BC, D'Amico TA, Berry MF, Harpole DH Jr. Adjuvant therapy for patients with early large cell lung neuroendocrine cancer: a National Analysis. Ann Thorac Surg. 2019;108:377–83.
68. Rossi G, Cavazza A, Marchioni A, Longo L, Migaldi M, Sartori G, Bigiani N, Schirosi L, Casali C, Morandi U, Facciolongo N, Maiorana A, Bavieri M, Fabbri LM, Brambilla E. Role of chemotherapy and the receptor tyrosine kinases KIT, PDGFRalpha, PDGFRbeta, and Met in large-cell neuroendocrine carcinoma of the lung. J Clin Oncol. 2005;23:8774–85.
69. Iyoda A, Hiroshima K, Moriya Y, Takiguchi Y, Sekine Y, Shibuya K, Iizasa T, Kimura H, Nakatani Y, Fujisawa T. Prospective study of adjuvant chemotherapy for pulmonary large cell neuroendocrine carcinoma. Ann Thorac Surg. 2006;82:1802–7.

Medullary Thyroid Cancer

14

Victor A. Gall and Amanda M. Laird

Introduction

Medullary thyroid cancer (MTC) was first histologically described in 1959 by Hazard et al. [1]. MTC is rare and, on a recent analysis of SEER data, accounts for only 1–2% of all thyroid cancers [2]. While papillary thyroid cancer originates from follicular cells, MTC originates from the parafollicular C-cells which have a distinct embryological origin [3]. During thyroid development, the majority of the gland arises from endodermal cells that migrate from the pharynx caudally over the trachea via the thyroglossal duct. These cells eventually form the follicular components of the thyroid and make up the bulk of the gland. Parafollicular C-cells are derived from neural crest cells that arise from the fourth and fifth pharyngeal pouches forming ultimobranchial bodies that fuse with the lateral thyroid at the superior dorsolateral aspects forming the tubercles of Zuckerkandl [4]. Once fully developed, these cells secrete calcitonin which is responsible for the regulation of serum calcium and serves as a biochemical marker in MTC [5]. Given this difference in physiology, the usual adjuncts to the treatment of thyroid cancer, including TSH suppression and radioactive iodine, are ineffective, and the management of MTC is mainly surgical. Over the course of this chapter, the etiologies of MTC are discussed, emphasizing the surgical management of this disease.

V. A. Gall
Rutgers Cancer Institute of New Jersey, New Brunswick, NJ, USA
e-mail: victor.gall@rutgers.edu

A. M. Laird (✉)
Rutgers Cancer Institute of New Jersey, Rutgers Robert Wood Johnson Medical School, New Brunswick, NJ, USA
e-mail: amanda.laird@cinj.rutgers.edu

© Springer Nature Switzerland AG 2021
J. M. Cloyd, T. M. Pawlik (eds.), *Neuroendocrine Tumors*,
https://doi.org/10.1007/978-3-030-62241-1_14

Etiology of MTC

Most MTC cases (75%) occur sporadically, and the remaining 25% of cases stem from hereditary syndromes [6]. In both, MTC is closely associated with the RET proto-oncogene (*RET*). This gene, found on chromosome 10q11.2, codes for a receptor in the tyrosine kinase family. Germline mutations in *RET* are present in all patients with hereditary forms of MTC [7, 8]. In sporadic cases of MTC, somatic mutations in *RET* have been found in about 69% of patients, while the remainder commonly have identifiable RAS mutations [9, 10]. As of the publication of this chapter, almost 200 different mutations have been identified in hereditary forms of MTC, and these distinct *RET* mutations present with characteristic disease phenotypes [11]. The particular genotype of an MTC patient can help predict the tumor's aggressiveness as well as its association with other tumor types including pheochromocytoma as genotype/phenotype relationships in MEN2 are well-established. The most recent American Thyroid Association (ATA) guidelines define groups of *RET* mutations by their aggressiveness. The redefined categories in the 2015 guidelines include HST (highest risk) which includes M918T mutations, H (high risk) which includes A833F and C634 mutations, as well as MOD (moderate risk) which encompasses all other known mutations [12] (Table 14.1).

Of these mutations, the highest risk is associated with a *RET* codon M918T mutation (HST). This mutation is found exclusively in MEN2B and leads to more aggressive tumors and a poorer prognosis and affects decision-making regarding

Table 14.1 Relationship of common *RET* mutations to risk of aggressive MTC in MEN and to the incidence of pheochromocytoma (PHEO) and hyperparathyroidism (HPTH)[12]

RET mutation	Exon	MTC risk level	Incidence of PHEO	Incidence of HPTH
G533C	8	MOD	*	–
C609F/G/R/S/Y	10	MOD	*/**	*
C611F/G/SA/W	10	MOD	*/**	*
C618F/R/S	10	MOD	*/**	*
C620F/R/S	10	MOD	*/**	*
C630R/Y	11	MOD	*/**	*
D631Y	11	MOD	***	–
C634F/G/R/S/W/Y	11	H	***	**
K666E	11	MOD	*	–
E7680	13	MOD	–	–
L790F	13	MOD	*	–
V804L	14	MOD	*	*
V804M	14	MOD	*	*
A883F	15	H	***	–
S891A	15	MOD	*	*
R912P	16	MOD	–	–
M918T	16	HST	***	–

Risk of aggressive MTC: *MOD* moderate, *H* high, *HST* highest
Incidence of PHEO and HPTH; * ~10%: ** ~20–30%; *** ~50%

early prophylactic thyroidectomy [13]. With somatic *RET* mutations, the M918T mutation is seen in varying degrees with a higher prevalence in larger tumors. Overall, the prevalence of the M918T mutation in sporadic MTC is 19.4%, but in tumors larger than 3 cm, the prevalence is as high as 58.3% [14]. It is unclear in sporadic cases if the *RET* proto-oncogene acts as the initiator of MTC or if it is activated downstream to stimulate tumor growth. In the case of sporadic MTC, prognosis is estimated based on the American Joint Committee on Cancer (AJCC) Tumor, Node, Metastasis (TNM) staging system.

Clinical Presentation

Sporadic MTC

In sporadic MTC, patients typically present with central neck masses between their fourth and sixth decades of life. Seventy percent of patients who present with a palpable mass have central or lateral cervical lymph node metastases, while 10% have distant metastases as well [15]. In a retrospective study evaluating the pattern of lymph node metastases in MTC, the risk of nodal involvement increased with increasing T stage. Central cervical node metastases were found 14%, 38%, and 86% of the time in T1, T2, and T4 tumors, respectively. Lateral cervical node metastases were found in 11%, 38%, and 93% of patients with T1, T2, and T4 tumors. In this particular study, T3 tumors were underrepresented but likely follow this pattern as well [16]. Other presenting symptoms in MTC can range from vague pain and soreness to dysphagia, dyspnea, and dysphonia in more locally aggressive disease. Given the neuroendocrine origins of MTC, patients can also present with ectopic Cushing's syndrome due to production of ACTH by tumor cells. MTC accounts for 2% of all cases of this paraneoplastic syndrome [17].

MTC in MEN2A

Hereditary MTC can present at a much earlier age and presents in various forms depending on the inherited genetic mutation. Multiple endocrine neoplasia (MEN)2A was first described in 1968 by Steiner and colleagues and was characterized by the presence of MTC, pheochromocytoma, and hyperparathyroidism in families [18]. It is most commonly associated with mutations in codons 609, 611, 618, or 620 of exon 10 or codon 634 of exon 11 (Table 14.1). All patients with MEN2A eventually develop MTC, but the incidence of pheochromocytoma varies with the inherited mutation [19]. It is highest in patients with codon 634 mutations (50% by age 50), and due to known genotype/phenotype relationships in MEN2A, occurrence is relatively predictable. Annual screening recommendations can then be tailored to the individual patient. Pheochromocytomas in the setting of this syndrome are typically benign and present as bilateral nodular hyperplasia. Hyperparathyroidism seen 30% of the time can also occur and has the potential to involve all four glands [20]. Familial medullary thyroid cancer (FMTC) is a variant of MEN2A in which there is an inherited form of MTC with *RET* mutation but none of the other manifestations of MEN. Overlap exists with *RET* mutations found in MEN2A and FMTC. To date, FMTC kindreds have had mutations identified in codons 609, 611, 618, 620, and 634. Mutations have also been found on codons 768 (E768D) and 804 (V804L) which have not been seen in MEN2 but have been associated with late-onset MTC [20–22].

MTC in MEN2B

MEN2B accounts for only 5% of hereditary MTC, and patients with this syndrome develop MTC, pheochromocytoma, and mucosal neuromas. In this rarer syndrome, MTC usually presents during the first years of life and is highly aggressive with early nodal metastases. About 95% of MEN2B patients have exon 13 (codon M918T) mutations, while the remaining 5% of patients will have exon 15 (codon A883F) mutations which tend to be less aggressive [23]. Half of all patients will develop pheochromocytomas later in life. Unlike MEN2A, hyperparathyroidism is not considered part of the syndrome, but patients can have distinct physical characteristics including a marfanoid habitus, skeletal abnormalities, and mucosal neuromas.

Diagnosis of Sporadic MTC

When MTC is diagnosed by thyroid FNA, further work-up is warranted in anticipation of surgery. Tumor markers, including calcitonin and CEA, are drawn to assess the extent of disease and establish a preoperative baseline. Despite the absence of a classic family history, de novo germline *RET* mutations, more commonly seen in familial disease, can be found in 7% of patients with presumed somatic MTC [24]. Given this high prevalence of *RET* mutations, all patients with sporadic MTC should also be screened for pheochromocytoma and hyperparathyroidism by preoperative testing of plasma metanephrines, calcium, and parathyroid hormone levels. Ultimately, all patients with MTC should undergo genetic testing, but mutation status should not delay initial surgical management. On the other hand, it is critical to evaluate for the possibility of pheochromocytoma prior to any surgery for MTC.

In addition to providing a biochemical baseline, preoperative calcitonin levels have been used to predict the risk of cervical lymph node and distant metastases. With respect to cervical lymph node metastases, in one study of 300 patients who underwent total thyroidectomy with lymph node dissection, it was noted that those with a preoperative calcitonin below 20 pg/mL had almost no risk of lymph node metastases. Calcitonin levels greater than 20 pg/mL were associated with metastases to the ipsilateral central and lateral neck, while levels greater than 50, 200, and 500 pg/mL were associated with metastases to the contralateral central neck, contralateral lateral neck, and upper mediastinal nodes, respectively [25]. It is important to note that, although extremely rare, cases of MTC without a detectable calcitonin elevation have been reported and prove to be a challenge to manage. Cases are often diagnosed at a more advanced stage and can be harder to surveil postoperatively. Several theories have been proposed for this atypical form of MTC including alterations in calcitonin secretion mechanisms or aberrant calcitonin precursors not recognized by testing antibodies [26, 27].

While calcitonin levels have been used to predict lymph node positivity, neck ultrasound is the most important preoperative imaging strategy to evaluate for local invasiveness and nodal involvement. All patients must undergo cervical lymph node mapping via ultrasound either by a dedicated radiologist or surgeon experienced in neck ultrasound prior to surgery. Neck ultrasound has limited sensitivity in the central neck compartment, but it is invaluable in evaluating the lateral neck. Sensitivity of ultrasound for cervical lymph node levels II–V is 98%. Lymph nodes with characteristic malignant appearance, that is, hypoechoic with loss of hilar architecture, taller than wide, hypervascular, and/or with posterior shadowing, must undergo fine needle aspiration (FNA) biopsy prior to thyroid surgery as a part of preoperative staging. If proven to contain metastases from the primary MTC, a lateral neck dissection should be included at the time of the initial operation. In patients with extensive disease in the neck, regional metastases, or serum calcitonin greater than 400 pg/mL, further work-up for distant disease is warranted. Distant metastases are best identified with contrast-enhanced CT of the chest, abdomen, and pelvis with a role for MRI as well to evaluate the liver. PET scans are less sensitive and have lower prognostic value [28]. In one study looking at patients with an elevated postoperative calcitonin, the overall sensitivity of an ^{18}F-FDG PET scan in detecting residual, recurrent, or metastatic disease was 62%. The sensitivity rose to 78% in patients with a calcitonin level greater than 1000 pg/mL. No true positives were identified in patient with calcitonin levels below 500 pg/mL suggesting limited utility in this group of patients [29]. Given the neuroendocrine nature of MTC, ^{68}Ga-DOTATATE PET scans have been utilized in the identification of recurrent MTC as well. Comparisons between these two modalities have shown similar lesion detection rates (sensitivity of 72% vs 78%). An added advantage to a DOTATATE scan would be the ability to identify patients who may benefit from targeted radionuclide somatostatin analogue therapy [30–31] (Fig. 14.1).

Surgery

The approach to surgical management of MTC depends upon whether it arises in sporadic form or as part of a hereditary syndrome. In known MEN2 kindreds, patients undergo prophylactic thyroidectomy in an effort to prevent distant metastatic spread. Age-based recommendations are outlined based on the *RET* mutation present (Fig. 14.2). In patients with sporadic MTC, recommendations are based on extent of disease as defined by imaging and serum calcitonin levels.

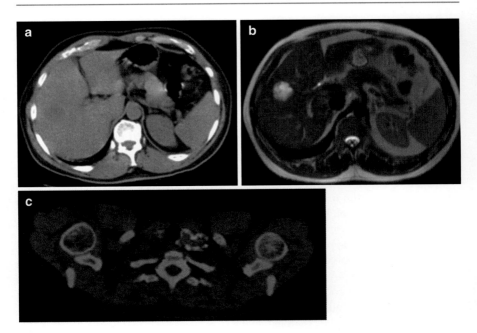

Fig. 14.1 CT (**a**) and MRI (**b**) imaging of the liver showing metastatic MTC. DOTATATE-PET CT showing uptake in the neck suggestive of disease recurrence (**c**)

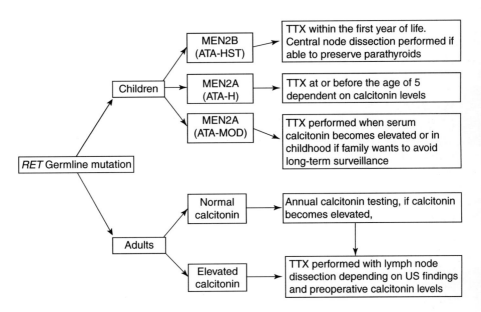

Fig. 14.2 Management of patients with *RET* germline mutations on genetic screening. ATA risk categories for aggressive MTC (HST – highest, H – high, MOD – moderate). TTX – total thyroidectomy[12]

Prophylactic Thyroidectomy in MEN2

In hereditary MTC, there remains the surgical management of those who have yet been affected by the disease but have tested positive for a germline *RET* mutation and remain at high risk. Classically, patients with hereditary forms of MTC progress from C-cell hyperplasia to MTC after which the disease can spread to both locoregional and distant sites [32]. This process can occur over a matter of months to years depending on the particular *RET* mutation in question. The goal of a prophylactic thyroidectomy is to remove all thyroid tissue prior to the development of MTC or, in some cases, while MTC is still subclinical and confined to the thyroid.

The decision on age for prophylactic thyroidectomy is based on multiple factors including direct DNA analysis to determine the mutation present as well as basal calcitonin levels [33]. Physicians must also balance the risks and benefits of undergoing thyroidectomy at an early age. Complication rates are known to be higher in children undergoing thyroidectomy with hypoparathyroidism being a particular risk given the difficulty in identifying parathyroid glands in young children [34]. In addition, there are potential detrimental effects in children requiring thyroid hormone replacement if replacement is insufficient due to noncompliance.

MEN2A

Children with MEN2A and an ATA-H (high-risk) *RET* mutation usually develop MTC within the first years of life. In these children, it is recommended that they receive annual examinations, neck US, and serum calcitonin levels beginning at 3 years of age. In children with *RET* mutations that fall under the ATA-MOD (moderate-risk) category, MTC typically develops at a later age and is less aggressive. For these patients, screening with physical exam, US, and serum calcitonin is recommended to start at age 5.

Eventually, all patients with MEN2A will require a thyroidectomy. Children with high-risk mutations (ATA-H) should have a thyroidectomy before the age of 5, while those with moderate-risk mutations (ATA-MOD) can have their thyroidectomies later in life up to young adulthood depending on serum calcitonin levels. In patients undergoing a prophylactic thyroidectomy, central neck dissection is not recommended as long as preoperative serum calcitonin levels are less than 40 pg/mL which was associated with low risk of nodal metastases in children with MTC.

The recommendations for surveillance with US and calcitonin are based on the ability of preoperative calcitonin levels to predict the presence of microcarcinoma and lymph node metastases as well as prognosticate the rate of biochemical remission after surgery. In an institutional series of 224 patients with MTC and elevated preoperative calcitonin levels, it was found that a basal calcitonin level greater than 500 pg/mL best predicted failure to achieve biochemical remission. Lymph node metastases began to be seen with basal calcitonin levels of 10–40 pg/mL. In patients with node-positive disease and a basal calcitonin above 3000 pg/mL, remission was not achieved [35].

MEN2B

Patients with MEN2B can carry the *RET* codon M918T mutation which is considered the highest-risk mutation in MTC (ATA-HST). Children with MEN2B can develop MTC with nodal metastases in the first year of life. For this reason, genetic testing should be done immediately after birth in those who are born to parents in known kindreds. In those who test positive for MEN2B, thyroidectomy should be performed within the first year. Serum calcitonin levels can be less reliable in the first months of life and are of limited utility in contributing to the timing of surgery [36]. Due to the aggressive nature of MTC in patients with MEN2B, central neck dissection should be considered even in the absence of suspicious nodes provided that the parathyroid glands can be identified and preserved [37].

Surgery in Sporadic MTC

After a diagnosis of sporadic MTC has been made, the minimum surgical treatment is a total thyroidectomy and a compartment-oriented central cervical lymph node dissection. Given the high rate of lymph node metastases in MTC and the low negative predictive value of intraoperative inspection by the operating surgeon, all patients undergo a compartment-oriented central lymph node dissection as part of their oncologic procedure regardless of whether lymph node metastases are present in the central compartment at time of surgery [38, 39]. The central compartment of the neck is also known as level VI and is bounded by the hyoid bone superiorly, the sternal notch inferiorly, and the carotid sheaths laterally and is anterior to the recurrent laryngeal nerves and deep cervical fascia. Extension of the inferior border to the innominate vein also includes level VII [40]. In addition, a lateral neck dissection, which includes lymph node levels II–V, is performed if there is proven disease by preoperative imaging and biopsy. Lymph node levels II–V correspond to the upper, middle, and lower jugular nodes (levels II, III, and IV) as well as the posterior triangle nodes (level V). The level II nodes are located along the upper third of the jugular vein extending from the skull base to the inferior border of the hyoid bone. Level III nodes follow the jugular vein between the hyoid bone and the inferior border of the cricoid cartilage. Level IV nodes are found along the lower third of the jugular vein located between the inferior border of the cricoid cartilage and the clavicle. The posterior boundary of the jugular nodes is the posterior border of the sternocleidomastoid (SCM). The level V nodes comprise the posterior triangle and are bounded anteriorly by the posterior border of the SCM and posteriorly by the trapezius muscle. The spinal accessory nerve can be encountered when operating in levels II or V of the neck, and care should be taken in this area as injury to this nerve can cause a debilitating shoulder droop [41].

Although controversial, some surgeons utilize preoperative calcitonin levels in patients with no sonographic evidence of disease in the lateral neck to select candidates for a prophylactic lateral neck dissection. For those with a baseline calcitonin level above 20 pg/mL, consideration has been given to a prophylactic ipsilateral lateral neck dissection. For those with basal calcitonin levels above 200 pg/mL, consideration is given to a contralateral lateral neck dissection [25]. In regard to prophylactic lateral lymph node dissections, no consensus has been reached by the ATA Task Force, and more evidence is needed to support its utility. It is the opinion of these surgeons that prophylactic lateral neck dissection should be avoided. We recommend that extent of surgery be guided by preoperative imaging and fine needle aspiration biopsy and that surgery should include removal of the thyroid gland, level VI lymph nodes bilaterally, and biopsy-proven lateral lymph node metastases in a compartment-oriented fashion. The lateral neck is a separate compartment from the central neck, and for persistently elevated calcitonin levels, the lateral neck may be addressed at a later time rather than at the initial operation.

Special Circumstances

Incomplete Thyroidectomy and Lymph Node Dissection

At times, a diagnosis of MTC is made following a hemithyroidectomy done either for diagnostic purposes or for a symptomatic nodule. In this situation, the management of the remainder of the neck is dependent on the etiology of the MTC. In hereditary MTC, the odds of MTC involving the opposite thyroid lobe or developing MTC in the future nears 100%, and patients should undergo completion thyroidectomy. In cases of sporadic MTC, the incidence of bilateral disease is 0–9%. In one study evaluating 15 patients with sporadic MTC managed with hemithyroidectomy, 12 (80%) patients were considered to be biochemically cured with postoperative calcitonin levels in the normal range following calcium and pentagastrin stimulation [42]. Per the most recent ATA guidelines, completion thyroidectomy following unilateral hemithyroidectomy is only indicated in patients with hereditary MTC (germline *RET* mutation), a calcitonin level above the normal range, or imaging studies (either US or CT) suggestive of residual disease [12]. Therefore, genetic testing following surgery is recommended as well as calcitonin, CEA, and neck ultrasonography to evaluate for additional disease to determine if completion thyroidectomy and additional lymphadenectomy are required.

In patients suspected to have residual lymph node metastases after their initial operation due to persistently elevated calcitonin levels, reoperation with the goal of removing regional cervical disease may be beneficial. One study evaluated 334 patients who underwent reoperation for persistent MTC determined by elevated postoperative calcitonin levels. Among these patients, central and lateral lymph node dissection led to biochemical cure in 44% of patients who had no lymph node metastases removed in their index operation. In those patients who had one to five positive lymph nodes removed with their original surgery, biochemical cure was only achieved 18% of the time with further lymph node dissection. This cure rate fell further as more positive lymph nodes were removed initially. As a result, reoperation for patients suspected to have residual lymph node disease after their initial operation is recommended for those patients who had five or fewer metastatic nodes removed initially and had a preoperative basal calcitonin level less than 1000 pg/mL

[43]. Surgery beyond these parameters is less likely to result in biochemical cure and is performed for local disease control in the neck. One study following patients who underwent reoperation for recurrent or persistent MTC for up to 10 years found that successful reoperations resulted in the lowering of calcitonin levels and of the patients who had levels reduced to less than 100 pg/mL (46.4%), none had shown radiographic recurrence [44].

Management of Locally Advanced or Metastatic Disease

In the setting of locally advanced disease, the goals of surgery for MTC become palliative in nature while attempting to minimize complications. When MTC begins to involve surrounding structures like the trachea, larynx, or esophagus, the extent of debulking surgery is dependent on an assessment of a patient's ability to maintain speech and swallowing function as well as on life expectancy. These factors are determined on a case-by-case basis. Less aggressive surgery can be acceptable in the central and lateral neck if the goal is to maintain speech, swallowing function, or shoulder mobility as aggressive debulking is unlikely to improve overall survival.

Distant metastases have been reported to the brain, bones, lungs, liver, and skin. Distant metastases portend a worse prognosis, and patients typically succumb to their disease within a year. According to the American Cancer Society (ACS), the 5-year relative survival rate for metastatic MTC falls around 39%, while 10-year survival falls to 21% [45, 46]. In the setting of solitary metastases to the liver, lungs, or skin, surgical resection is a generally accepted treatment strategy (Grade C recommendation) [12]. For more advanced metastatic disease, the goal is palliation with roles for adjunctive therapies like radiation, ablation, intratumoral injection, and chemoembolization for symptomatic metastases depending on the disease distribution and location.

A recent analysis of the SEER database followed trends in survival for MTC over the past 30 years. Over this period of time, 5-year disease-specific survival (DSS) had improved from 86% to 89% when comparing cases from the beginning to the end of this time period. The most dramatic increases in 5-year DSS occurred in patients with regional (82–91%) and distant (40–51%) disease [47]. This improvement in survival is largely attributable to medical advances in the treatment of advanced MTC. Different forms of targeted therapy have been studied in the treatment of MTC. Peptide receptor radionuclide therapy (PRRT) utilizes radiolabeled somatostatin analogues to deliver high-dose radiation to tumor cells. Its efficacy is limited to tumors that express somatostatin receptors and exhibit high uptake of somatostatin analogues. One study found about a 61% response rate to PRRT with improved response in lesions less than 2 cm in size and with a SUVmax less than 5 on FDG-PET [48]. Tyrosine kinase inhibitors (TKIs), including vandetanib and cabozantinib, have also shown promise in MTC by targeting the constitutively active *RET* receptor tyrosine kinase found in all hereditary MTC and half of sporadic MTC. Several TKIs have been studied with variable efficacy and a number of patients exhibiting prolonged stable disease. Vandetanib was studied in a phase III clinical trial of 331 patients with progressing or symptomatic metastatic MTC, and median progression-free survival (PFS) was improved in the treatment arm (30.5 months) compared to the placebo arm (19.3 months). A partial response was also noted in 45% of patients with associated improvements in quality of life [49]. Cabozantinib, another TKI, has also been FDA-approved for the treatment of advanced MTC having also shown improvements in PFS, response rates, and quality of life [50]. These treatments however have to be given daily to maintain disease control and can have significant short-term toxicities requiring dose reductions or withdrawal. Currently these therapies are reserved for patients with significant tumor burden or progressive disease. For patients with asymptomatic, stable disease, observation is preferred. Further study is needed to evaluate long-term survival outcomes with TKIs.

Postoperative Evaluation

After thyroidectomy, patients will require lifelong hormone replacement. Unlike with papillary thyroid cancer, there is no need to suppress thyroid-stimulating hormone (TSH) since MTC is not follicular in origin. The goal of thyroid hormone replacement is to maintain a euthyroid state. In addition, serum calcitonin level plays an important role in evaluating whether a thyroidectomy with or without lymphadenectomy of any type was curative. A study evaluating 124 patients after having a thyroidectomy for MTC found that 97% of patients had no detectable serum calcitonin after surgery. Those patients who had detectable levels either had residual thyroid tissue present or ectopic secretion of calcitonin from a non-thyroidal source [51]. Therefore, after appropriate surgery for MTC, calcitonin levels should be undetectable. Normalization of calcitonin postoperatively is associated with a favorable prognosis, and 3 months is about the amount of time given for calcitonin levels to reach their nadir [52]. Serum CEA and calcitonin levels should be measured at 3 months and if undetectable or within the normal range can be followed every 6 months for the first year and yearly thereafter. If the postoperative serum calcitonin is less than 150 pg/mL, patients should undergo examination and cervical ultrasound every 6 months because recurrence will typically be confined to the neck. If the calcitonin level is greater than 150 pg/mL, then further imaging including neck US and body imaging with CT and MRI is indicated to look for residual or distant disease.

Conclusion

MTC is a rare thyroid malignancy that is associated with a worse prognosis than follicular-derived thyroid cancers. It can occur sporadically or as part of a hereditary syndrome with various clinical phenotypes dependent on the tumor genotype. The mainstays for cure are early diagnosis and surgical removal of all disease. In the case of sporadic MTC, this is done with a total thyroidectomy and central lymph node dissection with a lateral dissection reserved for sonographic or biochemical evidence of disease. In patients with a hereditary form of MTC, the goal is for prophylactic surgery to improve future oncologic outcomes with the timing of surgery based on genotype and calcitonin level. Beyond the surgical management of MTC, further work is being done to identify systemic therapies, such as novel tyrosine kinase inhibitors, that improve outcomes in those who cannot be cured with surgery alone.

References

1. Hazard JB, Hawk WA, Crile G Jr. Medullary (solid) carcinoma of the thyroid; a clinicopathologic entity. J Clin Endocrinol Metab. 1959;19:152–61.
2. Surveillance, Epidemiology, and End Results (SEER) Program Populations (1969–2018). www.seer.cancer.gov/popdata, National Cancer Institute, DCCPS, surveillance research program, released December 2019.
3. Williams ED. Histogenesis of medullary carcinoma of the thyroid. J Clin Pathol. 1966;19:114–8.
4. Pearse AG, Polak JM. Cytochemical evidence for the neural crest origin of mammalian ultimobranchial C cells. Histochemie. 1971;27(2):96–102.
5. Foster GV. Calcitonin (thyrocalcitonin). N Engl J Med. 1968;279(7):349–60.
6. Block MA, Jackson CE, Greenawald KA, Yott JB, Tashjian AH Jr. Clinical characteristics distinguishing hereditary from sporadic medullary thyroid carcinoma. Treatment implications. Arch Surg. 1980;115:142–8.
7. Santoro M, Rosati R, Grieco M, et al. The ret proto-oncogene is consistently expressed in human pheochromocytomas and thyroid medullary carcinomas. Oncogene. 1990;5(10):1595–8.
8. Donis-Keller H, Dou S, Chi D, et al. Mutations in the RET proto-oncogene are associated with MEN 2A and FMTC. Hum Mol Genet. 1993;2(7):851–6.
9. Marsh DJ, Learoyd DL, Andrew SD, et al. Somatic mutations in the RET proto-oncogene in sporadic medullary thyroid carcinoma. Clin Endocrinol. 1996;44(3):249–57.
10. Agrawal N, Jiao Y, Sausen M, et al. Exomic sequencing of medullary thyroid cancer reveals dominant and mutually exclusive oncogenic mutations in RET and RAS. J Clin Endocrinol Metab. 2013;98(2):E364–9.
11. Margraf RL, Crockett DK, Krautscheid PM, et al. Multiple endocrine neoplasia type 2 RET protooncogene database: repository of MEN2-associated RET sequence variation and reference for genotype/phenotype correlations. Hum Mutat. 2009;30(4):548–56.
12. Wells SA Jr, Asa SL, Dralle H, et al. Revised American Thyroid Association guidelines for the management of medullary thyroid carcinoma. Thyroid. 2015;25(6):567–610.
13. Schilling T, Bürck J, Sinn HP, et al. Prognostic value of codon 918 (ATG-->ACG) RET protooncogene mutations in sporadic medullary thyroid carcinoma. Int J Cancer. 2001;95(1):62–6.
14. Romei C, Ugolini C, Cosci B, et al. Low prevalence of the somatic M918T RET mutation in micro-medullary thyroid cancer. Thyroid. 2012;22(5):476–81.
15. Moley JF. Medullary thyroid carcinoma: management of lymph node metastases. J Natl Compr Cancer Netw. 2010;8(5):549–56.
16. Machens A, Hinze R, Thomusch O, Dralle H. Pattern of nodal metastasis for primary and reoperative thyroid cancer. World J Surg. 2002;26(1):22–8.
17. Ilias I, Torpy DJ, Pacak K, Mullen N, Wesley RA, Nieman LK. Cushing's syndrome due to ectopic corticotropin secretion: twenty years' experience at the National Institutes of Health. J Clin Endocrinol Metab. 2005;90(8):4955–62.
18. Steiner AL, Goodman AD, Powers SR. Study of a kindred with pheochromocytoma, medullary thyroid carcinoma, hyperparathyroidism and Cushing's disease: multiple endocrine neoplasia, type 2. Medicine (Baltimore). 1968;47(5):371–409.

19. Raue F, Frank-Raue K. Genotype-phenotype correlation in multiple endocrine neoplasia type 2. Clinics (Sao Paulo). 2012;67(Suppl 1):69–75.
20. Eng C, Clayton D, Schuffenecker I, et al. The relationship between specific RET proto-oncogene mutations and disease phenotype in multiple endocrine neoplasia type 2. International RET mutation consortium analysis. JAMA. 1996;276(19):1575–9.
21. Dabir T, Hunter SJ, Russell CF, McCall D, Morrison PJ. The RET mutation E768D confers a late-onset familial medullary thyroid carcinoma – only phenotype with incomplete penetrance: implications for screening and management of carrier status. Familial Cancer. 2006;5(2):201–4.
22. Patócs A, Valkusz Z, Igaz P, et al. Segregation of the V804L mutation and S836S polymorphism of exon 14 of the RET gene in an extended kindred with familial medullary thyroid cancer. Clin Genet. 2003;63(3):219–23.
23. Gimm O, Marsh DJ, Andrew SD, et al. Germline dinucleotide mutation in codon 883 of the RET proto-oncogene in multiple endocrine neoplasia type 2B without codon 918 mutation. J Clin Endocrinol Metab. 1997;82(11):3902–4.
24. Elisei R, Romei C, Cosci B, et al. RET genetic screening in patients with medullary thyroid cancer and their relatives: experience with 807 individuals at one center. J Clin Endocrinol Metab. 2007;92(12):4725–9.
25. Machens A, Dralle H. Biomarker-based risk stratification for previously untreated medullary thyroid cancer. J Clin Endocrinol Metab. 2010;95(6):2655–63.
26. Gambardella C, Offi C, Patrone R, et al. Calcitonin negative medullary thyroid carcinoma: a challenging diagnosis or a medical dilemma? BMC Endocr Disord. 2019;19(Suppl 1):45. Published 2019 May 29
27. Brutsaert EF, Gersten AJ, Tassler AB, Surks MI. Medullary thyroid cancer with undetectable serum calcitonin. J Clin Endocrinol Metab. 2015;100(2):337–41.
28. Giraudet AL, Vanel D, Leboulleux S, et al. Imaging medullary thyroid carcinoma with persistent elevated calcitonin levels. J Clin Endocrinol Metab. 2007;92(11):4185–90.
29. Ong SC, Schöder H, Patel SG, et al. Diagnostic accuracy of 18F-FDG PET in restaging patients with medullary thyroid carcinoma and elevated calcitonin levels. J Nucl Med. 2007;48(4):501–7.
30. Treglia G, Tamburello A, Giovanella L. Detection rate of somatostatin receptor PET in patients with recurrent medullary thyroid carcinoma: a systematic review and a meta-analysis. Hormones (Athens). 2017;16(4):362–72.
31. Conry BG, Papathanasiou ND, Prakash V, et al. Comparison of 68Ga-DOTATATE and 18F-fluorodeoxyglucose PET/CT in the detection of recurrent medullary thyroid carcinoma. Eur J Nucl Med Mol Imaging. 2010;37:49.
32. Wolfe HJ, Melvin KE, Cervi-Skinner SJ, et al. C-cell hyperplasia preceding medullary thyroid carcinoma. N Engl J Med. 1973;289(9):437–41.
33. Machens A, Dralle H. Genotype-phenotype based surgical concept of hereditary medullary thyroid carcinoma. World J Surg. 2007;31(5):957–68.
34. Sosa JA, Tuggle CT, Wang TS, et al. Clinical and economic outcomes of thyroid and parathyroid surgery in children. J Clin Endocrinol Metab. 2008;93(8):3058–65.
35. Machens A, Schneyer U, Holzhausen HJ, Dralle H. Prospects of remission in medullary thyroid carcinoma according to basal calcitonin level. J Clin Endocrinol Metab. 2005;90(4):2029–34.
36. Klein GL, Wadlington EL, Collins ED, Catherwood BD, Deftos LJ. Calcitonin levels in sera of infants and children: relations to age and periods of bone growth. Calcif Tissue Int. 1984;36(6):635–8.
37. Zenaty D, Aigrain Y, Peuchmaur M, et al. Medullary thyroid carcinoma identified within the first year of life in children with hereditary multiple endocrine neoplasia type 2A (codon 634) and 2B. Eur J Endocrinol. 2009;160(5):807–13.
38. Laird AM, Gauger PG, Miller BS, Doherty GM. Evaluation of postoperative radioactive iodine scans in patients who underwent prophylactic central lymph node dissection. World J Surg. 2012;36(6):1268–73.

39. Moley JF, DeBenedetti MK. Patterns of nodal metastases in palpable medullary thyroid carcinoma: recommendations for extent of node dissection. Ann Surg. 1999;229(6):880–8.
40. American Thyroid Association Surgery Working Group. American Association of Endocrine Surgeons, American Academy of Otolaryngology-Head and Neck Surgery; consensus statement on the terminology and classification of central neck dissection for thyroid cancer. Thyroid. 2009;19(11):1153–8.
41. Stack BC Jr, Ferris RL, Goldenberg D, et al. American Thyroid Association consensus review and statement regarding the anatomy, terminology, and rationale for lateral neck dissection in differentiated thyroid cancer. Thyroid. 2012;22(5):501–8.
42. Miyauchi A, Matsuzuka F, Hirai K, et al. Prospective trial of unilateral surgery for nonhereditary medullary thyroid carcinoma in patients without germline RET mutations. World J Surg. 2002;26(8):1023–8.
43. Machens A, Dralle H. Benefit-risk balance of reoperation for persistent medullary thyroid cancer. Ann Surg. 2013;257(4):751–7.
44. Fialkowski E, DeBenedetti M, Moley J. Long-term outcome of reoperations for medullary thyroid carcinoma. World J Surg. 2008;32(5):754–65.
45. Modigliani E, Cohen R, Campos JM, et al. Prognostic factors for survival and for biochemical cure in medullary thyroid carcinoma: results in 899 patients. The GETC study group. Groupe d'étude des tumeurs à calcitonine. Clin Endocrinol. 1998;48(3):265–73.
46. Howlader N, Noone AM, Krapcho M, et al (eds). SEER cancer statistics review, 1975–2016, National Cancer Institute, Bethesda, MD. https://seer.cancer.gov/csr/1975_2016/, based on November 2018 SEER data submission, posted to the SEER website, April 2019.
47. Randle RW, Balentine CJ, Leverson GE, et al. Trends in the presentation, treatment, and survival of patients with medullary thyroid cancer over the past 30 years. Surgery. 2017;161(1):137–46.
48. Parghane RV, Naik C, Talole S, et al. Clinical utility of [177] Lu-DOTATATE PRRT in somatostatin receptor-positive metastatic medullary carcinoma of thyroid patients with assessment of efficacy, survival analysis, prognostic variables, and toxicity. Head Neck. 2020;42(3):401–16.
49. Wells SA Jr, Robinson BG, Gagel RF, et al. Vandetanib in patients with locally advanced or metastatic medullary thyroid cancer: a randomized, double-blind phase III trial [published correction appears in J Clin Oncol. 2013 Aug 20;31(24):3049]. J Clin Oncol. 2012;30(2):134–141.
50. Elisei R, Schlumberger MJ, Müller SP, et al. Cabozantinib in progressive medullary thyroid cancer [published correction appears in J Clin Oncol. 2014 Jun 10;32(17):1864]. J Clin Oncol. 2013;31(29):3639–3646.
51. Engelbach M, Görges R, Forst T, et al. Improved diagnostic methods in the follow-up of medullary thyroid carcinoma by highly specific calcitonin measurements. J Clin Endocrinol Metab. 2000;85(5):1890–4.
52. Ismailov SI, Piulatova NR. Postoperative calcitonin study in medullary thyroid carcinoma. Endocr Relat Cancer. 2004;11(2):357–63.

Paraganglioma and Pheochromocytoma

15

Maurizio Iacobone and Francesca Torresan

Introduction

Paraganglioma (PGL) and pheochromocytoma (PHEO) are rare neuroendocrine tumors arising from neural crest-derived chromaffin cells of the sympathetic and parasympathetic ganglia [1]. According to the World Health Organization (WHO) classification, the term PHEO is currently used for neuroendocrine chromaffin tumors of the adrenal medulla, and the term PGL for tumors of the extra-adrenal paraganglia. Parasympathetic-derived PGL arise from parasympathetic ganglia almost exclusively located along the branches of the cranial nerves in the neck and at the base of the skull (head and neck paraganglioma, HNPGL); sympathetic-derived PGL arise from extra-adrenal sympathetic ganglia of thorax, abdomen, and pelvis [2].

Usually, sympathetic PGL and PHEO tend to produce and secrete catecholamines, specifically epinephrine, norepinephrine, and dopamine. In contrast, around two-thirds of PGL of parasympathetic origin in the head and neck area are nonfunctional and present with mass-effect [1, 2].

Etiology

Even if most of PHEO/PGL are sporadic, about 40% are caused by specific germline mutation with a variable penetrance and clinical expressivity. In this setting PHEO/PGL may be also associated with other tumors (syndromic PHEO/PGL, Table 15.1) [3, 4]. Transcriptomic studies have shown that sporadic as well as

M. Iacobone (✉) · F. Torresan
Endocrine Surgery Unit, Department of Surgery, Oncology and Gastroenterology, University of Padua, Padua, Italy
e-mail: maurizio.iacobone@unipd.it

© Springer Nature Switzerland AG 2021
J. M. Cloyd, T. M. Pawlik (eds.), *Neuroendocrine Tumors*,
https://doi.org/10.1007/978-3-030-62241-1_15

Table 15.1 Genotype-phenotype correlation in syndromic pheochromocytomas/paragangliomas

Gene	Syndrome	Location	Rate of metastatic disease (%)	Multiple tumors (%)	Recurrence rate (%)	Associated tumors or clinical features
NF1,17q11.2	NF1	PHEO>> AT-PGL	1–9	25–50	11	Optic glioma, breast cancer MPNST, café-au-lait spots, freckles, and Lisch nodules
VHL,3p25.3	VHL	PHEO>> AT-PGL > HNPGL	1–9	>50	6	Hemangioblastoma, RCC, testicular tumors, pancreatic NET, and retinal abnormalities
RET, 10q11.2	MEN2	PHEO	<1	>50	17	MTC and primary hyperparathyroidism
SDHA,5p15.33	PGL5	HNPGL>PHEO+AT-PGL > PHEO	1–9	1–9	Unknown	GIST and pituitary tumors
SDHAF2,11q12.2	PGL2	HNPGL	Unknown	>50	Unknown	
SDHB,1p36.13	PGL4	AT-PGL > PHEO>HNPGL	25–50	10–24	20	RCC, GIST, and pituitary tumors
SDHC,1q23.3	PGL3	HNPGL>PHEO+AT-PGL	Unknown	10–24	Unknown	GIST and pituitary tumors
SDHD,11q23.1	PGL1	HNPGL>PHEO>AT-PGL	1–9	>50	58	RCC, GIST and pituitary tumors
TMEM127, 2q11.2	Familial PPGL TMEM 127-related	PHEO>> HNPGL	10–24	25–50	Unknown	
MAX	Familial PPGL MAX-related	PHEO	1–9	>50	Unknown	RCC
FH,1q42.1	HLRCC	PHEO and/or AT-PGL > HNPGL	3–5	3–5	Unknown	RCC and leiomyoma

MEN2 multiple endocrine neoplasia type 2; NF1 neurofibromatosis type 1; VHL Von Hippel-Lindau syndrome; PGL1–5 hereditary paraganglioma syndrome type 1–5; HLRCC hereditary leiomyomatosis and renal cell carcinoma; PHEO adrenal pheochromocytoma; AT-PGL abdomino-thoracic paraganglioma; HNPGL head and neck paraganglioma; MTC medullary thyroid cancer; MPNST malignant peripheral nerve sheath tumor; RCC renal cell carcinoma; NET neuroendocrine tumors hereditary PGL can be divided in two main clusters linked to two different signaling pathways. Cluster 1 tumors develop in presence of germline or somatic mutations of genes involved with the pseudo-hypoxic pathway response (including *VHL, EGLN1, SDH, IDH, HIF2A*, and *FH* genes). Cluster 2 tumors, including *RET, NF1, KIF1Bb, MAX*, and *TMEM127* mutated tumors, are associated with abnormal activation of kinase signaling pathways, leading to abnormal cell growth and diminished apoptosis capacity [5].

Pathology

PHEO and PGL originate from chief cells, which are neuroendocrine chromaffin cells expressing neuron-specific enolase (NSE), serotonin, and chromogranin. They often show enormous variability in cytologic and histologic pattern, and therefore must be distinguished from a variety of endocrine and non-endocrine tumors. In fact, the classic pattern of "zellballen" composed of clusters of chief cells surrounded by supportive sustentacular cells, is often not evident, and spindle cells, admixtures of large and small cells, and extreme cytologic atypia can be observed. For these reasons, the differential diagnosis of PHEO/PGL from other non-endocrine tumors may often require immunohistochemical staining of Chromogranin A (CgA), a major constituent of the matrix of catecholamine-containing secretory granules and the single most specific neuroendocrine marker for PHEO/PGL [6].

PHEO/PGL are usually benign tumors; malignancy occurs in 10–20% of cases. The diagnosis of malignancy may be challenging and no single histopathologic feature (including large tumor size, increased number of mitoses, DNA aneuploidy, extensive central necrosis of Zellballen, Ki67 labeling index, vascular and lymphatic invasion, and the presence of mitotic spindles) is alone able to identify malignant metastatic potential [7, 8].

Hence, several histologic algorithms have been developed to predict an aggressive behavior.

The Pheochromocytoma of Adrenal gland Scaled Score (PASS) first described in 2002 by Thompson [9] consists of 12 parameters, including large nests or diffuse growth, central or confluent necrosis, high cellularity, cellular monotony, tumor cell spindling, >3 mitotic figures/ten high- power fields, atypical mitotic figures, extension into adipose tissue, vascular invasion, capsular invasion, profound nuclear pleomorphism, and nuclear hyperchromasia. A maximum score of 20 points is obtained when all features are present. PHEO with a score <4 were considered to have no metastatic potential. Tumors with a score ≥4 were considered to have an increased metastatic potential. Thompson reported that all patients with a metastatic PHEO had PASS >4, but 34% of PASS >4 tumors did not metastasize in a follow-up period of approximately 5 years; one patient with a score of more than 15 did not metastasized in approximately 28 years. Moreover, it was further noted that a score of 3 or less does not guarantee that a patient will not develop metastases [9].

There is currently no agreement for the utility or reproducibility of the PASS score. A recent meta-analysis aiming to determine the value of the PASS algorithm in predicting malignancy found a sensitivity of 97% and a specificity of 68%. The positive predictive value (PPV) was 31%, and the negative predictive value (NPV) was 99%. These findings suggest that a PASS score <4 is highly indicative of a benign clinical course, but for tumors with PASS score ≥4, the predictive value with regard to disease course is limited [10].

In 2005 Kimura et al. [11] proposed the Grading of Adrenal Pheochromocytoma and Paraganglioma (GAPP) that can be applied for PHEO as well as PGL. It is based on histological pattern, cellularity, comedo-type necrosis, capsular invasion, vascular invasion, Ki67 labeling index, and catecholamine type. On the basis of a maximum score of 10 points, tumors are graded as well differentiated (0–2 points), moderately differentiated (3–6 points), and poorly differentiated (7–10 points). A sensitivity of 50% and specificity of 80% for detecting malignancy has been described for PHEO using GAPP classification. For PGL, the sensitivity was 100% and the specificity was 68%, with a PPV of 29% and a NPV of 100% [10]. Both PASS and GAPP have a low PPV but a high NPV, suggesting that these models are good at ruling out but poor at predicting metastatic potential.

In addition, a modified GAPP (M-GAPP) has been proposed, incorporating loss of Succinate Dehydrogenase Complex Iron Sulfur Subunit B *(SDHB)* staining as a criterion because of the increased metastatic risk related to *SDHB* mutations. Infact, recurrence and metastases are strongly associated with *SDHB* mutations. However, the loss of *SDHB* staining occurs with all SDHx mutations, and increased risk has not been noted for *SDHA, SDHC,* or *SDHD* mutations [12].

Due to the lack of standardized criteria for the prediction of biological behavior, according to the current WHO classification, malignancy is only diagnosed when metastasis to non-neuroendocrine tissue is demonstrated (e.g., lymph nodes, bone, liver, lung, and other distant metastatic sites) [2]. Therefore, since regional or distant metastases occur infrequently and often late after initial diagnosis, these tumors cannot be defined as benign by default and patients require continued lifelong surveillance.

Clinical Presentation

Pheochromocytoma and Extra-Adrenal Abdominal Paraganglioma

PHEO and sympathetic extra-adrenal abdominal PGL are usually characterized by clinical signs and symptoms that result from hemodynamic and metabolic actions of circulating catecholamines, or less frequently other amines and co-secreted neuropeptides (Table 15.2). Sustained or paroxysmal hypertension is the most common feature (85–90%). Paroxysmal signs and symptoms, due to the episodic nature of catecholamine secretion, such as hypertension, headache, spontaneous sweating, palpitations, and the presence of pallor are highly suggestive of PHEO/sympathetic PGL. Paroxysms can last minutes to hours and occur spontaneously or can be triggered by direct stimulation of the tumor (e.g.,

Table 15.2 Clinical symptoms and signs of pheochromocytoma and paraganglioma

Symptoms	Percentage
Headache	70–90
Palpitations ± tachycardia	50–70
Diaphoresis	60–70
Anxiety	20
Nervousness	35–40
Abdominal/chest pain	20–50
Nausea	26–43
Fatigue	15–40
Dyspnea	11–19
Dizziness	3–11
Heat intolerance	13–15
Pain/paresthesias	Up to 11
Visual symptoms	3–21
Constipation	10
Diarrhea	6
Signs	Percentage
Hypertension	90–100
Orthostatic hypotension	12
Pallor	30–60
Flushing	18
Fever	Up to 66
Hyperglycemia	42
Vomiting	26–43
Convulsions	3–5

palpation, a fall, and pregnancy), physical activity, ingestion of food or beverages containing tyramine (e.g., certain cheeses, beers, wines, bananas, and chocolate), diagnostic procedures, or certain drugs (e.g., anesthesia, metoclopramide, phenothiazine, methyldopa, monoamine oxidase inhibitors, tricyclic antidepressants, and opiates) [13].

Predominantly epinephrine or dopamine secreting PHEO/sympathetic PGL may also present with hypotension, particularly postural hypotension usually accompanied by orthostatic tachycardia. Other typical signs and symptoms are palpitations, due to the effect of catecholamines (especially epinephrine) on cardiac β-adrenergic receptors, pallor due to catecholamine-induced cutaneous vasoconstriction, more severe episodes of anxiety or panic attacks, fever, and constipation [14].

Some patients with PHEO have a subnormal level of plasma insulin that may cause hyperglycemia and diabetes mellitus, due to α2-adrenergic inhibition of insulin release, epinephrine-induced inhibition of glucose uptake by skeletal muscle, α-adrenergic stimulation of hepatic glucose production, and β-adrenergic receptor desensitization [15]. About 8–10% of patients with a small and non-significant catecholamine-secreting tumor may be completely asymptomatic and normotensive.

Parasympathetic HNPGL

The majority of HNPGL are non-secreting, benign, and slow-growing tumors. They may arise from parasympathetic head and neck paraganglia of the carotid body (60%), middle ear (30%), vagal (10%), and larynx (very rarely). The clinical presentation of HNPGL is often an asymptomatic incidentally detected neck mass, but considerable morbidity due to compression or infiltration of the adjacent structures and cranial nerve palsy with mass-effect symptoms may occur [16]. Carotid body HNPGL, located just anterior to the sternocleidomastoid muscle at the level of the hyoid, usually present as a slow-growing, nontender, painless cervical mass that may transmit the carotid pulse. Large compressive tumors that enlarge around the carotid vessels and the X–XII cranial nerves (30% of the cases) may result in cranial nerves paralysis and symptoms like dysphagia, odynophagia, or hoarseness of voice. Moreover, invasion or compression of cervical sympathetic chain and carotid sinus may lead to Horner's syndrome and syncope, respectively [17].

Tympanic and jugular foramen tumors most commonly present as a vascular middle ear mass causing pulsatile tinnitus and hearing loss. Vagal PGL are highly vascularized tumors that usually originate in the nodal ganglion, and are located behind the angle of the mandible and the internal carotid artery in the parapharyngeal space. Medial tumor growth can lead to voice changes, foreign body sensation, or dysphagia. Symptoms of lower cranial nerve deficits (IX, X, XI, and XII) like dysphagia and hoarseness and sympathetic deficits are frequent [18].

In a minority of cases, HNPGL are catecholamine-producing and lead to symptoms like fluctuating hypertension, blushing, obstructive sleep apnea, and palpitations.

Diagnosis

Pheochromocytoma and Extra-Adrenal abdominal Paraganglioma

Prerequisite prior to order biochemical testing is the exclusion of those conditions that can mimic a catecholamine-secreting tumor or cause falsely elevated test results, such as certain drugs like amphetamines or cocaine. Hence, a complete medical history including family history, physical examination, and the assessment of factors that may provoke paroxysmal crises should be firstly assessed [19]. Moreover, as PHEO/sympathetic PGL may be part of hereditary syndromes (e.g., von Hippel-Lindau disease and multiple endocrine neoplasia type 2 syndrome), the other clinical and biochemical features of these syndromes should be investigated.

According to the recommendations of the recent Endocrine Society guidelines, biochemical testing of plasma-free or urinary daily fractioned metanephrines are the tests of choice to screen for PHEO/sympathetic PGL, since metanephrines have a longer half-life and are produced continuously within the tumor [1]. Plasma-free metanephrines have higher sensitivity (96–100%) to rule out a diagnosis of catecholamine-secreting tumor compared to 24-h urine fractionated metanephrines (77–90%), but a lower specificity (85–89% vs. 93–98%). Metanephrines levels greater than 2–3 times the upper normal limit carry a near 100% positive predictive value for sympathetic PGL and PHEO. Similarly, a metanephrine level that is less than one time the upper normal limit has a very high negative predictive value [20]. Dopamine and its metabolite 3-methoxytyramine should be also tested, in particular in those patients with *SDHB* and *SDHD*-related PGL [21].

Computed tomography (CT) scanning and magnetic resonance imaging (MRI) are both considered gold standards for PHEO/sympathetic PGL localization. On CT, they usually present with a tissue density of more than ten Hounsfield Units (HU) with areas of low density that correspond to hemorrhage and necrosis (Fig. 15.1). On MRI, they present as a mass absent of fat, with a high signal on T2

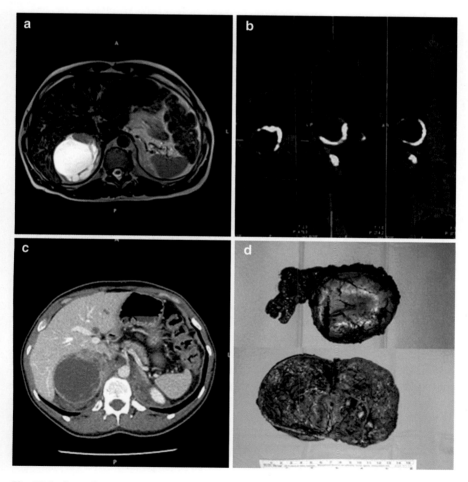

Fig. 15.1 Sporadic pheochromocytoma. (**a**) Abdominal Magnetic Resonance Imaging showing a 10 cm right adrenal mass with high signal on T2 sequences. (**b**) 18F-DOPA-PET uptake. (**c**) CT scan imaging. (**d**) surgical specimen, intact and sectioned

sequences as a result of their hypervascularity [22]. CT has a better spatial resolution than MRI, the latter been reserved for patients with metastatic disease, for lifelong screening, and for those patients in which CT should be avoided (allergy to CT contrast, children, and pregnant women).

The second and complementary imaging step is functional imaging that provides a higher specificity than radiological imaging and is particularly recommended for diagnosis of multifocal or metastatic disease. ^{123}I-metaiodobenzylguanidine (MIBG) single-photon emission computed tomography (SPECT) shows excellent sensitivity (nearly 100%) for detection of PHEO but low for extra-adrenal thoracic-abdominal PGL, metastases, and sympathetic SDHx-related PGL. In case of MIBG avid lesions, ^{123}I-MIBG is very useful to identify patients that may benefit from treatment with therapeutic doses of ^{131}I-MIBG.

More recently, novel functional imaging using ^{18}F-Fluorodihydroxyphenylalan ine (^{18}F-DOPA) (Fig. 15.2), ^{18}F-Fluorodeoxyglucose (^{18}F-FDG), and ^{68}Ga-labeled somatostatin analogues positron emission tomography (PET)-CT has achieved better sensitivity and resolution than SPECT scintigraphy. ^{18}F-DOPAPET-CT has a higher sensitivity for the localization of non-metastatic PGL (98–100%), while ^{18}F-FDG PET-CT for the detection of PGL metastases (97%), especially in *SDHB*-related cases [23, 24].

Parasympathetic HNPGL

Even if predominantly non-secreting tumors, some HNPGL secrete catecholamine metabolites and up to 32% of HNPGL are dopaminergic; symptoms in such cases may include palpitations, diaphoresis, and hypertension [23, 25]. Therefore, initial biochemical screening including measurements of plasma-free or urinary fractionated metanephrines and 3-methoxytyramine is also required for HNPGL. Anatomical imaging in HNPGL should include CT and/or MRI; nowadays, ultrasound has a limited diagnostic role but can be useful especially in carotid body PGL. MRI provides more diagnostic information than CT for evaluation of HNPGL, because of the better soft tissue contrast and characterization of tumor extension and vessel encasement. Angiography can be performed for preoperative endovascular embolization in order to minimize intraoperative blood loss [26].

Functional radionuclide imaging techniques are crucial and unavoidable to fully evaluate the extent of the disease and multifocality. Somatostatin receptor scintigraphy using ^{111}In-diethylene-triamine-pentaacetate acid-octreotide (Octreoscan) has been used to localize PGL, since they overexpress somatostatin receptors, with a sensitivity of 75–100%, even if small sized lesions are not detectable even by the best available cameras. More recently, ^{18}F-DOPAPET-CT and ^{68}Ga-labeled somatostatin analogues PET-CT have been introduced as an alternative to Octreoscan, with a sensitivity and specificity close to 100% [26, 27].

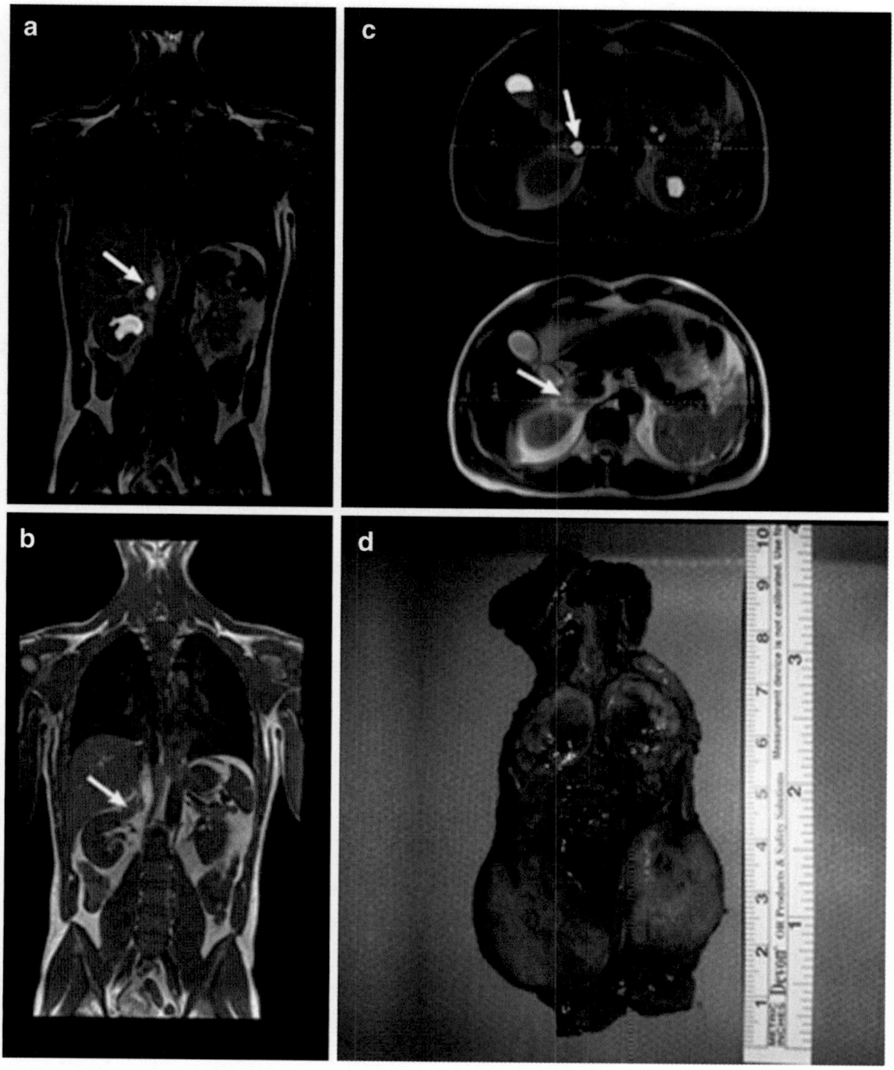

Fig. 15.2 Hereditary MEN-2A related pheochromocytoma. (**a–c**) 18F-DOPAPET/Magnetic Resonance Imaging showing a 2 cm right adrenal mass (arrow). (**d**) Surgical specimen showing multifocal pheochromocytoma, sectioned

Genetic Testing

Since about 40% of PHEO/PGL have a germline mutation in one of the 12 actually known susceptibility genes, genetic testing is strongly indicated in presence of a positive family history of PHEO/PGL, syndromic features, young patients or metastatic disease; however, it should probably be considered in all patients. The genes most frequently mutated are *SDHB* and *VHL* while *MAX, TMEM127, MDH2, SDHAF2*, and *FH* are less frequently mutated. Interestingly, the genotype of syndromic PHEO/PGL influences the phenotype in terms of secretion, age at onset, tumor aggressiveness, clinical presentation and associated diseases/neoplasia, and anatomic site of origin [28]. For example, mutations of *SDHB* gene are associated with an increased risk of development of metastatic disease (40–60%) [29, 30]. Identification of a gene mutation provides earlier detection of PHEO/PGL and other neoplasms, allowing a reduction of morbidity, more personalized approach, and an improvement of survival. Finally, all mutation carriers should receive at least annual biochemical surveillance for PHEO/PGL, and periodic radiological imaging of neck and/or thorax/abdomen, depending on the mutation, with additional functional imaging in selected cases [1].

Treatment and Outcome

Pheochromocytoma and Extra-Adrenal Abdominal Paraganglioma

Surgery is the treatment of choice for PHEO and extra-adrenal abdominal PGL. However, prior to surgery, a multidisciplinary evaluation and a proper medical treatment are essential and propaedeutic in order to avoid surgical complications and fatal sequelae. As pointed by the 2014 Endocrine Society guidelines, selective α-adrenergic receptor blockers (Doxazosin) are the recommended first choice drugs to avoid hypertensive crisis and arrhythmias [1]. However, a recent meta-analysis aiming to assess the potential benefit of preoperative α-blockade showed no differences in terms of systolic or diastolic BP, heart rate, cardiovascular complications, or mortality between patients treated or not with α-blockers [31]. Recent retrospective monocentric and multicentric studies seem to confirm these results [32, 33].

Even if some studies found calcium channel blockers effective as α-adrenergic receptor blockers, their use as monotherapy is not usually recommended [34, 35]. β-adrenoceptor blockers may be preoperatively used to control tachyarrhythmias only after administration of α-adrenergic receptor blockers, since hypertensive crisis due to unopposed stimulation of α-adrenergic receptors may occur.

Minimally invasive adrenalectomy, either through transperitoneal or through posterior retroperitoneal approach, is the preferred surgical technique for PHEO. Safety and efficacy of laparoscopic adrenalectomy, in terms of reduced pain, blood loss, hospital stay, and surgical morbidity, is well-documented in several large series [1, 3, 36–38]. Moreover, some studies provide evidence of significantly lower overall complication rates performing laparoscopic adrenalectomy (10.9% vs. 35.8% by open resections) [39].

First reported in 1995 [40], posterior retroperitoneoscopic adrenalectomy allows a direct approach to the adrenal glands. This approach provides an excellent exposure of adrenal gland avoiding the peritoneal cavity and, therefore, is often preferred for patients with a history of abdominal surgery. Other reported advantages to this technique are the decreased operative time, the low conversion rate, and the minimal dissection of surrounding tissues [41]. However, if retroperitoneoscopic approach is superior to laparoscopic approach remains unclear. In one prospective randomized controlled trial [42], operative time, blood loss, postoperative pain, and length of hospitalization were reported to be lower after retroperitoneoscopic than laparoscopic adrenalectomy. To the contrary, three prospective randomized controlled trials found no significant differences in these major outcome endpoints between the two techniques [43–45]. In the setting of bilateral disease, the theoretical advantage of posterior retroperitoneoscopic adrenalectomy is that the change in patient position is not required.

Minimally invasive adrenalectomy is also the preferred surgical approach for cortical-sparing adrenalectomy, a surgical technique in which at least one-third of vascularized adrenal gland is left to maintain the normal function of the adrenal cortex. The 2014 Endocrine Society guidelines [1] suggested cortical-sparing adrenalectomy for bilateral and hereditary PHEO because of the low risk of malignancy and the acceptably low rate of recurrence [1, 3, 46]. A recent retrospective series of 625 patients enrolled in 19 countries followed up for a median of eight years, showed a recurrence rate of PHEO in the spared ipsilateral adrenal gland of 13% (mostly in Von Hippel-Lindau [VHL] syndrome and multiple endocrine neoplasia type 2 [MEN2] patients), and adrenal insufficiency in 23% and at least one addisonian crisis in 18% of patients. Only three patients (5%) died of metastatic PHEO.

Evidence for surgery in the setting of metastatic PHEO is very limited. The resection of the primary tumors, when feasible, is generally advocated in order to reduce catecholamine-related cardiovascular mortality and may increase the efficacy of subsequent systemic therapies such as chemotherapy and radiopharmaceuticals. The preferred surgical approach for malignant PHEO is usually laparotomic. It facilitates the resection of the primary tumor, avoiding tumor rupture, and eventually locoregional and/or isolated resectable distant metastases.

Given the advances in preoperative localization, genetics, and laparoscopic techniques, minimally invasive surgery is nowadays considered the preferred surgical approach also for extra-adrenal abdominal PGL. The conversion rate from endoscopic to open surgery is about 5%, the reasons being large size of the tumor, malignancy, and bleeding. In some series, the retroperitoneal approach with "no touch technique" seemed to be better than transperitoneal in extra-adrenal PGL, in particular for suprarenal PGL, bilateral tumors and in the presence of previous abdominal surgery [47–49]. However, the minimally invasive approach to PGL is often challenged by tumor anatomical location and size. In fact, PGLs are often directly adjacent to structures that require protection, such as the ureter and/or the iliac vein in genitourinary PGL, or major vascular structures such as the inferior vena cava and aorta from which very short arterial vessels come off. For these reasons, the Endocrine Society guidelines suggest a conventional open approach for extra-adrenal abdominal PGL, reserving the endoscopic approach to experienced surgeons for small, noninvasive PGL in favorable anatomical sites [1]. Moreover, the endoscopic approach should be avoided in high-risk germline mutation carriers, such as *SDHB*, that present PGL in unfavorable location and/or with radiographic or clinical evidence of local invasion [50].

A postoperative lifelong annual follow-up to screen for locoregional or distant recurrence or new tumors should be performed, especially in patients with high-risk hereditary PGL [23].

Chemotherapy and radionuclide treatment using beta-emitting isotopes coupled with MIBG or somatostatin analogue may provide symptomatic and biochemical control in metastatic disease and unresectable lesions but are less effective in improving survival. External radiotherapy may be considered for treatment of inoperable PGL and especially for palliation of painful bone metastases [51]. Targeted therapy with receptor tyrosine kinase inhibitors has been tested in the treatment of malignant PGL, with some promising results [52].

Parasympathetic HNPGL

The management and treatment of HNPGL must take into consideration their location, tumor growth velocity and size, patient age and medical condition, multifocality, and genotype. Surgery is the treatment of choice, aiming to achieve and prevent local destruction of adjacent cranial nerves. However, even if mortality due to vascular complications is actually near 0% compared to 30–40% of historical series, surgical morbidity due to cranial nerve involvement remains significant [53].

Surgical resection of carotid body PGL is associated with cranial nerve (vagal, superior laryngeal, hypoglossal and accessory) or sympathetic trunk palsies, and vascular complications in more than 15% of cases. Hence, surgical treatment is usually planned according to the Shamblin classification [53]. Shamblin Class I carotid body PGL are usually small; Class II PGL usually surround the carotid vessels and are technically more difficult to resect; Class III PGL typically require the interruption of cerebral circulation since the tumor completely encases the carotid vessels. The reported rate of permanent nerve palsy and vascular injuries are significantly higher in Shamblin Class III compared to Class I/II carotid body (35.7% vs. 2.3%, respectively, $p < 0.001$) [54].

The preoperative transarterial embolization of these tumors has been reported but with debatable results [55]. Moreover, given the presence of multiple arteries and anastomoses between external and internal carotid arteries, the identification of the feeding arteries of the tumor can be complicated and the incidence of stroke is reported to be more than 10%.

Therefore, since most tumors grow slowly, a wait-and-scan policy and active surveillance is often advised.

Treatment strategies for jugulotympanic PGL include microsurgery, preoperative embolization followed by surgical resection, fractionated external beam radiotherapy, and gamma knife radiosurgery. Surgery for vagal PGL is the treatment of choice in young patients and in presence of intracranial extension, but radiotherapy may be considered in large unresectable tumors. Surgical resection of laryngeal PGL includes open resection, microlaryngoscopy with laser excision, and endoscopic removal [3].

Conclusions

In summary, PHEO and PGL are rare neuroendocrine tumors arising from adrenal medulla and extra-adrenal sympathetic or parasympathetic paraganglia, respectively. The diagnostic evaluation and optimal management require an experienced multidisciplinary team. Surgical resection is the only curative strategy for PHEO and PGL although given the significant morbidity in some HNPGL, a wait-and-scan policy is occasionally preferred. Minimally invasive approaches, either transperitoneal or retroperitoneoscopic, are now recommended for PHEO and most abdominal PGL and partial adrenalectomy should be considered for hereditary or bilateral PHEO. Given the risk of both locoregional or distant recurrent, lifelong surveillance is recommended.

References

1. Lenders JWM, Duh QY, Eisenhofer G, Gimenez-Roqueplo AP, Grebe SKG, Murad MH, Naruse M, Pacak K, Young WF. Pheochromocytoma and paraganglioma: an endocrine society clinical practice guideline. J Clin Endocrinol Metab. 2014;99:1915–42.
2. Lloyd RV, Osamura RY, Klöppel G, Rosai J. WHO Classification of Tumours of Endocrine Organs. 4th ed. Lyon: International Agency for Research on Cancer (IARC); 2017.
3. Iacobone M, Belluzzi A, Torresan F. Surgical approaches and results of treatment for hereditary paragangliomas. Best Pract Res Clin Endocrinol Metab. 2019;33:101298.
4. Neumann HPH, Young WF, Eng C. Pheochromocytoma and paraganglioma. N Engl J Med. 2019;381:552–65.
5. Yao L, Schiavi F, Cascon A, Qin Y, Inglada-Pérez L, King EE, Toledo RA, Ercolino T, Rapizzi E, Ricketts CJ, Mori L, Giacchè M, Mendola A, Taschin E, Boaretto F, Loli P, Iacobone M, Rossi GP, Biondi B, et al. Spectrum and prevalence of FP/TMEM127 gene mutations in pheochromocytomas and paragangliomas. JAMA 2010;304:2611–9.
6. Tischler AS. Pheochromocytoma and extra-adrenal paraganglioma: updates. Arch Pathol Lab Med. 2008;132:1272–84.
7. Scholz T, Schulz C, Klose S, Lehnert H. Diagnostic management of benign and malignant pheochromocytoma. Exp Clin Endocrinol Diabetes. 2007;115:155–9.
8. Ilona Linnoila R, Keiser HR, Steinberg SM, Lack EE. Histopathology of benign versus malignant sympathoadrenal paragangliomas: Clinicopathologic study of 120 cases including unusual histologic features. Hum Pathol. 1990;21:1168–80.
9. Thompson LDR. Pheochromocytoma of the adrenal gland scaled score (PASS) to separate benign from malignant neoplasms: a clinicopathologic and immunophenotypic study of 100 cases. Am J Surg Pathol. 2002;26:551–66.
10. Stenman A, Zedenius J, Juhlin CC. The value of histological algorithms to predict the malignancy potential of pheochromocytomas and abdominal paragangliomas – a meta-analysis and systematic review of the literature. Cancers (Basel). 2019;11:225.
11. Kimura N, Watanabe T, Noshiro T, Shizawa S, Miura Y. Histological grading of adrenal and extra-adrenal pheochromocytomas and relationship to prognosis: a clinicopathological analysis of 116 adrenal pheochromocytomas and 30 extra-adrenal sympathetic paragangliomas including 38 malignant tumors. Endocr Pathol. 2005;16:23–32.
12. Koh JM, Ahn SH, Kim H, Kim BJ, Sung TY, Kim YH, Hong SJ, Song DE, Lee SH. Validation of pathological grading systems for predicting metastatic potential in pheochromocytoma and paraganglioma. PLoS One. 2017;12:e0187398.

13. Lenders JWM, Eisenhofer G. Pathophysiology and diagnosis of disorders of the adrenal medulla: focus on pheochromocytoma. Compr Physiol. 2014;4:691–713.
14. Pacak K, Lenders JWM, Eisenhofer G. Pheochromocytoma: diagnosis, localization, and treatment. Malden, MA: Wiley-Blackwell; 2007.
15. Colwell JA. Inhibition of insulin secretion by catecholamines in pheochromocytoma. Ann Intern Med. 1969;71:251–6.
16. Taïeb D, Varoquaux A, Chen CC, Pacak K. Current and future trends in the anatomical and functional imaging of head and neck paragangliomas. Semin Nucl Med. 2013;43:462–73.
17. Patetsios P, Gable DR, Garrett WV, Lamont JP, Kuhn JA, Shutze WP, Kourlis H, Grimsley B, Pearl GJ, Smith BL, Talkington CM, Thompson JE. Management of carotid body paragangliomas and review of a 30-year experience. Ann Vasc Surg. 2002;16:331–8.
18. González-Orús Álvarez-Morujo R, Arístegui Ruiz M, Martin Oviedo C, Álvarez Palacios I, Scola Yurrita B. Management of vagal paragangliomas: review of 17 patients. Eur Arch Otorhinolaryngol. 2015;272:2403–14.
19. Lenders JWM, Eisenhofer G, Mannelli M, Pacak K. Phaeochromocytoma. Lancet. 2005;366:665–75.
20. Lenders JWM, Pacak K, Walther MM, Marston Linehan W, Mannelli M, Friberg P, Keiser HR, Goldstein DS, Eisenhofer G. Biochemical diagnosis of pheochromocytoma: which test is best? JAMA. 2002;287:1427–34.
21. Eisenhofer G, Peitzsch M. Laboratory evaluation of pheochromocytoma and paraganglioma. Clin Chem. 2014;60:1486–99.
22. Ilias I, Sahdev A, Reznek RH, Grossman AB, Pacak K. The optimal imaging of adrenal tumours: a comparison of different methods. Endocr Relat Cancer. 2007;14:587–99.
23. Plouin PF, Amar L, Dekkers OM, Fassnach M, Gimenez-Roqueplo AP, Lenders JWM, Lussey-Lepoutre C, Steichen O. European society of endocrinology clinical practice guideline for long-term follow-up of patients operated on for a phaeochromocytoma or a paraganglioma. Eur J Endocrinol. 2016;174:G1–10.
24. Barollo S, Bertazza L, Watutantrige-Fernando S, Censi S, Cavedon E, Galuppini F, Pennelli G, Fassina A, Citton M, Rubin B, Pezzani R, Benna C, Opocher G, Iacobone M, Mian C. Overexpression of L-type amino acid transporter 1 (LAT1) and 2 (LAT2): novel markers of neuroendocrine tumors. PLoS One. 2016;11:e0156044.
25. Williams MD. Paragangliomas of the head and neck: an overview from diagnosis to genetics. Head Neck Pathol. 2017;11:278–87.
26. Timmers HJLM, Taieb D, Pacak K. Current and future anatomical and functional imaging approaches to pheochromocytoma and paraganglioma. Horm Metab Res. 2012;44:367–72.
27. King KS, Chen CC, Alexopoulos DK, Whatley MA, Reynolds JC, Patronas N, Ling A, Adams KT, Xekouki P, Lando H, Stratakis CA, Pacak K. Functional imaging of SDHx-related head and neck paragangliomas: comparison of 18F-fluorodihydroxyphenylalanine, 18F-fluorodopamine, 18F-fluoro-2-deoxy-D-glucose PET, 123I-metaiodobenzylguanidine scintigraphy, and 111in-pentetreotide scintigraphy. J Clin Endocrinol Metab. 2011;96:2779–85.
28. Iacobone M, Citton M, Viel G, Schiavone D, Torresan F. Surgical approaches in hereditary endocrine tumors. Updat Surg. 2017;69:181–91.
29. Mannelli M, Castellano M, Schiavi F, Filetti S, Giacchè M, Mori L, Pignataro V, Bernini G, Giachè V, Bacca A, Biondi B, Corona G, Di Trapani G, Grossrubatscher E, Reimondo G, Arnaldi G, Giacchetti G, Veglio F, Loli P, et al. Clinically guided genetic screening in a large cohort of Italian patients with pheochromocytomas and/or functional or nonfunctional paragangliomas. J Clin Endocrinol Metab. 2009;94:1541–7.
30. Iacobone M, Schiavi F, Bottussi M, Taschin E, Bobisse S, Fassina A, Opocher G, Favia G. Is genetic screening indicated in apparently sporadic pheochromocytomas and paragangliomas? Surgery. 2011;150:1194–201.
31. Schimmack S, Kaiser J, Probst P, Kalkum E, Diener MK, Strobel O. Meta-analysis of α-blockade versus no blockade before adrenalectomy for phaeochromocytoma. Br J Surg. 2020;107:e102–8.

32. Groeben H, Walz MK, Nottebaum BJ, Alesina PF, Greenwald A, Schumann R, Hollmann MW, Schwarte L, Behrends M, Rössel T, Groeben C, Schäfer M, Lowery A, Hirata N, Yamakage M, Miller JA, Cherry TJ, Nelson A, Solorzano CC, et al. International multicentre review of perioperative management and outcome for catecholamine-producing tumours. Br J Surg. 2020;107:e170–8.

33. Buisset C, Guerin C, Cungi PJ, Gardette M, Paladino NC, Taïeb D, Cuny T, Castinetti F, Sebag F. Pheochromocytoma surgery without systematic preoperative pharmacological preparation: insights from a referral tertiary center experience. Surg Endosc. 2020. https://doi.org/10.1007/s00464-020-07439-1.

34. Siddiqi HK, Yang H, Laird AM, Fox AC, Doherty GM, Miller BS, Gauger PG, Sidell N, Verity MA, Nord EP. Utility of oral nicardipine and magnesium sulfate infusion during preparation and resection of pheochromocytomas. Surgery. 2012;152:1027–36.

35. Brunaud L, Boutami M, Nguyen-Thi P-L, Finnerty B, Germain A, Weryha G, Fahey TJ III, Mirallie E, Bresler L, Zarnegar R, Brunner U, Gensthaler BM, Bruno NA, Carver LA, Slate DL. Both preoperative alpha and calcium channel blockade impact intraoperative hemodynamic stability similarly in the management of pheochromocytoma. Surgery. 2014;156:1410–7.

36. Gagner M, Lacroix A, Prinz RA, Bolte E, Albala D, Potvin C, Hamet P, Querin S, Pomp A. Early experience with laparoscopic approach for adrenalectomy. Surgery. 1993;114:1120–5.

37. Gagner M, Pomp A, Todd Heniford B, Pharand D, Lacroix A. Laparoscopic adrenalectomy: lessons learned from 100 consecutive procedures. Ann Surg. 1997;226:238–47.

38. Brunt LM, Doherty GM, Norton JA, Soper NJ, Quasebarth MA, Moley JF. Laparoscopic adrenalectomy compared to open adrenalectomy for benign adrenal neoplasms. J Am Coll Surg. 1996;183:1–10.

39. Assalia A, Gagner M. Laparoscopic adrenalectomy. Br J Surg. 2004;91:1259–74.

40. Mercan S, Seven R, Ozarmagan S, Tezelman S. Endoscopic retroperitoneal adrenalectomy. Surgery. 1995;118:1071–5.

41. Walz MK, Alesina PF, Wenger FA, Deligiannis A, Szuczik E, Petersenn S, Ommer A, Groeben H, Peitgen K, Janssen OE, Philipp T, Neumann HPH, Schmid KW, Mann K. Posterior retroperitoneoscopic adrenalectomy-results of 560 procedures in 520 patients. Surgery. 2006;140:943–50.

42. Barczyński M, Konturek A, Nowak W. Randomized clinical trial of posterior retroperitoneoscopic adrenalectomy versus lateral transperitoneal laparoscopic adrenalectomy with a 5-year follow-up. Ann Surg. 2014;260:740–7.

43. Rubinstein M, Gill IS, Aron M, Kilciler M, Meraney AM, Finelli A, Moinzadeh A, Ukimura O, Desai MM, Kaouk J, Bravo E. Prospective, randomized comparison of transperitoneal versus retroperitoneal laparoscopic adrenalectomy. J Urol. 2005;174:442–5.

44. Mohammadi-Fallah MR, Mehdizadeh A, Badalzadeh A, Izadseresht B, Dadkhah N, Barbod A, Babaie M, Hamedanchi S. Comparison of transperitoneal versus retroperitoneal laparoscopic adrenalectomy in a prospective randomized study. J Laparoendosc Adv Surg Tech. 2013;23:362–6.

45. Chai YJ, Yu HW, Song R-Y, Kim S, Choi JY, Lee KE. Lateral transperitoneal adrenalectomy versus posterior retroperitoneoscopic adrenalectomy for benign adrenal gland disease. Ann Surg. 2019;269:842–8.

46. Castinetti F, Taieb D, Henry JF, Walz M, Guerin C, Brue T, Conte-Devolx B, Neumann HPH, Sebag F. Outcome of adrenal sparing surgery in heritable pheochromocytoma. Eur J Endocrinol. 2016;174:R9–R18.

47. Walz MK, Peitgen K, Neumann HPH, Janssen OE, Philipp T, Mann K. Endoscopic treatment of solitary, bilateral, multiple, and recurrent pheochromocytomas and paragangliomas. World J Surg. 2002;26:1005–12.

48. Mitchell J, Siperstein A, Milas M, Berber E. Laparoscopic resection of abdominal paragangliomas. Surg Laparosc Endosc Percutan Tech. 2011;21:e48-53.

49. Park JS, Lee KY, Kim JK, Yoon DS. The first laparoscopic resection of extra-adrenal pheochromocytoma using the da Vinci® robotic system. J Laparoendosc Adv Surg Tech. 2009;19:63–5.

50. Nockel P, El Lakis M, Gaitanidis A, Yang L, Merkel R, Patel D, Nilubol N, Prodanov T, Pacak K, Kebebew E. Preoperative genetic testing in pheochromocytomas and paragangliomas influences the surgical approach and the extent of adrenal surgery. Surgery. 2018;163:191–6.
51. Frilling A, Weber F, Saner F, Bockisch A, Hofmann M, Mueller-Brand J, Broelsch CE. Treatment with 90Y- and 177Lu-DOTATOC in patients with metastatic neuroendocrine tumors. Surgery. 2006;140:968–77.
52. Ferrara AM, Lombardi G, Pambuku A, Meringolo D, Bertorelle R, Nardin M, Schiavi F, Iacobone M, Opocher G, Zagonel V, Zovato S. Temozolomide treatment of a malignant pheochromocytoma and an unresectable MAX-related paraganglioma. Anti-Cancer Drugs. 2018;29:102–5.
53. Schneider R, Ukkat J, Nguyen-Thanh P, Lorenz K, Sekulla C, Dralle H, Plontke S, Behrmann C. Endocrine surgery for neck paraganglioma: operation, radiation therapy or wait and scan? Chirurg. 2012;83:1060–7.
54. Shamblin WR, ReMine WH, Sheps SG, Harrison EG. Carotid body tumor (chemodectoma). Clinicopathologic analysis of ninety cases. Am J Surg. 1971;122:732–9.
55. Abu-Ghanem S, Yehuda M, Carmel NN, et al. Impact of preoperative embolization on the outcomes of carotid body tumor surgery: a meta-analysis and review of the literature. Head Neck 2016;38(1):E2386e94.

Merkel Cell Carcinoma

16

Julie Howle and Michael Veness

Introduction

Merkel cell carcinoma (MCC) is an aggressive cutaneous malignancy first described in 1971 by Toker as a "trabecular carcinoma" originating in the dermis [1]. The exact cell of origin is not known and originally was thought to have arisen from Merkel cells, slowly adapting mechanoreceptors, located in the skin. However, more recent research has suggested alternative cells of origin, including epidermal or dermal stem cells or pre-/pro-B cells [2].

Epidemiology

Compared to malignant melanoma and other nonmelanoma skin cancers (NMSC), MCC is rare. Its incidence increases with age and is higher in men than women [3]. Australia has the highest reported incidence of MCC in the world with a rate of 1.6/100000/year [4].

The global incidence of MCC is increasing, and in the United States, the incidence almost doubled between 2000 and 2013 which may, in part, be due to improvements in diagnosis with the use of immunohistochemical stains, but, more importantly, an aging population and increasing levels of immunosuppression in the community [3].

MCC occurs most frequently in Caucasians, and its incidence is correlated with ultraviolet (UV) index [5]. Immunosuppression is also a risk factor for developing

J. Howle (✉)
Department of Surgery, Westmead Hospital, Sydney, NSW, Australia
e-mail: julie.howle@health.nsw.gov.au

M. Veness
Department of Radiation Oncology, Westmead Hospital, Sydney, NSW, Australia
e-mail: michael.veness@health.nsw.gov.au

© Springer Nature Switzerland AG 2021
J. M. Cloyd, T. M. Pawlik (eds.), *Neuroendocrine Tumors*,
https://doi.org/10.1007/978-3-030-62241-1_16

MCC [6]. MCC is more common in immunosuppressed patients than in the general population, with higher rates reported in patients with HIV [7] and hematological malignancies, such as chronic lymphocytic leukemia [8], and in solid organ transplant recipients [9]. Patients that are immunosuppressed make up 10% of all patients diagnosed with MCC and have a worse outcome, despite treatment, with a higher disease-specific mortality [10].

Pathogenesis

MCC carcinogenesis is thought to occur along two separate etiological pathways: one involving Merkel cell polyomavirus (MCV) infection and the other mediated by chronic UV radiation exposure. The MCV, first identified in 2008, is a double-stranded DNA virus that is clonally integrated in 80% of MCCs arising in patients in the Northern Hemisphere [11] but is present in only 20–25% of MCC in Southern Hemisphere countries such as Australia and New Zealand [12].

Unlike MCC, MCV infection is common with antibodies to the major capsid protein present in over 60% of the population [13]. It has been proposed that two events are required for MCC to develop: clonal integration of MCV and expression of viral oncoproteins (large T and small T antigens) [14]. Antibodies to MCV oncoprotein (T antigen) are found in approximately half of all viral positive MCC patients [15], and titers of these antibodies are an indicator of tumor burden and in seropositive patients may be measured to monitor for recurrence [16].

Viral-negative MCC is a consequence of chronic UV exposure and has a high mutation burden associated with a UV DNA damage signature [17]. Compared to MCV-associated MCC, viral-negative patients are thought to experience a higher risk of recurrence and a worse prognosis [18].

Clinical Presentation

MCC typically presents as a rapidly growing pink/purple cutaneous nodule arising in older Caucasian (median age 70–75 years) males on sun-exposed cutaneous sites, particularly in the head and neck region, but can also involve the trunk and extremities [6] (Fig. 16.1). It may be mistaken for another cutaneous malignancy such as basal cell carcinoma, dermal metastasis, and lymphoma or for a benign lesion such as a cyst or abscess.

Most patients (60–65%) will present with localized disease (stage I/II), with the remaining 20–35% presenting with clinically evident nodal disease [19]. Around 30% of patients presenting with stage I or II disease will have occult metastatic MCC identified following sentinel lymph node biopsy (SLNB) [20]. Distant sites of metastatic MCC at initial diagnosis are uncommon, occurring in <5% of patients, and the most common sites of distant metastases are the distant lymph nodes, lungs, liver, bone, and brain. Around 4% of all patients with MCC present with metastatic nodal disease of unknown primary [19]. This group of patients can account for up

Fig. 16.1 MCC typically presents as a pink nodule in sun-exposed skin

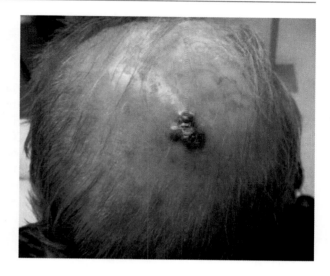

to half of patients who present with clinically evident nodal disease [21–23] and have a better prognosis than patients with a known primary [19].

Staging and Prognosis

The main determinants of prognosis are primary tumor diameter and nodal status [19]. Histologic factors associated with better prognosis include the absence of lymphovascular invasion, a nodular growth pattern, and a lower depth of invasion, [24] while immunosuppression and virus-negative tumors are associated with a worse prognosis [10, 18].

MCC is staged according to the American Joint Committee on Cancer (AJCC) TNM system. The eighth and most recent version of the AJCC system [25], based on analysis of over 9000 patients [19], separates clinical and pathological nodal stages; stages I and II represent local disease, stage III includes microscopic (IIIa) and macroscopic nodal disease, and stage IV represents distant disease.

The aggressive nature of MCC is reflected in the 5-year survival rates; even localized disease has a 5-year survival rate of only 35–63%, depending on tumor size and local invasion. Nodal disease has a 5-year survival of 40% for microscopic metastases and only 27% for macroscopic nodal disease. For those with distant disease, the 5-year survival is a dismal 13.5% [19].

Initial Assessment

As for any patient presenting with a cutaneous malignancy, a comprehensive history including medical comorbidities, in particular immunosuppression as well as previous surgery or radiotherapy, should be obtained. A full clinical examination of the skin and lymph node basins should be performed.

Biopsy

MCC often resembles other cutaneous lesions, and cannot be diagnosed based on clinical examination alone. Thus, biopsy, preferably excisional, should be performed to establish diagnosis. On hematoxylin and eosin staining, MCC appears as small round blue cells containing scant cytoplasm. Immunohistochemical stains should be performed to differentiate MCC from other tumors such as metastatic small cell lung cancer, melanoma, and lymphoma. MCC has a characteristic immunohistochemical profile. In most cases, it is cytokeratin 20-positive, typically in a paranuclear dot-like pattern. It also stains positive for many neuroendocrine markers such as chromogranin, synaptophysin, CD56, and neuron-specific enolase. Viral status can be assessed either by immunohistochemical stains or PCR. Confirmation of MCV enables MCC to be differentiated from other neuroendocrine tumors.

Imaging

At presentation, patients should undergo imaging (either CT chest, abdomen-pelvis, or PET-CT) for staging as clinically indicated. In patients who are node-positive (stage III), are immunosuppressed, or have large primary lesions, PET scans have been shown to upstage up to 30% of patients and impact management [26, 27]. Similarly, PET scans are useful in assessing posttreatment response, especially after RT alone and also in the setting of restaging following relapse [27]. PET scans should not be used as a substitute for SLNB as the resolution to identify macroscopic MCC is 4–5 mm and therefore unhelpful in setting microscopic nodal MCC [28]. As MCC expresses somatostatin receptors, PET scans utilizing somatostatin receptor analogues, for example, ^{68}Ga-DOTATATE, are also useful for staging MCC patients [29].

Management

Ideally, MCC patients should be discussed in a multidisciplinary setting which includes at least a surgeon, dermatologist, pathologist, radiation oncologist, and medical oncologist with expertise and interest in MCC. The appropriate management can then be tailored according to specific patient factors such as age and comorbidities including immunosuppression and the stage and location of their MCC.

Management of the Primary Tumor

In the majority of patients, localized MCC is treated with wide local excision +/− adjuvant RT. MCC is considered a very radioresponsive malignancy. There is debate in the literature regarding the optimal role and clear indications for RT, and there is no high-level evidence comparing patients undergoing surgery to patients undergoing surgery and adjuvant RT. The majority of the evidence regarding management of the primary tumor consists of small observational cancer registry-based cohort studies reporting retrospective and often heterogeneous data, and missing details such as extent of treatment, site of relapse, and cause of death. Patients either who are not fit for surgery or whose disease is deemed inoperable may be considered for RT alone in select circumstances.

Surgery

The National Comprehensive Cancer Network (NCCN) guidelines recommend excision margins of 1–2 cm peripherally, extending to the deep fascia or pericranium [30]. However, there have been no prospective studies that have defined what constitutes the most optimal excision margin. Many retrospective studies that analyzed the incidence of recurrence and outcome based on margin status have been confounded by the inclusion of patients who had also received adjuvant RT.

In a single institutional study of MCC in which only a small proportion of patients received adjuvant RT delivered to the primary site post-excision, there was no difference in local recurrence rate when excision margins of <1 cm and >1 cm were compared [31]. A more recent study also documented no difference in local recurrence rates and also that the extent of the excision margin did not impact overall- or disease-specific survival when comparing 1 cm, 1–1.9 cm, or 2 cm margins [32].

Data comparing Mohs micrographic surgery and wide local excision in a retrospective review of 1795 cases in the National Cancer Database (NCDB) could identify no difference in local recurrence rates between patients undergoing Mohs surgery and those undergoing wide local excision [33].

Adjuvant Radiotherapy

The NCCN guidelines recommend RT as an adjuvant therapy following excision of the primary tumor with negative margins, and this is currently the most common role for RT in the management of MCC [30]. There is an extensive body of evidence from both institutional and population-based studies supporting the addition of adjuvant RT to improve locoregional control. However, a proven benefit in overall survival (OS) from the addition of adjuvant RT remains controversial with any improvement in survival likely limited to patients with early-stage node-negative (stage I/II) MCC.

In an analysis of 6908 patients from the National Cancer Database (NCDB), patients with localized MCC (stage I/II) experienced a significant benefit in OS with the addition of adjuvant RT compared with surgery alone, and in contrast, patients with node-positive MCC (stage III) experienced no significant benefit in OS with the addition of adjuvant RT [34]. In a meta-analysis of over 17,000 patients, a significant benefit in OS was found with adjuvant RT compared to surgery alone. This study also reported a significant benefit in locoregional disease-specific survival but not in distant disease-free survival with the addition of adjuvant RT [35].

Sentinel Lymph Node Biopsy

Staging of the relevant lymph node basin is recommended as patients with clinically node-negative MCC have a worse prognosis than those confirmed as pathologically node-negative, as many will not undergo nodal treatment and subsequently develop nodal relapse [36]. SLNB, in which the first lymph node(s) that receives lymphatic drainage from the primary tumor site is identified, resected, and examined for the presence of metastatic disease, is a method by which the regional nodal basin can be pathologically assessed in patients with clinically node-negative MCC (Fig. 16.2).

Approximately 30% of clinically node-negative MCC patients will have occult nodal disease on SLNB [37], thus the utilization of SLNB results in many patients being upstaged. The SLNB result is also used to direct further management of the regional nodal basin with patients in whom micrometastatic nodal disease is identified proceeding to treatment of the relevant nodal basin, and

Fig. 16.2 An elderly patient with MCC of the nasal bridge with sentinel lymph nodes localized by lymphoscintigraphy to bilateral-level I lymph nodes

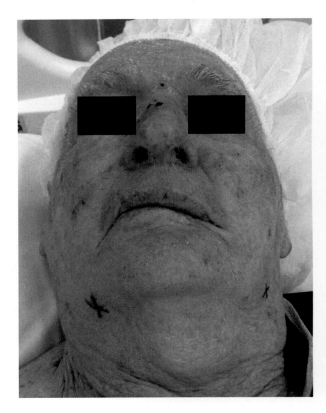

those who have a negative SLNB spared additional treatment of the nodal basin. In cases where an SLNB has not been, or could not have been performed, clinicians may consider elective treatment to the nodal basin or alternatively close observation.

There are no patients or tumor factors that allow clinically node-negative MCC patients to be categorized as low risk of having occult nodal metastatic disease. Even small (5–10 mm) MCC have the propensity to metastasize to sentinel nodes. Thus, SLNB is currently recommended for all suitable patients with clinically node-negative disease, provided they are fit for surgery, and should be performed at the time of the wide excision of the primary tumor in order to maximize accuracy of the technique [30].

Patients unable to undergo an SLNB may have lymphoscintigraphy performed to identify the draining lymph nodes with subsequent close observation with regular clinical examination and/or ultrasound or elective treatment of the nodal basin with RT.

There is conflicting evidence regarding the prognostic value of a positive SLNB in MCC. Some studies have shown that SLNB is not associated with survival [37, 38], while large retrospective analyses have demonstrated that survival is worse in patients with a positive SLNB than those with a negative SLNB [39, 40].

The reported false-negative rate of SLNB in MCC has ranged from 0% to 100% but was found to be 17% in a systematic review of SLNB in MCC patients [20]. Thus those patients who have a negative SLNB should undergo regular observation of the nodal basin. It has been suggested that select higher-risk patients may benefit from adjuvant RT to the nodal basin following a negative SLNB, for example, those who are immunosuppressed and those who are at higher risk of a false-negative SLNB (head and neck primary tumor and wide excision of the primary tumor prior to SLNB) [30].

Management of SLNB-Positive Disease

Patients with a positive SLNB should proceed to treatment of the nodal basin in the form of completion lymphadenectomy (CLND) and/or RT, as there may be further microscopic nodal metastases in the remaining lymph nodes that left untreated will become clinically evident with time.

There is limited and conflicting evidence as to which treatment modality is the most beneficial. Studies of patients undergoing CLND alone, RT alone, or CLND and RT, following a positive SLNB, found outcomes were similar regardless of the treatment modality used [41–43]. In a study of 71 patients with a positive SLNB undergoing various treatment modalities including CLND, CLND and adjuvant RT, and RT alone, all treatment groups had a risk of regional recurrence <10%, and there was no significant difference in DFS or OS [41].

Completion lymphadenectomy can be used to obtain prognostic information such as the number of nodes involved and the presence of extranodal spread, but it is unclear how this information contributes to further management and outcome.

Management of Clinically/Radiologically Evident Nodal Disease

Patients who present with palpable regional nodes should have the diagnosis of metastatic MCC confirmed by fine needle aspiration or core biopsy and imaging to exclude distant metastatic disease.

Patients with clinically evident lymph node metastases may be treated with surgery (therapeutic lymphadenectomy) and/or RT [30], and similar to the management of SLNB-positive patients, it is unclear from the literature which treatment modality offers the best outcome. A small study of 50 patients with metastatic nodal disease found no difference in DFS when definitive RT versus surgery and adjuvant RT were compared [43]. And while one large retrospective analysis of the NCDB suggested that patients who underwent surgery with or without adjuvant RT had a better OS than those patients who underwent definitive RT [44], another large retrospective analysis of the same database demonstrated no difference in survival in patients treated with surgery and RT compared to surgery alone [45].

Definitive Radiotherapy

In many patients, surgery is contraindicated due to age and/or comorbidities, and in these cases, RT alone may be considered. The radioresponsiveness of MCC provides the option of RT alone with doses in the range of 45–55 Gy achieving almost a 90% in-field control rate, even in the setting of large primary lesions and/or nodal metastasis [46]. Many patients eventually die from distant recurrence, or unrelated comorbidity, but up to 40–60% may be cured [47].

Systemic Therapy in MCC

MCC is considered to be a chemosensitive malignancy, and in the past, patients with distant metastatic disease have been treated with agents such as carboplatin, cisplatin, etoposide, cyclophosphamide, and doxorubicin as monotherapy or in combinations, with response rates ranging from 20% to 61% [48]. However, responses to these agents are rarely durable (median duration 5–8 months), and treatment toxicity limits their use in the elderly MCC patient population.

More recently, the focus of systemic therapy for metastatic MCC has shifted to the use of immune checkpoint inhibitors. Compared to conventional chemotherapeutic agents, immune checkpoint inhibitors are often well tolerated by the elderly and have a greater and more durable response rate. Avelumab, an anti-PDL1 antibody, was the first such agent to be used in the treatment of metastatic MCC. The JAVELIN trial in which patients were treated with avelumab as a second-line agent, demonstrated an overall response rate of 33% and a median survival of just over 12 months [49]. Pembrolizumab, an anti-PD-1 antibody, when used as first-line treatment for metastatic MCC, has been associated with an overall response rate of 56% [50]. Recently it has been demonstrated that nivolumab, another anti-PD-1 antibody, elicited a 47% pathologic complete response when used in the neoadjuvant setting [51]. Interestingly, response to immunotherapy appears to be independent of the viral status of the tumor.

Although the use of immune checkpoint inhibitors shows promising results, meaningful responses only occur in about 50% of patients. Thus there is a need for the development of other agents or treatment combinations. Areas of continued investigation include the use of combination immune therapies, targeted therapies such as somatostatin analogues, mTor inhibitors as single agents or in combination with immune checkpoint inhibitors, and combining immune therapy with radiotherapy.

Avelumab, pembrolizumab, and nivolumab are currently recommended as treatment options for stage IV MCC [30]. In stage III disease, adjuvant systemic therapy is currently not recommended. There is a need for an effective adjuvant systemic therapy in the setting of stage III disease, as around 50% of these patients go on to develop distant metastatic disease [52]. There are clinical trials in progress that are investigating the use of immune checkpoint inhibitors such as avelumab in order to attempt to address the need to reduce the rate of distant recurrence in these patients.

Recurrence and Follow-Up

Around 50% of patients develop recurrent disease, which generally occurs within the first 2 years following treatment [51]. Most commonly, the regional nodal basin is the first site of metastatic disease, and around 1/3 patients will develop distant metastatic disease [37, 51].

Due to the high risk of recurrence, patients treated for MCC should undergo regular surveillance. However, there is no evidence regarding what constitutes the most appropriate follow-up of MCC patients. The NCCN recommends that patients be followed up every 3–6 months for 3 years and then every 6–12 months [30]. Follow-up should consist of regular clinical examination of the skin and lymph node basins. Routine imaging can be performed if clinically indicated or in patients at higher risk of recurrence, for example, the immunosuppressed or those with stage III disease at diagnosis. MCV oncoprotein antibody levels can be measured in patients who are seropositive at baseline, as rising titers can be a sign of early recurrence. It has been suggested that unless there is clinical suspicion of recurrence or an increase in MCV oncoprotein antibody titer, routine imaging could be omitted in seropositive patients [16].

Conclusion

In summary, MCC is an aggressive cutaneous neuroendocrine tumor. Significant advances in our understanding of the pathogenesis and management of this rare tumor have occurred in recent years. However, its prognosis remains poor, and translational and clinical research investigating its behavior and what constitutes the most appropriate management is ongoing.

References

1. Toker C. Trabecular carcinoma of the skin. Arch Dermatol. 1972;105:107–10.
2. Sauer C, Haugg A, Chteinberg E, Rennspiess D, Winnepenninck V, Speel E-J, Becker J, Kurz A, Hausen A. Reviewing the current evidence supporting early B cells as the cellular origin of Merkel cell carcinoma. Crit Rev Oncol Haematol. 2017;116:99–105.
3. Paulson K, Park S, Vandeven N, Lachance K, Thomas H, Chapuis A, Harms K, Thompson J, Bhatia S, Stang A, Nghiem P. Merkel cell carcinoma: current United States incidence and projected increases based on changing demographics. J Am Acad Dermatol. 2018;78:457–63.
4. Youlden D, Soyer H, Youl P, Fritschi L, Baade P. Incidence and survival for Merkel cell carcinoma in Queensland, Australia, 1993–2010. JAMA Dermatol. 2014;150:864–72.
5. Agelli M, Clegg L. Epidemiology of primary Merkel cell carcinoma in the United States. J Am Acad Dermatol. 2003;49:832–41.
6. Heath M, Jaimes N, Lemos B, Mostaghimi A, Wang L, Penas P, Nghiem P. Clinical characteristics of Merkel cell carcinoma at diagnosis in 195 patients: the "AEIOU" features. J Am Acad Dermatol. 2008;58:375–81.
7. Engels E, Goedert J, Biggar R, Miller R. Merkel cell carcinoma and HIV infection. Lancet. 2002;359:497–8.
8. Koljone V, Kukko H, Pukkala E, Bohling T, Tukainen E, Sihto H, Joensuu H. Chronic lymphocytic leukemia patients have a high risk of Merkel cell polyomavirus DNA-positive Merkel cell carcinoma. Br J Cancer. 2009;101:1444–7.
9. Penn I, First M. Merkel cell carcinoma in organ transplant recipients: report of 41 cases. Transplantation. 1999;68:1717–21.
10. Asgari M, Sokil M, Warton M, Iyer J, Paulson K, Nghiem P. Effect of host, tumor, diagnostic and treatment variables on outcomes in a large cohort with Merkel cell carcinoma. JAMA Dermatol. 2014;150:716–23.
11. Feng H, Shuda M, Chang Y, Moore P. Clonal integration of a polyomavirus in human Merkel cell carcinoma. Science. 2008;319:1096–100.
12. Garneski K, Warcola A, Feng Q, Kiviat N, Leonard H, Nghiem P. Merkel cell polyomavirus is more frequently present in North American than Australian Merkel cell tumors. J Invest Dermatol. 2009;129:246–8.
13. Tolstov Y, Pastrana D, Feng H, Becker J, Jenkins F, Moschos S, Chang Y, Buck C, Moore P. Human Merkel cell polyomavirus infection II. MCV is a common human infection that can be detected by conformational capsid epitope immunoassays. Int J Cancer. 2009;125:1250–6.
14. Houben R, Shuda M, Weinkam R, Schrama D, Feng H, Chang Y, Moore P, Becker J. Merkel cell polyomavirus-infected Merkel cell carcinoma cells require expression of viral T antigens. J Virol. 2010;84:7064–72.
15. Paulson KG, Carter JJ, Johnson LG, Cahill K, Iyer J, Schrama D, Becker J, Madeleine M, Nghiem P, Galloway D. Antibodies to Merkel cell polyomavirus T antigen oncoproteins reflect tumor burden in Merkel cell carcinoma patients. Cancer Res. 2010;70:8388–97.
16. Paulson K, Lewis c RM, Simonson W, Lisberg A, Ritter D, Morishima C, Hutchinson K, Mudgistrativa L, Blom A, Iyer J, Moshiri A, Tarabadkar E, Carter J, Bhatia S, Karawumi M, Galloway D, Wener M, Nghiem P. Viral oncoprotein antibodies as a marker for recurrence of Merkel cell carcinoma: a prospective validation study. Cancer. 2017;123:1464–74.
17. Wong S, Waldeck K, Vergara I, Schroder J, Madore J, Wilmott J, Colebatch A, De Paoli-Iseppi R, Li J, Lupat R, Semple T, Arnau G, Fellowes A, Leonard J, Hruby G, Mann G, Thompson J, Cullinane C, Johnston M, Shackleton M, Sandhu S, Bowtell D, Johnstone R, Fox S, McArthur G, Papenfuss A, Scolyer R, Gill A, Hicks R, Tothill R. UV-associated mutations underlie the etiology of MCV-negative Merkel cell carcinomas. Cancer Res. 2015;75:5228–34.
18. Moshiri A, Doumani R, Yelistratova L, Blom A, Lachance K, Shinohara M, Delaney M, Chang O, McArdle S, Thomas H, Asgari M, Huang M-L, Schwartz S, Nghiem P. Polyomavirus-negative Merkel cell carcinoma: a more aggressive subtype based on analysis of 282 cases using multimodal tumor virus detection. J Invest Dermatol. 2017;137:819–27.

19. Harms K, Healy M, Nghiem P, Sober A, Johnson T, Bichakjian C, Wong S. Analysis of prognostic factors from 9387 Merkel cell carcinoma cases forms the basis for the new 8th edition AJCC staging system. Ann Surg Oncol. 2016;23:3564–71.
20. Gunaratne D, Howle J, Veness M. Sentinel lymph node biopsy in Merkel cell carcinoma: a 15-year institutional experience and statistical analysis. Br J Dermatol. 2016;174:273–81.
21. Chen K, Papvasiliou P, Edwards K, Perlis C, Wu H, Turaka A, Berger A, Farma J. A better prognosis for Merkel cell carcinoma of unknown primary. Am J Surg. 2013;206:752–7.
22. Foote M, Veness M, Zarate D, Poulsen M. Merkel cell carcinoma: the prognostic implications of an occult primary in stage IIIB (nodal) disease. J Am Acad Dermatol. 2012;67:395–9.
23. Fields RC, Busam KJ, Chou JF, Panageas K, Pulitzer M, Allen P, Kraus D, Brady M, Coit D. Five hundred patients with Merkel cell carcinoma evaluated at a single institution. Ann Surg. 2011;254:465–73.
24. Andea AA, Coit DG, Amin B, Busam KJ. Merkel cell carcinoma Cancer. 2008;113:2549–58.
25. Edge SB, Edge SB. AJCC cancer staging manual. 8th ed. New York: Springer; 2017.
26. Poulsen M, Macfarlane D, Veness M, Estall V, Hruby G, Kumar M, Pullar A, Tripcony L, RIschin D. Prospective analysis of the utility of 18-FDG PET in Merkel cell carcinoma of the skin: a Trans Tasman Radiation Oncology Group Study, TROG 09:03. J Med Imaging Radiat Oncol. 2018;62(3):412–9.
27. Byrne K, Siva S, Chait L, Callahan J, Seel M, MacManus M, Hicks R. 15-year experience of 18F-FDG PET imaging in response assessment and restaging after definitive treatment of Merkel cell carcinoma. J Nucl Med. 2015;56(9):1328–33.
28. Liu J, Larcos G, Howle J, Veness M. Lack of clinical impact of 18F-fluorodeoxyglucose positron emission tomography with simultaneous computed tomography for stage I and II Merkel cell carcinoma with concurrent sentinel lymph node biopsy staging: a single institutional experience from Westmead Hospital, Sydney. Aust J Dermatol. 2017;58:99–105.
29. Buder K, Lapa C, Kreissl MC, Schirbel A, Herrmann K, Schnack A, Brocker E, Goebeler M, Buck A, Becker J. Somatostatin receptor expression in Merkel cell carcinoma as target for molecular imaging. BMC Cancer. 2014;14:268.
30. Bichakjian CK, Olencki T, Aasi SZ, et al. Merkel cell carcinoma. Version 1.2018, NCCN clinical practice guidelines in oncology. J Natl Compr Cancer Netw. 2018;16:1043–7.
31. Allen P, Browne W, Jaques D, Brennan M, Busam K, Coit D. Merkel cell carcinoma: prognosis and treatment of patients from a single institution. J Clin Oncol. 2005;23:2300–9.
32. Perez M, de Pinho F, Holstein A, Oliver D, Naqvi S, Younchul K, Messina J, Burke E, Gonzalez R, Sarnaik A, Cruse W, Wuthrick E, Harrison L, Sondak V, Zager J. Resection margins in Merkel cell carcinoma: is a 1cm margin wide enough? Ann Surg Oncol. 2018;25:3334–40.
33. Singh B, Qureshi M, Truong M, Sahni D. Demographics and outcomes of stage I and II Merkel cell carcinoma treated with Mohs micrographic surgery compared with wide local excision in the National Cancer Database. J Am Acad Dermatol. 2018;79:126–34.
34. Bhatia S, Storer B, Iyer J, Moshiri A, Parvathaneni U, Byrd D, Sober A, Sondak V, Gershenwald J, Nghiem P. Adjuvant radiation therapy and chemotherapy in Merkel cell carcinoma: survival analyses of 6908 cases from the National Cancer Data Base. J Natl Cancer Inst. 2016;108: 09 pii:pjwo42.
35. Petrelli F, Ghidini A, Torchio M, Prinzi N, Trevisan F, Dallera P, De Stefani A, Russo A, Vitali E, Bruschieri L, Costanzo A, Seghezzi S, Ghidini M, Varricchio A, Cabiddu M, Barni S, de BRaud F, Pusceddu S. Adjuvant radiotherapy for Merkel cell carcinoma: a systematic review and meta-analysis. Radiother Oncol. 2019;134:211–9.
36. Lemos B, Storer B, Iyer J, Phillips J, Bichakjian C, Fang C, Johnson T, Liegeois-Kwon N, Otley C, Paulson K, Ross M, Yu S, Zeitouni N, Byrd D, Sondak V, Gershenwald J, Sober A, Nghiem P. Pathologic nodal evaluation improves prognostic accuracy in Merkel cell carcinoma: analysis of 5,823 cases as the basis of the first consensus staging system for this cancer. J Am Acad Dermatol. 2010;63:751–61.
37. Fields R, Busam K, Chou J, Pulitzer M, Kraus D, Brady M, Coit D. Recurrence and survival in patients undergoing sentinel lymph node biopsy for Merkel cell carcinoma: analysis of 153 patients from a single institution. Ann Surg Oncol. 2011;18:2529–37.

38. Fritsch V, Camp E, Lentsch E. Sentinel lymph node status in Merkel cell carcinoma of the head and neck: not a predictor of survival. Head Neck. 2014;36:571–4.
39. Conic R, Ko J, Saridakis S, Damiani G, Funchain P, Vidimos A, Gastman B. Sentinel lymph node biopsy in Merkel cell carcinoma: predictors of sentinel lymph node positivity and association with overall survival. J Am Acad Dermatol. 2019;81:364–72.
40. Sridharan V, Muralidhar V, Margalit D, Tishler R, DeCaprio J, THakuria M, Rabinowits G, Schoenfeld J. Merkel cell carcinoma: a population analysis on survival. J Natl Compr Cancer Netw. 2016;14:1247–57.
41. Perez M, Oliver D, Weitman E, Boulware D, Messina J, Torres-Roca J, Cruse W, Gnozalez R, Sarnail A, Sondak V, Wuthrick E, Harrison L, Zager J. Management of sentinel lymph node metastasis in Merkel cell carcinoma: completion lymphadenectomy, radiation or both? Ann Surg Oncol. 2019;26:379–85.
42. Lee J, Durham A, Bichakjian C, Harms P, Hayman J, McLean S, Harms K, Burns W. Completion lymph node dissection or radiation therapy for sentinel node metastasis in Merkel cell carcinoma. Ann Surg Oncol. 2019;26:386–94.
43. Fang L, Lemos B, Douglas J, Iyer J, Nghiem P. Radiation monotherapy as regional treatment for lymph node positive Merkel cell carcinoma. Cancer. 2010;116:1783–90.
44. Wright G, Hotlzman M. Surgical resection improves median overall survival with marginal improvement in long-term survival when compared with definitive radiotherapy in Merkel cell carcinoma: a propensity score matched analysis of the National Cancer Database. Am J Surg. 2018;215:384–7.
45. Bhatia S, Storer B, Iyer J, Moshiri A, Parvathaneni U, Byrd D, Sober A, Sondak V, Gershenwald J, Nghiem P. Adjuvant radiation therapy and chemotherapy in Merkel cell carcinoma: survival analyses of 6908 cases from the National Cancer Database. J Natl Cancer Inst. 2016;108:(9):djw042.
46. Gunaratne D, Howle J, Veness M. Definitive radiotherapy for Merkel cell carcinoma confers clinically meaningful in-field locoregional control: a review and analysis of the literature. J Am Acad Dermatol. 2017;77:142–148e1.
47. Sundaresan P, Hruby G, Hamilton A, et al. Definitive radiotherapy or chemoradiotherapy in the treatment of Merkel cell carcinoma. Clin Oncol. 2012;24:e131–6.
48. Nghiem P, Kaufman H, Bharmal M, Mahnke L, Phatak H, Becker JC. Systematic literature review of efficacy, safety and tolerability outcomes of chemotherapy regimens in patients with metastatic Merkel cell carcinoma. Future Oncol. 2017;13:1263–79.
49. Kaufman H, Russel J, Hamid O, Bhatia S, Terheyden P, D'Angelo S, Shih K, Lebbe C, Milella M, Brownel I, Lewis K, Lorch J, von Heydebreck A, Henessy M, Nghiem P. Updated efficacy of avelumab in patients with previously treated metastatic Merkel cell carcinoma after >=1 year of follow-up: JAVELIN Merkel 200, a phase 2 clinical trial. J Immunother Cancer. 2018;6:7.
50. Nghiem P, Bhatia S, Lipson E, Sharfman W, Kudchadkar R, Brohl A, Friedlander P, Daud A, Kluger H, Reddy S, Boulmay B, Riker A, Burgess M, Hanks B, Olencki T, Margolin K, Lundgren L, Soni A, Ramchurren N, CHaurch C, Park S, Shinohara M, Salim B, Taube J, Bird S, Ibrahim N, Fling S, Moreno B, Sharon E, Cheever M, Topalian S. Durable tumor regression and overall survival in patients with advanced Merkel cell carcinoma receiving pembrolizumab as first-line therapy. J Clin Oncol. 2018;37:693–702.
51. Topalian S, Bhatia S, Amin A, Kudchadkar R, Sharfman W, Lebbe C, Delord J-P, Dunn L, Shinohara M, Kulikauskas R, Chung C, Martens U, Ferris R, Stein J, Engle E, Devriese L, Lao C, Gu J, Li B, Chen T, Barrows A, Horvath A, Taube J, Nghiem P. Neoadjuvant nivolumab for patients with resectable Merkel cell carcinoma in the CheckMate 358 trial. J Clin Oncol. 2020;38:2476–87.
52. Song Y, Azari F, Tang R, Shannon A, Miura J, Fraker D, Karakousis. Patterns of metastasis in Merkel cell carcinoma. Ann Surg Oncol 2020. https://doi-org.ezproxy.surgeons.org/10.1245/s10434-020-08587-3.

Part IV

Metastatic Disease

Neuroendocrine Liver Metastases

Ashley Kieran Clift and Andrea Frilling

Introduction

Neuroendocrine neoplasms (NEN) represent a clinically challenging bevy of variegated tumours that develop from widely dispersed neuroendocrine cells, with florid diversity in their primary organs of origin, hormone secretory activity, symptomatology and clinical behaviour and aggressiveness [1]. The most common sites of origin are the gastroenteropancreatic and bronchopulmonary tracts [2], although pituitary, thyroid and dermatological forms of the disease are also encountered. Whilst generally exhibiting more favourable outcomes as compared to adenocarcinomas derived from the same organs, traditional perspectives of rarity and indolence are wholly inappropriate given the evolving epidemiology of several NEN types demonstrating marked increments in incidence [2] and also observations that the majority of small bowel NEN, for example, present with at least nodal metastases at initial diagnosis [3].

Neuroendocrine neoplasms harbour a predilection for hepatic metastases [4], particularly those from the small bowel and pancreas [5]. They also exert stark prognostic risk, and most are not resectable using standard surgical approaches due to their oft bilobar, multifocal distribution which is not fully captured by even gold standard imaging [6]. Liver metastases therefore represent a fundamental aspect of the effective multidisciplinary care of patients with NEN, and given that surgery provides the only opportunity for cure (by complete resection of the primary and attendant metastatic deposits), robust evaluation of the presence, and technical and oncological resectability, of liver metastases is crucial [4].

In this chapter, we provide an overview of the radiological assessment of patients with neuroendocrine liver metastases (NELM) whilst emphasising methods to assess the resectability of hepatic deposits. Thereafter, we review the surgical

A. K. Clift · A. Frilling (✉)
Department of Surgery & Cancer, Imperial College London, London, UK
e-mail: a.frilling@imperial.ac.uk

© Springer Nature Switzerland AG 2021
J. M. Cloyd, T. M. Pawlik (eds.), *Neuroendocrine Tumors*,
https://doi.org/10.1007/978-3-030-62241-1_17

strategies that may be employed in appropriately selected patients, namely, hepatectomy with curative intent, palliative debulking, advanced procedures such as two-step resections and transplantation. Crucially, however, in addition to reviewing the evidence base for surgical intervention in NELM, we include a review of the novel paradigms offered by discussing neoadjuvant and adjuvant approaches that include surgical intervention as part of advanced surgical procedures, multimodal treatment concepts or novel tools to aid future surgical decision-making. Throughout, there is emphasis on the limitations of currently available literature, and we posit future avenues for progress in refining the role of surgery in the treatment of this exigent class of tumours.

Radiological Assessment of Liver Metastases

A suite of morphological and functional radiological imaging modalities may be employed in the interrogation of NELM [8]. A major focus of the radiological workup of patients with NELM is the assessment of both the oncological resectability, which considers the extent/stage of disease, and the technical resectability, which refers to the feasibility of operative intervention on anatomic factors such as proximity of lesions to vascular or other structures. Briefly, three major morphological categories of neuroendocrine liver metastases have been described (Table 17.1). Type 1 disease consists of a single liver metastasis of any size or location; type 2 disease manifests as the bulk of deposits in one lobe with smaller lesions in the other; type 3 disease corresponds to diffuse disease spread characterised by multifocal tumour burden and is not amenable to hepatectomy (encountered in approximately 70% of individuals) [7]. This classification not only informs the amenability of hepatic neuroendocrine disease burden to a surgical approach but also has prognostic implications. Briefly, patients with type 1 or type 2 disease may be candidate for hepatic resection, whereas those with type 3 disease are usually directed towards systemic or liver-directed palliative therapies or may be considered for liver transplantation depending on the extent and resectability of extrahepatic metastases. Thus, whilst there is an incumbent duty to evaluate the distribution of hepatic deposits within the liver to ascertain the adequacy and appropriateness of a surgical approach, evaluation of the presence and extent of extrahepatic disease is also key.

Neuroendocrine liver metastases are typically hypervascular, which may be elucidated on Doppler ultrasound and contrast-enhanced ultrasound (arterial enhancement) [9] or particularly during the hepatic arterial phase of standard oncological

Table 17.1 Types of neuroendocrine liver metastases as described by Frilling et al. [7]

Type	Description	Prevalence
I	Single metastasis of any size	19%
II	Metastases predominantly involving one lobe with smaller lesions in the other	15%
III	Disseminated bilobar metastases	66%

computed tomography imaging, which depicts more liver lesions than contrast-enhanced ultrasound [10]. The highest degree of lesion detection can be obtained using magnetic resonance imaging (MRI), particularly with hepatic arterial phase liver MRI or fat-suppressed T2-weighted imaging [11], although for sub-centimetric deposits (which should always be assumed) diffusion-weighted MRI has the highest specificity [12] and is advised to be a component of the workup of all individuals evaluated in terms of NELM.

Aside from the standard modalities of CT and MRI, nuclear imaging is a cornerstone of disease evaluation and targets the expression of somatostatin receptors (SSTRs) on the cell membranes using radiolabelled agonists or antagonists. The gold standard form of imaging for G1/G2 NEN is positron emission tomography (PET) combined with CT using gallium-68 radiolabelled 'DOTA' peptides (^{68}Ga-DOTA PET/CT) [13]. These radiopharmaceuticals supersede the traditional approach of SSTR-targeted scintigraphy with ^{111}In-octreotide as they may be able to visualise lesions <5 mm in size [14], offer high sensitivity (82–100%) and specificity (67–100%) for NELM and have excellent sensitivity (85–100%) and specificity (67–90%) for extrahepatic disease [15]. The power of this approach has been highlighted in institutional series that demonstrated its propensity to alter initially intended treatment strategies in up to 60% of cases, in terms of modifying surgical approach or deselecting patients from hepatic surgery [16]. There is also the potential role of combining somatostatin receptor-targeted PET with the archetypal oncological radiotracer, ^{18}F-FDG PET [17]. This relatively recent 'tandem' approach facilitates an assessment of the metabolic activity of tumour deposits, more successfully depicts higher-grade lesions (grade 2/3) that have a lower level of SSTR expression, may have prognostic implications [18] and is increasingly advocated.

Overall, the radiological armamentarium for NELM is broad, and the use of gold standard imaging modalities, especially MRI and ^{68}Ga-DOTA PET/CT, is crucial for adequate treatment selection, regardless of intended modality. Nevertheless, the Achilles' heel of radiological or nuclear medicine imaging in NELM is the presence of oft miliary liver metastases, in which even such optimal imaging often under-stages by up to 50% [6]. Recent developments in the imaging of neuroendocrine metastases include novel radiotracers which have been excellently reviewed elsewhere but include radiolabelled antagonists for insulinoma [19] and the use of copper-64 as an alternative to gallium-68 [20].

Hepatic Resection: Curative Intent

Hepatectomy with microscopically clear margins (R0) represents the only modality at present that confers the possibility of cure. It should be the first-choice strategy for individuals with grade 1 or 2 disease (KI67 < 20%) with type 1 LM burden and no extrahepatic disease (or limited disease outside the liver that can be effectively managed) [4]. Generally accepted principles include the consideration of Couinaud segmental anatomy and preservation of adequate functional liver volume post-surgery.

Table 17.2 Summary of results from selected case series regarding hepatectomy for neuroendocrine liver metastases

Series	Number of patients	R0/R1 resection and overall survival	R0/R1 resection and progression-free survival	Number of patients	R2 resection and overall survival	R2 resection and progression-free survival
Fairweather et al. [21]	58 (649 total)	90% at 5 years 70% at 10 years	Not reported	–	–	–
Maxwell et al. [22]		–	–	108	76.1% at 5 years Median 10.5 years	30.2% at 5 years Median 2.2 years
Saxena et al. [23]	48 (74 total)	Median 98 months	Median 48 months	26	Median 27 months	Median 24 months
Scigliano et al. [24]	37 (41 total)	88% for R0 82% for R1	31% for R0 9% for R1	4	50%	0%
Frilling et al. [7]	23 (119 total)	100%	96%	–	–	–
Gomez et al. [25]	15 (18 total)	86%	90%	3	–	25%
Elias et al. [26]	37 (47 total)	74% for R0 70% for R1	66% for R0 46% for R1	10	47%	30%

R0 resection is often promulgated as having 'curative intent', yet the operative word is 'intent' rather than 'curative'. There are to date no randomised controlled trials of surgery versus other modalities, with the evidence base consisting solely of retrospective case series with meticulously selected patients (Table 17.2). However, these data starkly demonstrate that disease recurrence occurs post-resection in the overwhelming majority of patients. In a salient systematic review that identified 29 case series [27], median 1-year, 5-year and 10-year overall survival after resection were 94% (range: 79% to 100%), 70.5% (range: 31% to 100%) and 42% (range: 0% to 100%), respectively, yet the recurrence-free survival rates at the same time points were 63% (range: 50% to 80%), 29% (range: 6% to 66%) and 1% (range: 0% to 11%), respectively [27].

Post-resection recurrence should therefore be actively anticipated, but the optimal strategy for dealing with this is not yet clear. Post-curative hepatectomy recurrence is predominantly in the liver: intrahepatic-only recurrence is observed in approximately 66% of patients, with extrahepatic-only recurrence seen in 11%, with a 'mixed' extrahepatic/intrahepatic pattern seen in 23% [28]. Repeat surgery for individuals with resectable recurrent disease may be suitable as is often practiced in hepatocellular carcinomas, colorectal cancer metastases and intrahepatic cholangiocarcinoma. One multi-institutional series observed that repeat resection was used in 36.6% of individuals, with intra-arterial therapy (transarterial embolisation/chemoembolisation or radioembolisation) in 21.4% [28]. The 10-year overall survival for those undergoing repeat resection was 60.3%, compared to 52% for IAT [28].

An interesting conceptual divergence from the seemingly generally accepted principles that resection is for low grade, low-burden NELM is a recent Nordic study that examined intended curative resection +/− radiofrequency ablation in LM from neuroendocrine carcinomas (grade 3, poorly differentiated NEN), which are rapidly progressive and usually reserved for purely palliative cytotoxic chemotherapy (median OS 11 months) [29]. In a case series of 32 patients with gastroenteropancreatic NELM, 20 of which had Ki67 ≥ 55%, the 3-year and 5-year overall survival following hepatic resection/RFA was 47% and 43%, respectively, with a median post-surgery progression-free survival of 8.4 months. A Ki67 < 50% and adjuvant chemotherapy were associated with favourable OS [29].

A further divergence or refinement in perspective may also arise when transferring from disease-free survival outcome-based definitions to statistical modelling. An important recent multicentric case series utilised cure fraction modelling in 376 patients undergoing hepatectomy with curative intent [30]. Whilst the concept of cure from hepatectomy for NELM may appear very unlikely from the perspective of the median 10-year recurrence-free survival of 1%, 'cure models' statistically define cure as when the mortality of treated patients (the sum of excess and expected hazards of death) returns to the same level as that of the general population. This utilised non-mixture cure models, which are parametric models that estimate an asymptote for the survival 'function'. Time to cure was also modelled, defined statistically as when the survival time tends towards infinity. Whilst the observed 5-year disease-free survival was 46.3%, the probability of being cured after hepatectomy (according to the cure model approach) was 43.9%, with a time to cure of 5.1 years, and a median survival of non-cured patients was 1.7 years. Several factors were observed to significantly impact the cure probability on univariate analyses, which include but were not limited to primary tumour location (lower in pancreatic), tumour differentiation (higher in well-differentiated disease) and presence of extrahepatic disease (higher in absence thereof). In the multivariable model, however, NET type (gastrointestinal, non-functional pancreatic, functional pancreatic and 'other'), grade of differentiation (well, moderate, poor) and degree of liver involvement possessed independent predictive capabilities regarding cure probability. It was observed that the excess hazards of death in the patient cohort decreased to a 99% confidence level in the general (US) population at 5.1 years posthepatectomy, which is interpreted as follows: if an individual is without disease recurrence at 5.1 years after hepatectomy, they can be deemed as 'cured' with 99% certainty. The authors concluded that in accordance with their cure model, up to 40% of patients may be considered as 'cured' following R0 resection [30].

Overall, hepatic resection with curative intent is suitable for a diminutive proportion of patients with neuroendocrine liver metastases, and the evidence base predicating the perspective that it is the gold standard is subject to grand limitations, specifically solely consisting of retrospective, noncontrolled case series of patients that were highly selected (had lower-volume disease, probably younger with fewer comorbidities). There is evidence that although complete resection of NELM confers benefit at 5 years in terms of overall survival, this is not translated into any meaningful effect at 10 years [31]. Moreover, the criteria used for such selection are poorly documented, if at all. Therefore, the extent to which outcomes (in terms of overall survival) are biased due to selection or attributable to the treatment is to be disentangled. Emergent from this complex situation are the following observations:

1. Hepatectomy with microscopically complete resection almost always ultimately fails and despite its 'curative' moniker is in reality palliative in the long term by offering a longer duration of transient disease control. Although statistical cure modelling may indicate that a statistically defined cure is obtainable in an almost counterintuitively high proportion of patients, the majority of individuals do develop recurrent disease evident on imaging. Even accepting results from statistical modelling, with the caveat that imaging-based recurrence and mortality hazards are not directly comparable, at least more than half of patients undergoing surgery with curative intent will not attain cure [30].
2. This is inherently due to the nature of NELM being understaged by even best standard imaging [6]. It is probable that in the majority of patients, there are miliary micrometastases that fall below the sensitivity thresholds of current modalities and are not detected or resected. These slow-growing tumours then drive later relapse, which isn't necessarily recurrence of resected disease but rather emergence of hitherto unidentified lesions that proliferate past the threshold of detectability.
3. Recurrent disease may be considered for repeat resection [28], but perhaps a more effective strategy in future practice is the use of multimodal therapy strategies that combined the macro-disease control of surgery with the micro-control afforded by non-surgical systemic treatments.
4. Despite the limitations in terms of evidence as discussed above, in appropriately selected patients, hepatectomy with R0 resection still has a fundamental role to play and should be considered in all patients with G1/G2, low-burden NELM as it probably confers the strongest conduit for long-term disease control. Issues with recurrence mean that it is a modality that should be supplemented and better reported, rather than disregarded.

Two-Step Advanced Surgical Approaches for Hepatectomy

Although the overwhelming majority of patients are ineligible for hepatic surgery with curative intent, a small suite of advanced surgical procedures is available which has the capability to 'convert' patients with traditionally unresectable liver metastases to having resectable disease [32–35].

One approach, associating liver partition and portal vein ligation (ALPPS), was evaluated using an international registry; herein, of 954 procedures undertaken in 135 international centres, 24 (2.5%) were performed with NELM as an indication, and 21 were included in the final analysis [32]. Here, R0 resection was attained in 90% of cases (n = 19) at the second stage, and median 2-year disease-free survival was 41.8%. However, given the observation of 5% 90-day mortality rate and an incidence of 27% grade 3b or higher morbidity after stage 2, the procedure should be undertaken with some caution and specialist centres [32].

Other two-step approaches in oncological hepatic resection reported in the literature include preoperative portal vein embolisation [34] or radiation lobectomy in those not initially suitable for resection due to small future liver remnant [33]. The latter uses unilobar infusion of radiolabelled microspheres via the hepatic artery, which preferentially lodge in the metastatic tumour vasculature and results in hypertrophy of the contralateral liver lobe.

Hepatic Resection: Debulking

Liver resection with the intent to 'debulk' hepatic metastatic burden (R2, macroscopically incomplete) may be an option for symptomatic patients or those with hormonally hypersecreting tumours that induce symptoms poorly controlled with medical approaches. The traditional target for these approaches is to extirpate 90% of the extant liver tumour burden. However, this was derived from older work that was not solely pertaining to NEN, and the first studies that examined NEN in this context were before the effective symptom control from somatostatin analogues was introduced. Therefore, this cut-off is rooted not in intent to attain improved oncological outcomes, but rather attain symptomatic relief prior to availability of effective medical adjuncts for the same [36]. This slightly fallaciously grounded but often expounded '90% rule' has generally persisted, may exclude up to 90% of individuals considered for debulking [37] and may in actuality not confer a significant 'penalty' in terms of outcomes based on data from some centres [38]. In one series, 42 patients undergoing a total of 44 debulking procedures were stratified into those in whom ≥70%, ≥90% and 100% of the total gross LM burden were resected; no significant association was found between the extent of cytoreduction and hepatic progression of disease [38]. Furthermore, in another series of 108 patients with pancreatic or small intestinal NELM, 70% debulking was attained in 64% and ≥ 90% debulking in only 39% [22]. Here, patients with NELM of pancreatic origin had both PFS and OS prolonged when ≥70% of burden was resected, whereas this effect was not seen in those with small bowel primaries, and there was no benefit for OS in patients that had ≥90% cytoreduction [22].

Overall, the following can be surmised regarding cytoreductive/debulking hepatic resection:

1. The distinction between resection with 'curative' and purely 'palliative' extent may be somewhat artificial and is better considered as two approaches both offering transient disease control, but of differing durations. Recurrence is inevitable regardless of margin status. A more refined conceptualisation of the role of debulking surgery should focus on its role to palliatively ameliorate symptoms of hormone hypersecretion, rather than as a 'second rate' short shrift attempt at cure.

2. Traditional 'cut-offs' for selecting patients for debulking surgery on the basis of 'anticipated percentage extirpation' may be overly exclusive if the goal is symptom control and are based on experience preceding modern clinical practice, where somatostatin analogues are now standard of care.

3. With the advent of trans-arterial liver-directed interventional procedures and systemic radiolabelled therapy such as PRRT, the role for debulking surgery should be carefully scrutinised and continuously (re)evaluated, as these modalities arguably may confer valuable opportunities for disease control but avoid the need for major surgery. Indeed, with the caveat that the data are nonrandomised, there is no evidence that cytoreduction/debulking offers better outcomes over and above intra-arterial liver-directed therapies in NELM.

Liver or Multivisceral Transplantation

The concept of 'transplant oncology' outside of the realm of hepatocellular carcinoma (HCC), for which there are validated selection criteria, is somewhat controversial but has been applied to over 700 individuals with NELM [39], albeit representing probably only 0.2% of all liver transplants [40]. Over the past decades, its role in patients with NELM has spanned 'upfront' curative intent with radical resection of both primary tumour and associated hepatic metastatic burden to a more 'ultima ratio' attempt at the same, but after failure of other therapies. Multivisceral transplantation (stomach, small bowel, pancreas and liver) has been utilised in a very small number of cases [41, 42], mostly those with pancreatic primaries where bulky metastatic burden threatens the mesenteric root and thus vascularity of the gut.

As is the case with hepatectomy, the role of liver transplantation, either as an isolated procedure or more rarely as part of a multi-organ allograft, is characterised by mostly mono-institutional, nonrandomised studies where (barring one exception) [43] selection criteria are poorly documented (Table 17.3). A recent systematic

Table 17.3 Results from selected case series regarding liver transplantation for neuroendocrine liver metastases

Series	Patients	Overall survival				Disease-free survival			
		1 yr	3 yrs.	5 yrs.	10 yrs.	1 yr.	3 yrs.	5 yrs.	10 yrs.
Mazzaferro et al. [43]	42			97.2%	88.8%			86.9%	86.9%
Bonaccorsi-Riani et al. [44]	9	88%	77%	33%		67%	33%	11%	
Olausson et al. [42]	15[a]			90%			70%	20%	
van Vilsteren et al. [45]	19	88%				80%			
Frilling et al. [46]	15[b]	78.3%		67.2%		69.4%		48.3%	

[a]Includes five patients undergoing multivisceral transplantation
[b]Includes one patient undergoing multivisceral transplantation

review documented 1-year OS of 89%, 3-year OS of 69% and 5-year OS of 63%, with disease recurrence ranging between 17.7% and 38.7% [47]. Furthermore, and importantly, the outcomes of OLT for NELM do not appear to be worse than that observed in HCC [40, 48].

The largest registry-based study to date is that of 213 European patients with NELM undergoing orthotopic liver transplantation between 1982 and 2009, which retrospectively catalogued outcomes and factors associated with the said outcomes and devised a point-based scoring system [49]. Five-year OS and disease-free survival were 52% and 30%, respectively, but there appeared to be a temporal effect, with those receiving allografts after 2000 experiencing a 59% OS rate. In this same more 'contemporary' subpopulation, age > 45 years, hepatomegaly and concomitant resection (at time of transplant) were negatively associated with outcomes. These three negative prognostic factors were used as a basis for a scoring system which was retrospectively applied to the same cohort: patients with scores of 0 or 1 had 5-year overall survival of 79% and 5-year disease-free survival of 57%, whereas those with scores of 2 or more have 5-year overall survival of 35% and 5-year disease-free survival of 19%. The validity of age as a significant prognosticator has been debated in other studies, and experience from the United States [40] suggests that higher recipient bilirubin or lower recipient albumin are associated with poorer survival outcomes, as well as higher donor creatinine.

The one notable exception to the poor reporting of liver transplantation selection criteria for NELM is the 'Milan criteria', which were adapted from guidelines for HCC to NEN. Several updates to the prospective follow-up of patients treated by Mazzaferro et al. have been published, evaluating the outcomes pursuant to compliance with the following strict criteria: low-grade NEN (clinical syndrome irrelevant), primary tumour drained by portal venous system, aged 55 years or younger, 50% or less liver involvement, complete resection of the primary tumour and any extrahepatic disease and at least 6 months of stable disease/response to treatment prior to transplantation [43]. Of 280 patients evaluated for possible OLT for NELM in their centre, 88 were deemed eligible, and 42 were transplanted. There were no differences in terms of the extent of liver metastases, tumour differentiation or primary tumour site, but those who did receive a transplant were significantly younger on average, had lower tumour grade and received more loco-regional treatments, and fewer has SSA therapy. Cognisant of these selection biases and the observation that in many centres such patients would be selected for hepatectomy rather than OLT, the 10-year OS and PFS for those transplanted were 88.8% and 86.9%, respectively, compared to 22.4% and 11%, respectively, for non-transplanted individuals [43].

Overall, whilst excellent results are obtainable with ardently strict selection criteria, the nonrandomised evidence base regarding transplantation for NELM is beset by non-uniform reporting, collation of probably heterogeneous case mixes and heterogeneity in the timing of transplantation. As is the case with hepatectomy, the risk of recurrence (albeit apparently only outside of Milan criteria) is high, and there is sparse evidence regarding combining transplantation with other non-surgical modalities to suppress this. In short:

1. Generally accepted contraindications for OLT include higher tumour grade, non-portal primary tumour drainage, unresectable extrahepatic metastases and advanced carcinoid heart disease, but the Milan criteria are more restrictive.
2. The extent to which favourable outcomes with stringently selected patients are attributable to bias over and above the procedure itself is difficult to ascertain.
3. Future work in this arena should focus on clear reporting of selection criteria, collaboration across centres for large registries to pool individual-level data and, eventually, preferably, a randomised trial comparing OLT according to a priori criteria and hepatectomy.

Novel Strategies in Treatment, Clinical Decision-Making and Follow-Up

The combination of surgical and medical therapeutic strategies within multimodal neoadjuvant/adjuvant treatment concepts may offer possibilities for long-term disease control by comprehensively treating macroscopic and microscopic neuroendocrine disease. Experience with such modalities is as of yet limited to relatively small case series but has promising rationale and results [50, 51].

In patients with initially unresectable or borderline resectable NELM, neoadjuvant peptide receptor radionuclide therapy (PRRT) may downstage disease sufficiently to act as a bridging therapy to resection and be used in the adjuvant setting to minimise risk of disease recurrence (Fig. 17.1) or even as a retreatment in cases of post-surgical relapse [52–54]. An additional approach undertaken by some

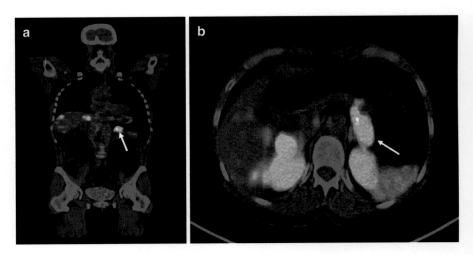

Fig. 17.1 Sagittal (A, *left*) and transverse view (B, *right*) of ^{68}Ga-NODAGA-LM3 PET/CT in a 40-year-old patient with a G2 NEN localised in the pancreatic tail (*arrow*) and multiple liver metastases. The patient underwent a two-stage approach: in stage 1 neoadjuvant peptide receptor radionuclide therapy and in stage 2 distal pancreatectomy and debulking of liver metastases (with courtesy of R. Baum and D. Kämmerer)

centres is the use of somatostatin analogues (SSA) in the adjuvant setting after liver resection: in one recent case series, the 5-year overall survival in patients with metastatic pancreatic NEN who underwent surgical treatment alone was 34%, whereas in those who received adjuvant SSA, it was 79% (p < 0.01). The side-effect profile was minimal, and quality of life was preserved, suggesting that wider utilisation of this approach may be warranted [55].

Treatment selection and sequencing are aspects of clinical decision-making that may be informed by multivariate clinical risk prediction models, which seek to mathematically assimilate predictor variable values to output either an estimation of the percentage risk of an event of interest occurring or stratifying a population in terms of risk [56]. Given the particular heterogeneity of NEN, although grading and staging criteria are well established, the behaviour of seemingly heterogeneous tumours can be markedly divergent, and thus the precision of any inference one can make regarding an individual patient's disease course purely based on reductionist, unidimensional metrics will be incomplete. Prognostic or predictive scores may have utility in selecting patients for (and designing) clinical trials or directing patients towards more aggressive, earlier therapy for aggressive tumours versus monitoring for indolent disease or closer follow-up depending on their risk profile.

Risk prediction models, although generally not specifically generated for surgical selection, have been generated and to varying extents validated in the field of NEN, such as predicting overall survival in patients with small intestinal NEN [52], disease recurrence after surgery [53] or overall survival in metastatic, well-differentiated NEN [54]. These are typically based on similar regression methodology as used to identify 'risk factors' or 'risk associations' but output relative or absolute risk estimate of the event probability.

One such system, the Neuroendocrine Score ('NEP Score') classification incorporates age, primary tumour site, timing of metastases (synchronous or metachronous), Ki67, functional status and occurrence of primary surgery to classify patients with well-differentiated NEN into high-, intermediate- or low-risk groups, which correspond to 10-year overall survival of ≥70%, 30–70% and <30%, respectively [54]. However, whilst this score was developed and validated on datasets considered large for the NEN literature (n = 1387), the discrimination of the model was not excellent (c-index 0.661 in training set, 0.601 to 0.626 in the validation data), and in the validation set, calibration was rather poor [54]. Further work should be undertaken to develop more robust risk models that have strong discrimination, calibration and decision-informing capabilities, which are capable of providing more precise estimations of clinical risk, either across wide-ranging groups of NEN, but probably more reliably so in well-defined subsets, given the diversity of behaviour even within tumour classes.

In contrast to risk scores that may infer relative or absolute risk of a clinical endpoint to stratify patients, another novel theme in NEN is the use of multi-analyte biomarkers that are capable of determining completeness of resection, detecting disease relapse or quantifying disease burden with far higher sensitivity than traditional assays such as chromogranin A. The NETest is a PCR-based 51-gene blood-based analysis that has been demonstrated to not only significantly outperform CgA in diagnosis of NEN [57] but also delineate between complete resection and cytoreduction, predict response to radionuclide therapy and identify recurrent disease up to 6 months before gold standard imaging does [58]. Given the marked propensity of NELM to recur after surgery, one opportunity may be to use such blood-based multi-analyte assays to assess radicality of resection, monitor for recurrence to direct earlier intervention and prolongation of survival in relapse or even perhaps select individuals for surgical treatment, although these require further research.

Conclusions

The literature regarding NELM advocates the benefits of a surgical approach to the management of these complex tumours – however, the evidence is clearly subject to a significant degree of bias in terms of patient selection and also demonstrates that even in the small proportion (<20%) of patients with NELM that can be treated with curative intent, cure is rarely attained. The best outcomes have been observed in patients either undergoing R0 'curative resection' (where margin status has an at times disputed effect on prognosis and the term 'curative' approximates a misnomer) or with OLT according to the Milan NET criteria (which should be heavily caveated with selection bias). In combination with the outdated perspective that cytoreduction requires 90% extirpation to be oncologically/symptomatically worthwhile, the traditional surgical thinking in this arena should be challenged. Surgery certainly is the keystone in the management of NELM and does possess opportunity to cure, but it should be embedded within a multimodal concept where surgery and medical/interventional strategies combine to obtain protracted long-term disease control or a genuine cure.

As is the established case with the treatment of liver metastases from colorectal liver metastases, future efforts in advancing the care of patients with neuroendocrine liver metastases should focus on the implementation of neoadjuvant and adjuvant treatment concepts. The integration of novel molecular and mathematical strategies to risk stratify and longitudinally assess surgical candidates/patients is eagerly awaited in a much-needed divergence from 'established' pauci-variable scores or eminence-based criteria, insensitive mono-analytes and constraint to a focus on clinicopathological features that imprecisely capitulate the true complexities of NEN biology.

References

1. Frilling A, et al. Recommendations for management of patients with neuroendocrine liver metastases. Lancet Oncol. 2014;15:e8–21.
2. Dasari A, et al. Trends in the incidence, prevalence, and survival outcomes in patients with neuroendocrine tumors in the United States. JAMA Oncol. 2017;3:1335.
3. Pavel M, et al. ENETS consensus guidelines update for the Management of Distant Metastatic Disease of intestinal, pancreatic, bronchial Neuroendocrine Neoplasms (NEN) and NEN of unknown primary site. Neuroendocrinology. 2016;103:172–85.

4. Frilling A, Clift AK. Therapeutic strategies for neuroendocrine liver metastases. Cancer. 2015;121:1172–86.
5. Clift AK, et al. Neuroendocrine neoplasms of the small bowel and pancreas. Neuroendocrinology. 2019. https://doi.org/10.1159/000503721.
6. Elias D, et al. Hepatic metastases from neuroendocrine tumors with a 'thin slice' pathological examination: they are many more than you think. Ann Surg. 2010;251:307–10.
7. Frilling A, et al. Treatment of liver metastases from neuroendocrine tumours in relation to the extent of hepatic disease. Br J Surg. 2009;96:175–84.
8. Ronot M, et al. Morphological and functional imaging for detecting and assessing the resectability of neuroendocrine liver metastases. Neuroendocrinology. 2017. https://doi.org/10.1159/000479293.
9. Mörk H, Ignee A, Schuessler G, Ott M, Dietrich CF. Analysis of neuroendocrine tumour metastases in the liver using contrast enhanced ultrasonography. Scand J Gastroenterol. 2007;42:652–62.
10. Ronot M, et al. Morphological and functional imaging for detecting and assessing the resectability of neuroendocrine liver metastases. Neuroendocrinology. 2018;106:74–88.
11. d'Assignies G, et al. High sensitivity of diffusion-weighted MR imaging for the detection of liver metastases from neuroendocrine tumors: comparison with T2-weighted and dynamic gadolinium-enhanced MR imaging. Radiology. 2013;268:390–9.
12. Vilgrain V, et al. A meta-analysis of diffusion-weighted and gadoxetic acid-enhanced MR imaging for the detection of colorectal liver metastases. Eur Radiol. 2016;26:4595–615.
13. Schraml C, et al. Staging of neuroendocrine tumours: comparison of [68Ga]DOTATOC multiphase PET/CT and whole-body MRI. Cancer Imaging. 2013;13:63–72.
14. Ronot M, Clift AK, Vilgrain V, Frilling A. Functional imaging in liver tumours. J Hepatol. 2016;65:1017–30.
15. Breeman WAP, et al. (68)Ga-labeled DOTA-peptides and (68)Ga-labeled radiopharmaceuticals for positron emission tomography: current status of research, clinical applications, and future perspectives. Semin Nucl Med. 2011;41:314–21.
16. Frilling A, et al. The impact of 68Ga-DOTATOC positron emission tomography/computed tomography on the multimodal management of patients with neuroendocrine tumors. Ann Surg. 2010;252:850–6.
17. Kayani I, et al. Functional imaging of neuroendocrine tumors with combined PET/CT using 68Ga-DOTATATE (DOTA-DPhe1,Tyr3-octreotate) and 18F-FDG. Cancer. 2008;112:2447–55.
18. Binderup T, Knigge U, Loft A, Federspiel B, Kjaer A. 18F-fluorodeoxyglucose positron emission tomography predicts survival of patients with neuroendocrine tumors. Clin Cancer Res. 2010;16:978–85.
19. Christ E, et al. Glucagon-like peptide-1 receptor imaging for the localisation of insulinomas: a prospective multicentre imaging study. Lancet Diabetes Endocrinol. 2013;1:115–22.
20. Pfeifer A, et al. 64Cu-DOTATATE PET for neuroendocrine Tumors: a prospective head-to-head comparison with 111In-DTPA-octreotide in 112 patients. J Nucl Med. 2015;56:847–54.
21. Fairweather M, et al. Management of Neuroendocrine Tumor Liver Metastases: long-term outcomes and prognostic factors from a large prospective database. Ann Surg Oncol. 2017;24:2319–25.
22. Maxwell JE, Sherman SK, O'Dorisio TM, Bellizzi AM, Howe JR. Liver-directed surgery of neuroendocrine metastases: what is the optimal strategy? Surgery. 2016;159:320–35.
23. Saxena A, et al. Progression and survival results after radical hepatic metastasectomy of indolent advanced neuroendocrine neoplasms (NENs) supports an aggressive surgical approach. Surgery. 2011;149:209–20.
24. Scigliano S, et al. Clinical and imaging follow-up after exhaustive liver resection of endocrine metastases: a 15-year monocentric experience. Endocr Relat Cancer. 2009;16:977–90.
25. Gomez D, et al. Hepatic resection for metastatic gastrointestinal and pancreatic neuroendocrine tumours: outcome and prognostic predictors. HPB (Oxford). 2007;9:345–51.
26. Elias D, et al. Liver resection (and associated extrahepatic resections) for metastatic well-differentiated endocrine tumors: a 15-year single center prospective study. Surgery. 2003;133:375–82.

27. Saxena A, Chua TC, Perera M, Chu F, Morris DL. Surgical resection of hepatic metastases from neuroendocrine neoplasms: a systematic review. Surg Oncol. 2012;21:e131–41.
28. Spolverato G, et al. Management and outcomes of patients with recurrent neuroendocrine liver metastasis after curative surgery: an international multi-institutional analysis. J Surg Oncol. 2017;116:298–306.
29. Galleberg RB, et al. Results after surgical treatment of liver metastases in patients with high-grade gastroenteropancreatic neuroendocrine carcinomas. Eur J Surg Oncol. 2017;43:1682–9.
30. Bagante F, et al. Neuroendocrine liver metastasis: the chance to be cured after liver surgery. J Surg Oncol. 2017;115:687–95.
31. Manguso N, et al. Prognostic factors influencing survival in small bowel neuroendocrine tumor with liver metastases. J Surg Oncol. 2019;120:926–31.
32. Linecker M, et al. ALPPS in neuroendocrine liver metastases not amenable for conventional resection – lessons learned from an interim analysis of the international ALPPS registry. HPB. 2020;22:537–44.
33. Vouche M, et al. Radiation lobectomy: time-dependent analysis of future liver remnant volume in unresectable liver cancer as a bridge to resection. J Hepatol. 2013;59:1029–36.
34. Kianmanesh R, et al. Two-step surgery for synchronous bilobar liver metastases from digestive endocrine tumors: a safe approach for radical resection. Ann Surg. 2008;247:659–65.
35. Schnitzbauer AA, et al. Right portal vein ligation combined with in situ splitting induces rapid left lateral liver lobe hypertrophy enabling 2-staged extended right hepatic resection in small-for-size settings. Ann Surg. 2012;255:405–14.
36. McEntee GP, Nagorney DM, Kvols LK, Moertel CG, Grant CS. Cytoreductive hepatic surgery for neuroendocrine tumors. Surgery. 1990;108:1091–6.
37. Sarmiento JM, et al. Surgical treatment of neuroendocrine metastases to the liver: a plea for resection to increase survival. J Am Coll Surg. 2003;197:29–37.
38. Morgan RE, Pommier SJ, Pommier RF. Expanded criteria for debulking of liver metastasis also apply to pancreatic neuroendocrine tumors. Surgery. 2018;163:218–25.
39. Fan ST, et al. Liver transplantation for neuroendocrine tumour liver metastases. HPB (Oxford). 2015;17:23–8.
40. Gedaly R, et al. Liver transplantation for the treatment of liver metastases from neuroendocrine tumors: an analysis of the UNOS database. Arch Surg. 2011;146:953–8.
41. Mangus RS, Tector AJ, Kubal CA, Fridell JA, Vianna RM. Multivisceral transplantation: expanding indications and improving outcomes. J Gastrointest Surg. 2013;17:179–86; discussion p. 186–7.
42. Olausson M, et al. Orthotopic liver or multivisceral transplantation as treatment of metastatic neuroendocrine tumors. Liver Transpl. 2007;13:327–33.
43. Mazzaferro V, et al. The long-term benefit of liver transplantation for hepatic metastases from neuroendocrine tumors. Am J Transplant. 2016;16:2892–902.
44. Bonaccorsi-Riani E, et al. Liver transplantation and neuroendocrine tumors: lessons from a single Centre experience and from the literature review. Transpl Int. 2010;23:668–78.
45. van Vilsteren FGI, et al. Liver transplantation for gastroenteropancreatic neuroendocrine cancers: defining selection criteria to improve survival. Liver Transpl. 2006;12:448–56.
46. Frilling A, et al. Liver transplantation for patients with metastatic endocrine tumors: single-center experience with 15 patients. Liver Transpl. 2006;12:1089–96.
47. Moris D, et al. Liver transplantation in patients with liver metastases from neuroendocrine tumors: a systematic review. Surgery. 2017;162:525–36.
48. Nguyen NTT, Harring TR, Goss JA, O'Mahony CA. Neuroendocrine liver metastases and orthotopic liver transplantation: the US experience. Int J Hepatol. 2011;2011:742890.
49. Le Treut YP, et al. Liver transplantation for neuroendocrine tumors in Europe-results and trends in patient selection: a 213-case European liver transplant registry study. Ann Surg. 2013;257:807–15.
50. Kaemmerer D, et al. Neoadjuvant peptide receptor radionuclide therapy for an inoperable neuroendocrine pancreatic tumor. World J Gastroenterol. 2009;15:5867–70.

51. Partelli S, et al. Peptide receptor radionuclide therapy as neoadjuvant therapy for resectable or potentially resectable pancreatic neuroendocrine neoplasms. Surgery. 2017. https://doi.org/10.1016/j.surg.2017.11.007.

52. Clift AK, et al. Predicting the survival of patients with small bowel neuroendocrine tumours: comparison of 3 systems. Endocr Connect. 2017;6:71–81.

53. Genç CG, et al. A new scoring system to predict recurrent disease in grade 1 and 2 nonfunctional pancreatic neuroendocrine tumors. Ann Surg. 2018;267:1148–54.

54. Pusceddu S, et al. A classification prognostic score to predict OS in stage IV well-differentiated neuroendocrine tumors. Endocr Relat Cancer. 2018;25:607–18.

55. Fisher AT, et al. Management of ileal neuroendocrine tumors with liver metastases. J Gastrointest Surg. 2019:1–10. https://doi.org/10.1007/s11605-019-04309-7.

56. Steyerberg EW, Harrell FE. Prediction models need appropriate internal, internal-external, and external validation. J Clin Epidemiol. 2016;69:245–7.

57. Öberg K, et al. A meta-analysis of the accuracy of a neuroendocrine tumor mRNA genomic biomarker (NETest) in blood. Ann Oncol. 2020;31:202–12.

58. Ćwikła JB, et al. Circulating transcript analysis (NETest) in GEP-NETs treated with somatostatin analogs defines therapy. J Clin Endocrinol Metab. 2015;100:E1437–45.

Neuroendocrine Peritoneal Metastases

18

Jennifer L. Leiting and Travis E. Grotz

Epidemiology

Approximately 10–33% of patients with neuroendocrine tumors (NETs) will develop peritoneal carcinomatosis (PC) [1–4]. The predilection for NETs to develop PC depends on the origin of the primary tumor. Patients with midgut (primary jejunoileal and appendiceal) NETs have higher rates of PC compared to patients with foregut (primary pancreatic or duodenal) or hindgut (primary rectal) NETs [4]. One study found that up to 62% of patients with PC from a NET had a primary tumor that originated in the small intestine, and another found 81% of patients had a primary tumor in the ileum or the appendix [3, 5]. The prevalence of PC also appears to be higher (19–33%) in well-differentiated NET. The incidence of both well-differentiated and midgut NETs are increasing in frequency in the United States, and it is therefore possible we will see an increase in peritoneal metastasis from NETs in the future [6].

Association with Other Metastatic Disease

PC from NET is frequently associated with synchronous metastasis to other sites such as the liver and lymph nodes. One study showed a 100% correlation between PC and synchronous liver metastases [3]. Others found that 11–25% of patients with PC had no evidence of liver metastases [3, 7]. The frequency of other metastatic sites is likely related to the extent of preoperative evaluation, specifically the use of contemporary imaging modalities. A comprehensive evaluation strategy is necessary not only for accurate staging and prognostication of patients with PC from NET but also for establishing the optimal treatment strategy.

J. L. Leiting (✉) · T. E. Grotz
Hepatobiliary and Pancreatic Surgery, Mayo Clinic, Rochester, MN, USA
e-mail: Leiting.jennifer@mayo.edu; Grotz.travis@mayo.edu

© Springer Nature Switzerland AG 2021
J. M. Cloyd, T. M. Pawlik (eds.), *Neuroendocrine Tumors*,
https://doi.org/10.1007/978-3-030-62241-1_18

Genetics

The genetic alterations in patients with NETs have been investigated, with some effort to distinguish differences in patients with PC and those without PC. The most common genetic alteration seen in patients with NETs, particularly midgut NETs, is on chromosome 18 with loss of heterozygosity (LOH) or deletion, with the percentage of tumors affected ranging from 67 to 88% [8–10]. This LOH was not seen in lung NETs, further differentiating the two tumor types [9]. One study found that the primary tumors of patients with PC from NETs showed complete or partial loss of heterozygosity (LOH) on chromosome 18 compared to limited or no LOH in patients without PC [7]. Therefore, this may prove a useful biomarker in the future for distinguishing patients who are at high risk for developing PC from NETs.

Preoperative Assessment

The preoperative workup to assess patients for PC from NETs is varied and is dependent on the provider and available resources. In a survey of experts, a computed tomography (CT) scan was the preferred imaging modality with only 24% and 19% saying that they would obtain an MRI or a PET scan, respectively [11]. Additionally, only 38% said they would perform a diagnostic laparoscopy [11]. The Chicago Consensus on Peritoneal Surface Malignancies recommends multidisciplinary tumor board review with pathologic review, assessment of carcinoid symptoms, laboratory studies such as urine 5-HIAA and chromogranin A, and imaging with either CT, MRI, or PET/CT scan [12]. If disease is considered resectable by imaging, then a laparoscopy could be considered. Recently, octreotide scans have been replaced by Gallium-68 DOTATATE PET/CT (Fig. 18.1). The reported sensitivity and specificity of Gallium-68 DOTATATE PET/CT is 82–100% and 88–100%, respectively [13]. Crown et al. reported that DOTATATE PET/CT scans identified new nodal, bone, liver, pleural, and peritoneal metastasis missed by conventional imaging in 48% (37 of 77) of patients with metastatic NETs. This resulted in a change in management in 35% of patients [14]. However, there are some potential pitfalls the surgeon must be aware of, in relation to false-positive results related to prominent pancreatic uncinate process, inflammation, degenerative bone disease, fracture, accessory splenunculi/splenosis, and benign meningioma [15].

Only 10% of patients with carcinoid heart disease are symptomatic. Therefore, all patients with carcinoid syndrome should be evaluated with a cardiac ultrasound to diagnose/exclude carcinoid heart disease. Right heart valve damage typically in the form of tricuspid insufficiency and pulmonary stenosis can be found in 50% of patients with carcinoid syndrome [16, 17]. Undiagnosed right heart failure can lead to significant postoperative complications and should be repaired prior to surgical debulking, particularly if hepatic resection is involved [18, 19].

Patients with carcinoid syndrome should be given long-acting octreotide preoperatively to control carcinoid syndrome. Once clinical control is stabilized, elective cytoreductive surgery can be undertaken. In patients where carcinoid syndrome is

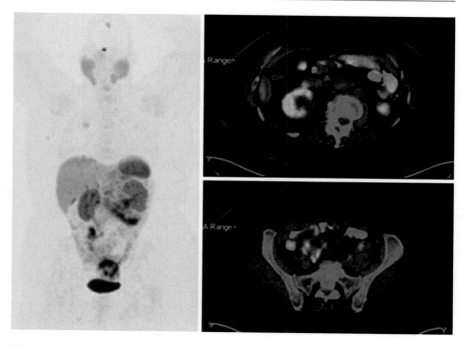

Fig. 18.1 Representative images from Gallium-68 DOTATATE PET/CT demonstrating peritoneal carcinomatosis from grade 2 well-differentiated small bowel neuroendocrine tumor

incompletely controlled, a bolus injection of short-acting octreotide should be given preoperatively to decrease any induction-associated hormone release. Short-acting octreotide should be immediately available for patients with metastatic NET undergoing cytoreductive surgery; however, true perioperative carcinoid crisis is rare in our experience [20].

Surgery

There is insufficient data regarding the optimal surgical management because neuroendocrine PC still remains relatively rare. Most of the evidence is level 2 or level 3 in quality. In 2010, the European Neuroendocrine Tumor Society (ENETS) published consensus guidelines for the management of NET-associated PC [21]. However, most recommendations are extrapolated from larger studies of neuroendocrine liver metastases. As a result, the surgical management of PC from NETs is far from standardized.

Several grading systems have been proposed to quantify the extent of disease for patient selection and prognostication. The Lyon prognostic index, or Gilly classification, a staging system first described by Gilly and colleagues, was proposed by the ENETS as a way to retrospectively classify PC from NETS by both size and distribution (Table 18.1) [21, 22]. The Peritoneal Carcinomatosis Index (PCI) is a

Table 18.1 Lyon prognostic index

Stage 0	No macroscopic disease
Stage I	Malignant nodules <5 mm in size in one part of the abdomen
Stage II	Malignant nodules <5 mm in size diffuse to the whole abdomen
Stage III	Malignant nodules 5–20 mm in size
Stage IV	Malignant nodules >20 mm

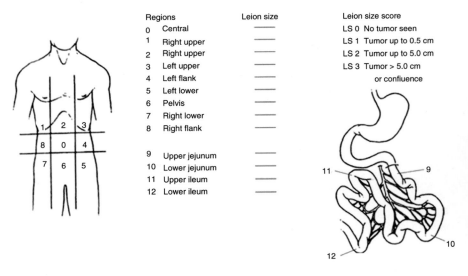

Regions	Leion size	Leion size score
0 Central	———	LS 0 No tumor seen
1 Right upper	———	LS 1 Tumor up to 0.5 cm
2 Right upper	———	LS 2 Tumor up to 5.0 cm
3 Left upper	———	LS 3 Tumor > 5.0 cm
4 Left flank	———	or confiuence
5 Left lower	———	
6 Pelvis	———	
7 Right lower	———	
8 Right flank	———	
9 Upper jejunum	———	
10 Lower jejunum	———	
11 Upper ileum	———	
12 Lower ileum	———	

Fig. 18.2 Peritoneal Carcinomatosis Index. (Cotte et al. [46])

widely used classification system that quantifies the extent of PC in the abdomen and has been found to be predictive of survival and ability to achieve a complete cytoreduction in many cancer subtypes (Fig. 18.2) [23–25]. Patients are scored intraoperatively via a thorough examination of the peritoneal cavity and receive a score of 0 to 39. This system takes into account both size and location of the tumor nodules.

The Gravity PC Score (GPS) was proposed by the ENETS and incorporates both the extent of peritoneal disease and other intra-abdominal metastases, particularly the liver and lymph nodes [21]. Patients are scored from 0 to 9 with lower numbers indicating a low risk for abdominal spread (Table 18.2).

Cytoreduction is defined as the complete removal or fulguration of all visible cancer in the abdomen and pelvis in the form of peritonectomy, visceral resection, and resection of tumor implants. Complete resection of the primary tumor and metastasis remains the only potentially curable treatment for PC from NET. Furthermore, several retrospective series have demonstrated symptomatic and survival improvement with debulking of 70–90% of the entire tumor burden [26, 27]. For example, Wonn and colleagues identified 98 patients with PC from NET

Table 18.2 Gravity Peritoneal Carcinomatosis Score (GPS)

	0 points	1 point	2 points	3 points
Lymph node metastases	Local	Regional	Distant abdominal[a]	Extra-abdominal
Liver metastases	No macroscopic nodule	One lobe < 5 nodules	Both lobes 5–10 nodules	Both lobes > 10 nodules
PC	No macroscopic nodule	Gilly I–II Resectable	Gilly III–IV Resectable	Any Gilly Unresectable

[a]Retroperitoneal or hepatic pedicle
Grade A: 0–3 points
Grade B: 4–6 points
Grade C: 7–9 points

and demonstrated that survival was unaffected by Lyon score prior to surgery but was directly correlated to the level of cytoreduction able to be achieved [28]. Complete or near complete clearance of all macroscopic disease (Lyon Stage 0–1) correlated with a median overall survival following cytoreduction of 76 months compared to patients with Lyon Stage 3 or greater whose median survival was only 32 months [28]. Furthermore, synchronous liver metastasis, which was common, did not portend a worse survival as long as debulking of >70% of the liver metastasis was achieved [28].

The addition of hyperthermic intraperitoneal chemotherapy (HIPEC) to cytoreductive surgery has been explored in NET throughout the world [29]. However, unlike PC from other histologies like ovarian, appendiceal, and gastric cancer, there does not appear to be any benefit to the addition of intraperitoneal chemotherapy to cytoreductive surgery. Elias and colleagues looked at the impact of cytoreductive surgery with and without hyperthermic intraperitoneal chemotherapy (HIPEC) for patients with peritoneal metastases from NETs [30]. They reported a 2% postoperative mortality and 56% major postoperative morbidity with Grades III–V complications. The 5-year and 10-year overall survival rates were 69% and 52%, respectively [30]. The disease-free survival rates were much lower, just 17% and 6% at 5 years and 10 years [30]. In their comparison between patients who received HIPEC and those that did not, they found no difference in survival outcomes despite the increased morbidity and duration of hospital stay in patients who received HIPEC [30]. As a result, in 2020, the Chicago Consensus on Peritoneal Surface Malignancies put forth recommendations for cytoreductive surgery alone without the use of intraperitoneal chemotherapy [12].

Debulking (removal of 70–90%) or cytoreduction (complete resection of all known tumor) of PC is a complex procedure with a prolonged learning curve. It should therefore be pursued at centers and by surgeons with experience with the surgical techniques of parietal and visceral peritonectomy procedures which include visceral resections [31–33]. Many of these surgical tenets and techniques have been well described by several experts and are beyond the scope of this chapter [34–36].

Nonsurgical Alternatives

The systemic treatment of metastatic NETs is described elsewhere in this book. Briefly, the PROMID and CLARINET phase III RCT established the role of somatostatin analogs for first line for advanced of progressive NETs [37, 38]. More recently, the NETTER-1 trial demonstrated improved progression-free survival using peptide receptor radionuclide therapy (PRRT) which targets and treats NETs with radiolabeled somatostatin analogs [39]. No study of systemic treatment that the authors are aware of have included subgroup analysis or specifically enrolled NET patients with PC.

Given the important role VEGF has in the development of peritoneal metastasis, ascites, as well as prognostication in other histologies such as gastric and ovarian cancer, targeted therapies that inhibit angiogenesis are of particular interest [40, 41]. Sunitinib is a multi-targeted receptor tyrosine kinase inhibitor that blocks VEGFR as well as PDGFR. It has been demonstrated in a multinational phase III study to improve progression-free and overall survival in pancreatic NETS [42, 43]. This drug and others like it have not been studied as of yet in PC from NETs but could be of interest.

Survival Outcomes

The impact of PC on patient survival has historically been overlooked and underreported with some studies suggesting that the presence of PC did not negatively influence survival [4]. More recent evidence would suggest the opposite. Elias and colleagues found that PC was the cause of death in up to 40% of patients [3]. Norlen and colleagues found PC to be an independent predictor for worse outcomes in patients with small intestine (SI) NETs, in addition to advanced age, liver tumor load, and Ki-67 [2]. In another study, Norlen and colleagues compared survival in patients with PC from SI NETs to those without PC. They found significantly decreased overall survival (OS) and disease-specific survival (DSS) in patients with PC, only 5.1 years and 5.8 years, respectively, compared to 11.1 years and 12.6 years in patients without PC [7]. This correlates with most other malignancies with worse prognoses seen in patients with PC [44, 45]. Thus, there is an unmet need to improve the medical and surgical treatment of these patients. Although neuroendocrine PC is a risk factor for reduced OSNET, the survival at 5 years is still around 50% which remains better than PC from most other histologies, and a nihilistic approach is not warranted. Appropriate treatment of patients with metastatic NET, including PC, can result in improved quality of life and prolonged survival.

References

1. Elias D, Lasser P, Ducreux M, Duvillard P, Ouellet JF, Dromain C, et al. Liver resection (and associated extrahepatic resections) for metastatic well-differentiated endocrine tumors: a 15-year single center prospective study. Surgery. 2003;133(4):375–82.

2. Norlen O, Stalberg P, Oberg K, Eriksson J, Hedberg J, Hessman O, et al. Long-term results of surgery for small intestinal neuroendocrine tumors at a tertiary referral center. World J Surg. 2012;36(6):1419–31.
3. Elias D, Sideris L, Liberale G, Ducreux M, Malka D, Lasser P, et al. Surgical treatment of peritoneal carcinomatosis from well-differentiated digestive endocrine carcinomas. Surgery. 2005;137(4):411–6.
4. Vasseur B, Cadiot G, Zins M, Flejou JF, Belghiti J, Marmuse JP, et al. Peritoneal carcinomatosis in patients with digestive endocrine tumors. Cancer. 1996;78(8):1686–92.
5. Modlin IM, Lye KD, Kidd M. A 5-decade analysis of 13,715 carcinoid tumors. Cancer. 2003;97(4):934–59.
6. Lee MR, Harris C, Baeg KJ, Aronson A, Wisnivesky JP, Kim MK. Incidence trends of gastroenteropancreatic neuroendocrine tumors in the United States. Clin Gastroenterol Hepatol. 2019;17(11):2212–2217.e1.
7. Norlen O, Edfeldt K, Akerstrom G, Westin G, Hellman P, Bjorklund P, et al. Peritoneal carcinomatosis from small intestinal neuroendocrine tumors: clinical course and genetic profiling. Surgery. 2014;156(6):1512. https://doi.org/10.1016/j.surg.2014.08.090.
8. Lollgen RM, Hessman O, Szabo E, Westin G, Akerstrom G. Chromosome 18 deletions are common events in classical midgut carcinoid tumors. Int J Cancer. 2001;92(6):812–5. https://doi.org/10.1002/ijc.1276.
9. Kytola S, Hoog A, Nord B, Cedermark B, Frisk T, Larsson C, et al. Comparative genomic hybridization identifies loss of 18q22-qter as an early and specific event in tumorigenesis of midgut carcinoids. Am J Pathol. 2001;158(5):1803–8.
10. Andersson E, Sward C, Stenman G, Ahlman H, Nilsson O. High-resolution genomic profiling reveals gain of chromosome 14 as a predictor of poor outcome in ileal carcinoids. Endocr Relat Cancer. 2009;16(3):953–66.
11. Au JT, Levine J, Aytaman A, Weber T, Serafini F. Management of peritoneal metastasis from neuroendocrine tumors. J Surg Oncol. 2013;108(6):385–6.
12. Schuitevoerder D, Plana A, Izquierdo FJ, Lambert LA, Keutgen XM, Deneve JL, et al. The Chicago consensus on peritoneal surface malignancies: Management of Neuroendocrine Tumors. Ann Surg Oncol. 2020;27(6):1788–92.
13. Tirosh A, Kebebew E. The utility of 68Ga-DOTATATE positron-emission tomography/computed tomography in the diagnosis, management, follow-up and prognosis of neuroendocrine tumors. Future Oncol. 2018;14(2):111–22.
14. Crown A, Rocha FG, Raghu P, Lin B, Funk G, Alseidi A, et al. Impact of initial imaging with gallium-68 dotatate PET/CT on diagnosis and management of patients with neuroendocrine tumors. J Surg Oncol. 2020;121(3):480–5.
15. Hofman MS, Eddie Lau WF, Hicks RJ. Somatostatin receptor imaging with68Ga DOTATATE PET/CT: clinical utility, normal patterns, pearls, and pitfalls in interpretation1. Radiographics. 2015;35(2):500–16.
16. Fox DJ, Khattar RS. Carcinoid heart disease: presentation, diagnosis, and management. Heart. 2004;90(10):1224–8.
17. Mansencal N, Mitry E, Bachet JB, Rougier P, Dubourg O. Echocardiographic follow-up of treated patients with carcinoid syndrome. Am J Cardiol. 2010;105(11):1588–91.
18. Lillegard JB, Fisher JE, McKenzie TJ, Que FG, Farnell MB, Kendrick ML, et al. Hepatic resection for the carcinoid syndrome in patients with severe carcinoid heart disease: does valve replacement permit safe hepatic resection? J Am Coll Surg. 2011;213(1):130–6.
19. Kinney MA, Warner ME, Nagorney DM, Rubin J, Schroeder DR, Maxson PM, et al. Perianaesthetic risks and outcomes of abdominal surgery for metastatic carcinoid tumours. Br J Anaesth. 2001;87(3):447–52.
20. Kinney MA, Nagorney DM, Clark DF, O'Brien TD, Turner JD, Marienau ME, et al. Partial hepatic resections for metastatic neuroendocrine tumors: perioperative outcomes. J Clin Anesth. 2018;51:93–6.
21. Kianmanesh R, Ruszniewski P, Rindi G, Kwekkeboom D, Pape UF, Kulke M, et al. ENETS consensus guidelines for the management of peritoneal carcinomatosis from neuroendocrine tumors. Neuroendocrinology. 2010;91(4):333–40.

22. Gilly FN, Carry PY, Sayag AC, Brachet A, Panteix G, Salle B, et al. Regional chemotherapy (with mitomycin C) and intra-operative hyperthermia for digestive cancers with peritoneal carcinomatosis. Hepato-Gastroenterology. 1994;41(2):124–9.
23. Llueca A, Serra A, Rivadulla I, Gomez L, Escrig J, Multidisciplinary Unit of Abdominal Pelvic Oncology Surgery. Prediction of suboptimal cytoreductive surgery in patients with advanced ovarian cancer based on preoperative and intraoperative determination of the peritoneal carcinomatosis index. World J Surg Oncol. 2018;16(1):37.
24. Chia CS, You B, Decullier E, Vaudoyer D, Lorimier G, Abboud K, et al. Patients with peritoneal carcinomatosis from gastric cancer treated with cytoreductive surgery and hyperthermic intraperitoneal chemotherapy: is cure a possibility? Ann Surg Oncol. 2016;23(6):1971–9.
25. Ng JL, Ong WS, Chia CS, Tan GH, Soo KC, Teo MC. Prognostic relevance of the peritoneal surface disease severity score compared to the peritoneal cancer index for colorectal peritoneal carcinomatosis. Int J Surg Oncol. 2016;2016:2495131.
26. Chan DL, Dixon M, Law CH, Koujanian S, Beyfuss KA, Singh S, et al. Outcomes of cytoreductive surgery for metastatic low-grade neuroendocrine tumors in the setting of Extrahepatic metastases. Ann Surg Oncol. 2018;25(6):1768–74.
27. Tsang ES, McConnell YJ, Schaeffer DF, Lee L, Yin Y, Zerhouni S, et al. Outcomes of surgical and chemotherapeutic treatments of goblet cell carcinoid Tumors of the appendix. Ann Surg Oncol. 2018;25(8):2391–9.
28. Wonn SM, Limbach KE, Pommier SJ, Ratzlaff AN, Leon EJ, McCully BH, et al. Outcomes of cytoreductive operations for peritoneal carcinomatosis with or without liver cytoreduction in patients with small bowel neuroendocrine tumors. Surgery. 2020;S0039-6060(20):30174–30174.
29. Goéré D, Passot G, Gelli M, Levine EA, Bartlett DL, Sugarbaker PH, et al. Complete cytoreductive surgery plus HIPEC for peritoneal metastases from unusual cancer sites of origin: results from a worldwide analysis issue of the Peritoneal Surface Oncology Group International (PSOGI). Int J Hyperth. 2017;33(5):520–7.
30. Elias D, David A, Sourrouille I, Honore C, Goere D, Dumont F, et al. Neuroendocrine carcinomas: optimal surgery of peritoneal metastases (and associated intra-abdominal metastases). Surgery. 2014;155(1):5–12.
31. Kuijpers AM, Hauptmann M, Aalbers AG, Nienhuijs SW, de Hingh IH, Wiezer MJ, et al. Cytoreduction and hyperthermic intraperitoneal chemotherapy: the learning curve reassessed. Eur J Surg Oncol. 2016;42(2):244–50.
32. Polanco PM, Ding Y, Knox JM, Ramalingam L, Jones H, Hogg ME, et al. Institutional learning curve of cytoreductive surgery and hyperthermic intraperitoneal chemoperfusion for peritoneal malignancies. Ann Surg Oncol. 2015;22(5):1673–9.
33. Kusamura S, Baratti D, Virzì S, Bonomi S, Iusco DR, Grassi A, et al. Learning curve for cytoreductive surgery and hyperthermic intraperitoneal chemotherapy in peritoneal surface malignancies: analysis of two centres. J Surg Oncol. 2013;107(4):312–9.
34. Bao P, Bartlett D. Surgical techniques in visceral resection and peritonectomy procedures. Cancer J. 2009;15(3):204–11.
35. Mehta SS, Bhatt A, Glehen O. Cytoreductive surgery and peritonectomy procedures. Indian J Surg Oncol. 2016;7(2):139–51.
36. Sugarbaker PH. Cytoreductive surgery & perioperative chemotherapy for peritoneal surface malignancy: textbook and video atlas. 2nd ed. Woodury: Cine-Med Publishing; 2012.
37. Rinke A, Müller HH, Schade-Brittinger C, Klose KJ, Barth P, Wied M, et al. Placebo-controlled, double-blind, prospective, randomized study on the effect of octreotide LAR in the control of tumor growth in patients with metastatic neuroendocrine midgut tumors: a report from the PROMID study group. J Clin Oncol. 2009;27(28):4656–63.
38. Caplin ME, Pavel M, Ćwikła JB, Phan AT, Faderer M, Sedlackova E, et al. Lanreotide in metastatic enteropancreatic neuroendocrine tumors. N Engl J Med. 2014;371(3):224–33.
39. Strosberg J, El-Haddad G, Wolin E, Hendifar A, Yao J, Chasen B, et al. Phase 3 trial of 177 Lu-dotatate for midgut neuroendocrine tumors. N Engl J Med. 2017;376(2):125–35.

40. Bekes I, Friedl TWP, Köhler T, Mobus V, Janni W, Wockel A, et al. Does VEGF facilitate local tumor growth and spread into the abdominal cavity by suppressing endothelial cell adhesion, thus increasing vascular peritoneal permeability followed by ascites production in ovarian cancer? Mol Cancer. 2016;15:13.
41. Fushida S, Oyama K, Kinoshita J, Yagi Y, Okamoto K, Tajima H, et al. VEGF is a target molecule for peritoneal metastasis and malignant ascites in gastric cancer: prognostic significance of VEGF in ascites and efficacy of anti-VEGF monoclonal antibody. Onco Targets Ther. 2013;6:1445–51.
42. Raymond E, Dahan L, Raoul JL, Bang YJ, Borbath I, Lombard-Bohas C, et al. Sunitinib malate for the treatment of pancreatic neuroendocrine Tumors. N Engl J Med. 2011;364(6):501–13.
43. Faivre S, Niccoli P, Castellano D, Valle JW, Hammel P, Raoul JL. et al. Sunitinib in pancreatic neuroendocrine tumors: updated progression-free survival and final overall survival from a phase III randomized study. Ann Oncol. 2017;28(2):339–43.
44. Shiozaki H. Elimova E, Slack RS, Chen HC, Staerkel GA, Sneige N, et al. Prognosis of gastric adenocarcinoma patients with various burdens of peritoneal metastases. J Surg Oncol. 2016;113(1):29–35.
45. Glockzin G, Schlitt HJ, Piso P. Peritoneal carcinomatosis: patients selection, perioperative complications and quality of life related to cytoreductive surgery and hyperthermic intraperitoneal chemotherapy. World J Surg Oncol. 2009;7:5.
46. Cotte E, Passot G, Gilly FN, Glehen O. Selection of patients and staging of peritoneal surface malignancies. World J Gastrointest Oncol. 2010;2(1):31–5.

Palliative Interventions for Metastatic Neuroendocrine Tumors

19

Caitlin Hodge and Bridget N. Fahy

Introduction

The World Health Organization defines palliative care as "an approach that improves the quality of life of patients and their families facing the problem associated with life-threatening illness, for the prevention and relief of suffering by means of identification and impeccable assessment and treatment of pain and other problems, physical, psychosocial and spiritual" [1]. In general, "palliative surgery focuses on improving quality of life and relief of symptoms, and can be combined with other therapies with curative intent" [2].

While most appendiceal, gastric, and rectal neuroendocrine tumors (NETs) are localized, 65–95% of other gastroenteropancreatic NETs, such as small intestine and pancreatic, are metastatic at the time of diagnosis [3]. In addition, only 10% of patients with liver metastases have disease that is amenable to curative resection [4]. Furthermore, approximately 20% of patients who undergo exploration are found to have peritoneal carcinomatosis [5]. While it is difficult to study treatment for metastatic NETs given the relatively rare incidence and the heterogeneity of presentation and tumor biology [6], these tumors are often indolent in nature and can have lengthy survival even in the setting of metastatic disease [7].

The combination of frequent metastatic disease and indolent nature creates a unique scenario for palliation in the treatment of NETs. This requires a thoughtful approach to quality of life and symptom control in the setting of long-term

C. Hodge
Department of Surgery, Abington Hospital-Jefferson Health, Abington, PA, USA

B. N. Fahy (✉)
Department of Surgery, Division of Surgical Oncology, University of New Mexico, Albuquerque, NM, USA
e-mail: bfahy@salud.unm.edu

© Springer Nature Switzerland AG 2021
J. M. Cloyd, T. M. Pawlik (eds.), *Neuroendocrine Tumors*,
https://doi.org/10.1007/978-3-030-62241-1_19

metastatic disease. For NETs that are not amenable to resection with curative intent, interventions can be aimed at prolonging survival and/or relieving symptoms. While the strictest definition of palliation is focused solely on symptom management without the goal of life prolongation, most studies that discuss palliative surgery in NETs define it as non-curative surgery or surgery that leaves gross residual disease [8–11]. This type of surgery can be aimed at prolonging survival or at reducing disease burden to allow other treatments to be more effective.

Symptoms

Symptoms from NETs fall into two categories: symptoms caused by excess hormones released by the tumor and nonhormonal symptoms caused by the tumor itself. Hormonal symptoms are typically related to carcinoid syndrome secondary to metastasis to the liver [6]. The syndrome is characterized by diarrhea, flushing, and fatigue and can lead to complications such as carcinoid heart disease (which does not improve with the treatment of the hormone excess state [12, 13]), carcinoid fibrosis, and carcinoid crisis (which can be precipitated by surgery or other procedures [13, 14]).

Pancreatic NETs can also present with one of nine functional syndromes: insulinoma, gastrinoma, glucagonoma, somatostatinoma, VIPoma (vasoactive intestinal peptide), PPoma (pancreatic polypeptide), ACTHoma (adrenocorticotropic hormone), GHRoma (growth hormone-releasing factor), and PTHrPoma (parathyroid hormone-related peptide) [15–17]. While insulinomas are the most common type of functional pancreatic NETs, accounting for 35% to 40% of all cases, they rarely metastasize [15–17]. On the other hand, gastrinomas, the second most common type, are metastatic in 62–70% of cases. These syndromes lead to the need for life-long treatment of the excess hormone state greater than 60% of patients [13].

Nonhormonal symptoms are related to the physical effects of the tumor itself. The most common of these are abdominal pain, compressive symptoms, and weight loss [14, 18]. Gastric NETs can cause bleeding, while intestinal NETs can cause perforation or obstruction that can lead to the need for emergent surgery [19]. Large plaques on the colon can cause obstruction, leading to long-term nausea, vomiting, crampy abdominal pain, or obstruction leading to a need for diverting ostomy [5]. For small intestine NETs, the primary tumor is often small, but metastatic lymph nodes can be bulky and become more problematic than the primary [20]. Mesenteric and peritumoral fibrosis can lead to bowel ischemia, obstruction, or ileus. Tumor infiltration of the root of the mesentery can lead to vascular ischemia and subsequent malnutrition and cachexia [5, 14, 20, 21]. Most nonfunctional pancreatic NETs are found incidentally, but they can cause abdominal pain, jaundice, and weight loss [22, 23]. Hepatic metastases can lead to nausea, early satiety, pain, and impaired liver function [10, 21]. A summary of the various sites of NETs and their associated symptoms is listed in Table 19.1.

Table 19.1 Symptoms associated with tumor locations

Tumor location	Associated symptoms
Stomach	Bleeding, obstruction
Small or large intestine	Partial or complete obstruction, perforation
Pancreas	Pain, jaundice, weight loss Functional: associated hormonal syndrome
Lymph nodes (metastases)	Mesenteric fibrosis → bowel ischemia, bowel obstruction, ileus Retroperitoneal fibrosis → obstructive uropathy
Liver (metastases)	Pain, nausea, early satiety, liver failure Functional: carcinoid syndrome

Quality of Life

Studies on the impact of symptoms from NETs on quality of life (QoL) are heterogeneous. A systematic review of studies on quality of life in well-differentiated metastatic NETs found 49 studies that used 27 different questionnaires to assess various symptoms [24]. The authors found that symptom relief is common even in the absence of objective change in tumor burden. However, patients reported concerns about their family's future, exacerbation of their disease, distressing medical tests, and treatment toxicity [24]. An online, anonymous survey offered to all NET patients via support groups used the Short Form-36 (SF-36) and PROMIS-29 questionnaires to assess QoL [25, 26]. Patients with NETs had worse QoL than the general population standard for these tests. Furthermore, patients with current disease (i.e., disease either that has not been surgically removed or that has recurred), carcinoid syndrome, or increased bowel movements or flushing episodes had worse QoL than other NET patients [25]. In fact, flushing symptoms occurring even as little as once per 14 days contributed to worse QoL [26]. Patients with recurrent disease reported increased anxiety as well as worse physical, social, and mental function. Most notably, they reported impaired overall physical function, compromised sleep, and significant fatigue [26]. Another study that focused specifically on patients with small intestine NETs found worse health-related QoL (HRQoL) on the QoL 15D and SF-36 questionnaires in the NET group compared to controls for these tools [27]. Specifically, scores for sleep, excretion, depression, distress, vitality, sexual activity, breathing, usual activities, discomfort, and symptoms were worse. Among patients with NETs, patients with excretion-related symptoms had worse HRQoL than those without. A Canadian retrospective cohort study of prospectively collected Edmonton Symptom Assessment Scale scores for all NET patients found moderate to severe scores were most common for the domains of tiredness, well-being, lack of appetite, drowsiness, and anxiety [28]. For patients who survived at least 1 year, the proportion of patients with symptoms was stable over time, up to 5 years, suggesting that these symptoms often remained unmitigated [28]. Higher symptom burden was associated with primary tumor site, metastatic disease, younger age, higher comorbidities, lower socioeconomic status, and receipt of therapy within 30 days of assessment [28]. Furthermore, patients who died had the highest risk of moderate to severe symptoms along with a steep increase in reported symptoms in the last 2 months of life [29]. Interestingly, women reported a higher risk of anxiety, nausea, and pain [28].

Selecting Patients for Palliative Interventions

Selecting patients for curative-intent procedures is often straightforward, whereas selecting patients for surgical intervention in the palliative or non-curative setting is more challenging. Surgical decision-making is particularly difficult in the case of NETs due to the heterogeneous nature of these tumors and the prolonged survival of many patients, including those with metastatic disease. Additionally, there is a paucity of literature that specifically addresses the impact of surgical or other procedural interventions on the symptoms commonly associated with NETs. In order to guide surgical decision-making for palliation of NETs, it is helpful to consider three key factors: patient-related, procedure-related, and tumor-related.

Patient Factors

Patient selection is the single most important factor in surgical decision-making, and this is particularly true when considering surgical palliation [30]. The data on patient selection for palliative surgery is heterogeneous, and no single instrument has been defined as the best metric. A systematic review of selection criteria for evaluation of patients for palliative surgery found 17 studies that proposed various criteria for patient selection [31]. The criteria for evaluation included symptom control, prognosis, preoperative performance, quality of life, tumor burden amenable to palliation, procedure-related morbidity and mortality, feasibility of nonsurgical options, anticipated duration of hospitalization, requirement for additional palliation, and cost [31].

Studies have provided mixed results regarding the predictive value of biochemical markers in palliative surgery, and all studies to date on this topic have assessed heterogeneous groups of patients [30]. Markers that have been associated with poor outcomes following palliative surgery include anemia, hypoalbuminemia, elevated C-reactive protein, elevated creatinine, leukocytosis, and neutrophil-to-lymphocyte ratio. Several composite scores have been created by combining various lab values and measures of functional status; these include the Palliative Index, University of California, Davis nomogram, Glasgow prognostic score, and LENT score [30]. Other functional assessments include Eastern Cooperative Oncology Group (ECOG) performance status, American Society of Anesthesiologists (ASA) classification, and National Cancer Institute Fatigue Scale [30]. None of these assessment tools have specifically been applied to patients with NETs. The unique biology and natural history of NETs limit the ability to apply the findings when utilizing these tools for selecting patients for palliative procedures with other tumor types to patients with NETs.

With proper patient selection for palliative surgery, good results can be achieved. An early study by Miner et al. in 2004 of a series of 1022 patients who underwent a variety of palliative procedures for various tumor-related symptoms showed 80% symptom relief with a median duration of symptom control of 135 days [32]. However, these procedures were associated with significant 30-day morbidity and mortality of 29% and 11%, respectively. The authors subsequently proposed the palliative triangle as a framework for selecting patients for palliative interventions [33]. This framework engages the patient, family, and surgeon in a shared decision-making process that evaluates treatment options through the lens of the patient's symptoms and values as well as the likelihood of the intervention to resolve these symptoms and risks of the procedure [33]. A review of all palliative surgeries at a single institution found that for patients who underwent a palliative intervention after participating in discussions based on the palliative triangle framework, palliative surgery achieved 90% symptom resolution with a 30-day morbidity of 20% and mortality of 4%, with no difference in palliative surgery after initial nonoperative management [33].

When considering previously reported outcomes following palliative procedures for NETs, it is important to consider that most studies are retrospective and thus include bias. A systematic review of pancreatic NETs by Zhou et al. found likely bias within studies favoring resection in patients with better performance status, less advanced disease, and tumors in the body or tail [34]. Furthermore, many studies do not measure QoL directly but use symptom control as a surrogate measure. When this is considered along with the indolent nature of NETs and possible long life expectancy even in metastatic disease, the cost and benefit of palliative intervention must be weighed carefully. Patient goals for intervention should be determined preoperatively, as morbidity and mortality alone may not be representative of the patient's values or expectations.

Procedural Factors

Morbidity and Mortality of Procedure

Given the patient population, palliative procedures can be associated with high morbidity and mortality [32, 33]. A specific challenge is the difficulty in predicting outcomes for palliative procedures, as no available tool specifies surgical intent. For example, the American College of Surgeons National Surgical Quality Improvement Program (ACS-NSQIP) risk calculator was found to significantly overestimate complications from palliative procedures (31% versus predicted 59%) and significantly underestimate length of stay (actual 5.4 days versus predicted 2.1 days) [35]. In addition, the number of patients within the ACS-NSQIP pool who received palliative surgery is very small. In a review of a single institution's ACS-NSQIP database, only 1.8% of the 7763 patients had disseminated cancer, and less than 1/4 of those patients received palliative surgery [36].

While palliative procedures in general have a high risk of morbidity and mortality, several factors impact the risk of procedures for NETs specifically. A review of a European surgical quality registry for gastroenteropancreatic NETs from 2015 to 2018 found that severe complications (defined as Clavien-Dindo > III) were more common for duodenal and pancreatic lesions (22%) than for small intestine lesions (11%) [37]. In addition, functional tumors had higher rates of complications (23%) than nonfunctional tumors (14%). Interestingly, resection with curative intent of lymph nodes had a higher complication rate (21%) than resection for patients either without lymph node metastasis or with palliative intent (12%). The most common complications in this cohort were bleeding, surgical site infections, and pancreatic fistulas (which was most common with enucleation) [37].

Resection of the primary tumor in the setting of metastatic disease remains controversial [38]. However, reported mortality is low. For midgut NETs, a systematic review found that for studies that reported perioperative mortality, the rates ranged from 1.6% to 2.0% [12]. However, in one study, the mortality rate after the first resection was 0.5% and then increased to 2.0% with resection of recurrent disease [12, 20]. There is more controversy surrounding resection of primary pancreatic NETs in the setting of metastatic disease, given the increased morbidity and mortality for pancreatic resections [6]. However, a systematic review found that for studies reporting these data, mortality was 0%, and morbidity was 16–42% [34]. This likely reflects a combination of selection bias, including increased likelihood of resection of tumors in the body and tail of the pancreas, and performance of these procedures at specialized centers. A systematic review of resection of liver metastases in NETs found similarly low mortality rates [39]. Resection alone had reported mortality rates of 0–9% (median < 1%), and resection plus ablation had reported mortality rates of 0–5% (median 1%). Morbidity ranged from 3% to 45% (median 23%) and included intra-abdominal abscess formation (0–11%), wound infection (0–13%), bile leak (0–12%), hepatic failure (0–6%), and postoperative bleeding (0–11%).

Clinical Outcomes

The efficacy of a palliative procedure is measured by improvement in symptoms and/or quality of life. In the case of NETs, decreased tumor burden leads to decreased hormone secretion, which in turn leads to a decrease in or resolution of symptoms [14, 19]. The burden of liver disease and associated hormonal secretion from liver metastases makes liver-directed therapies a major focus of palliative interventions. Symptomatic relief after treatment of liver metastases occurred in 50–100% (median 93%) of patients according to a systematic review by Saxena et al. [39]. The 5-year symptom-free survival ranged from 15% to 46% (median 37%). The included studies all reported symptom relief based on patient reports and chart reviews [8–11, 40–46]. One study also reported ECOG performance status, which significantly decreased in patients undergoing embolization compared to their own pre-treatment scores as well as posttreatment scores of the surgery group [8]. Another study reported Karnofsky functional status, which improved by postoperative month three and maintained in survivors for up to 54 months [41]. Watzka et al. found that patients with NETs and hepatic metastases showed partial or complete control of symptoms for all patients following surgery for functioning tumors, with the location of the primary tumor having no effect on the outcome [47]. Following treatment of liver metastases, Spolverato et al. found that the proportion of patients reporting diarrhea decreased from 41% to 26% and flushing decreased from 34% to 11% [48]. However, less than 25% of patients experienced improved QoL after treatment, as evaluated by their own assessment tool. Patients with poor pre-treatment QoL were more likely to experience improvement. Despite the lack of objective difference in QoL, fewer patients in the surgery group than the nonsurgery group were dissatisfied with their outcomes [48].

The benefit of surgical intervention in patients with metastatic NETs and asymptomatic primary intestinal tumors is unclear. Watchful waiting with intervention at the time that patients become symptomatic has similar outcomes to prophylactic intervention. Furthermore, asymptomatic patients do not share the survival benefit as those who were symptomatic [14]. In addition, early intervention may increase risk of subsequent intestinal obstructions. A retrospective cohort review found that upfront resection of the primary tumor for patients with asymptomatic stage IV small intestine NETs showed no survival benefit over delayed surgery and was associated with more reoperations for intestinal obstructions [49]. One systematic review and meta-analysis found that for patients with midgut NETs without liver debulking surgery, there were conflicting findings regarding the effects of primary tumor resection on subsequent bowel complications [50]. One study showed a higher rate of bowel obstruction in the resected group along with higher rate of infarction in the non-resected group, while another noted that small bowel obstruction-related cachexia was more common in the non-resected group [50].

Tumor-Related Considerations

Recommending surgical palliation for well-differentiated NETs also requires the surgeon to consider the biology of the underlying tumor. The indolent nature of many NETs poses a unique challenge for the surgeon in this regard since many patients will live with their disease, and associated tumor-related symptoms, for many months to years. Surgical palliation under these circumstances may be very beneficial, whereas the same would not be true for a different histology (e.g., small cell carcinoma, adenocarcinoma). Knowledge regarding overall survival, risk of recurrence, and poor prognostic factors should guide decision-making for palliative interventions.

Overall Survival

Reports of overall survival (OS) in NETs vary widely. In a Surveillance, Epidemiology, and End Results (SEER) analysis, median OS for all NETs was 9.3 years, with stage, grade, age at diagnosis, primary site, and year of diagnosis associated with differences in 5-year OS [51]. OS has improved over time, especially for distant gastrointestinal and pancreatic disease [51]. Hill et al. found a median OS of 114 months for patients across all groups (local, regional, metastatic) undergoing surgery versus 35 months for patients in whom surgery was recommended but did not receive it [52]. The factors significantly associated with decreased OS include the inability to undergo complete surgical resection, presence of extrahepatic disease, nonfunctional tumors, pancreatic primary tumors, and poorly differentiated tumors [39, 53, 54]. When present, these factors should be considered when selecting patients for palliative interventions in order to balance the potential benefits of the palliative procedure against the patient's OS.

Risk of Recurrence

Similar to OS, risk of recurrent disease is an important factor when considering a patient for a palliative intervention; patients at high risk of recurrence may be less likely to experience the full benefit of a palliative intervention, particularly if the palliative procedure is associated with significant morbidity or a prolonged recovery. Recurrence of metastatic disease is common, even after complete resection [20, 55]. This often leads to the need for reoperation or other inventions [20]. A Canadian cohort study found recurrence after complete resection of gastroenteropancreatic NETs in 23% of patients at 3 years, 34% at 5 years, and 49% at 10 years [56]. Pancreatic NETs recurred earliest, with a median time to recurrence of 7.2 years [56]. For pancreatic NETs, Ki67 > 5%, larger tumors (>2.1–4 cm), lymph node metastasis, advanced stage, higher grade, and vascular infiltration have been shown to predict recurrence of disease [17, 57–61]. Small intestine NETs recurred at a median of 8.7 years, and the overall median time to recurrence for all gastroenteropancreatic NETs was 9.5 years [56]. Stage significantly influences recurrence rates. One group found recurrence rates for midgut NETs of 50% at 5 years and 85% at 10 years, with no recurrence in stage I disease and equal rates of recurrence in stages II and III disease [62]. Another group found that median recurrence-free survival after complete resection of ileojejunal NETs decreased from 53 months for stage I/II to 36 months in stage III and only 9 months in stage IV disease [63]. NETs usually recurred in the liver, mesentery, and pelvic lymph nodes [62].

Recurrence rates are higher for metastatic disease, and the liver is the primary site of progression in most patients [39]. A multi-institutional database looking at neuroendocrine liver metastases showed a recurrence rate of 65% within a median follow-up of 4.5 years for patients who had received curative-intent liver surgery [55]. In this study, the disease-free survival was 76% at 1 year, 40% at 5 years, and 32% at 10 years. Nonanatomic liver resection is also associated with increased recurrence [64]. The US Neuroendocrine Study Group found an eventual 95% recurrence after treatment of metastatic NETs [53].

Predictors of Poor Prognosis

Several factors have been shown to correlate with poor prognosis. A retrospective study using the SEER database found that stage, primary tumor site, grade, sex, race, age, and year of diagnosis correlated with prognosis [54]. The median survival by grade in the study was 124 months for grade I, 64 months for grade II, and 10 months for grades III and IV tumors [54]. The US Neuroendocrine Study Group found high-grade tumors to have worse OS, with median survival of 13.5 months versus 63 months for intermediate and 132 months for low-grade tumors [53]. Similarly, poorly differentiated tumors had a median OS of 4.7 months versus 68 months for moderately and 116 months for well-differentiated tumors [53]. Preoperative imaging findings associated with poor prognosis include calcifications and hypoenhancement on CT scan, PET avidity, and lack of uptake on octreotide scan [23].

Availability of Other Treatment Options

The decision to offer a palliative operation for NETs is also impacted by the availability of nonsurgical therapies and their efficacy in treating NET-associated symptoms. Somatostatin analogues (SSAs) are the first-line therapy for management of symptoms from most functional NETs and can control carcinoid-related diarrhea and flushing [17]. They are generally well-tolerated and have also been shown to decrease tumor proliferation [17]. A recent systematic review and meta-analysis found that SSAs control diarrhea and flushing associated with carcinoid syndrome in 66–70% of patients, with similar results between octreotide and lanreotide [65]. For patients with refractory symptoms on SSAs, dose escalation controls diarrhea and flushing in 72–84% of patients [65]. A newer therapy for refractory diarrhea is telotristat ethyl (a tryptophan hydroxylase inhibitor) [66]. Studies of the effects of interferon on carcinoid symptoms have showed mixed results, but a meta-analysis showed improvement of diarrhea in 45% and flushing in 61% of patients [65]. The use of interferon is limited by its side effect profile, including flu-like symptoms and fatigue [66]. Chemotherapy has largely been studied in poorly differentiated and progressive NETs, and data on its effects on symptom control are lacking [17, 65]. A systematic review and network analysis found seven studies that used the European Organization for Research and Treatment of Cancer (EORTC) Quality of Life Questionnaire (QLQ) C30 to evaluate changes in QoL for SSAs, interferon, sunitinib, two chemotherapy regimens, and telotristat [67]. They found that telotristat followed by SSAs had the greatest effect on improving QoL scores using this metric [67].

Targeted therapies include sunitinib (a tyrosine kinase inhibitor) and everolimus (mammalian target of rapamycin inhibitor), which have both been shown to improve progression-free survival (PFS) [13]. Sunitinib has largely been studied in pancreatic NETs, and everolimus has been studied in both pancreatic and gastrointestinal NETs [13]. Data on symptom control are limited to small series and case reports, which have shown control of insulinoma symptoms with everolimus and sunitinib and control of VIPoma symptoms with sunitinib [13]. A small series reported that everolimus controlled symptoms of carcinoid symptoms for 7 out of 10 patients with symptomatic NETs, with a mean duration of improvement of 13.9 months (range 1–39 months) [68]. A study of sunitinib versus placebo using the EORTC-QLQ C30 questionnaire showed no significant change in HRQoL categories or symptoms in patients with pancreatic NETs, with the sole exception of worsening diarrhea in the sunitinib group [69]. A phase IV study of nonfunctional tumors treated with everolimus showed no change from baseline HRQoL scores using the FACT-G questionnaire [70]. Another study of everolimus for advanced progressive pancreatic NETs using the EORTC-QLQ C30 showed a decrease from baseline physical functioning after 3 months and an improvement from baseline in disease-related worries, with all other domains remaining similar before and after treatment [71]. While the data is not robust, sunitinib and everolimus seem to have little effect on overall HRQoL but may be used to control specific refractory symptoms of functional NETs.

Outcomes Following Palliative Procedures

Lymph Node

Lymph node metastases are common in small intestine NETs and can lead to a desmoplastic reaction in the mesentery that causes decreased bowel perfusion and resulting abdominal pain [19]. Thus, the initial surgical approach for small intestine NETs may initially include extensive mesenteric dissection for removal of mesenteric lymph nodes [20]. Many patients develop collaterals to avoid life-threatening ischemia but still may develop chronic mesenteric ischemia and ultimately require bowel resection for symptom control [5]. Segmental resection with nodal resection may be helpful in this scenario. Mesenteric fibrosis causing symptomatic obstruction of the mesenteric vessels can be treated with surgical removal or superior mesenteric vein (SMV) stenting [14]. A retrospective review found that SMV stenting was equivalent to surgical resection of central mesenteric metastases in regard to subjective symptom alleviation but had less morbidity [49]. Retroperitoneal fibrosis causing ureteral obstruction can also occur, and this can be treated with percutaneous nephrostomy or placement of stents [49]. Intestinal bypass is another option for obstructing small intestine NETs but may not provide effective relief of intestinal angina symptoms that occur secondary to chronic mesenteric ischemia.

Liver

Liver metastases are common in both small intestine and pancreatic NETs [3] and are present in 50–95% of patients at presentation [4, 47]. They are usually multiple and bilobar [19]. Treatment of liver lesions can not only improve survival but also decrease hormonal symptoms and thus improve QOL. Intervention is indicated to reduce hormonally functioning tumor burden refractory to medical therapy [3]. There are a variety of treatment options for liver metastases, including surgery, radiofrequency ablation (RFA), transarterial embolization/transarterial chemoembolization (TAE/TACE), selective internal radiotherapy (SIRT), and peptide receptor radionucleotide therapy (PRRT) [14, 63]. Aggressive locoregional control may be beneficial for symptom control even for high-grade NETs. In a retrospective review of 36 patients with grade III gastroenteropancreatic NETs, patients receiving aggressive locoregional control (cytoreductive surgery, RFA, intra-arterial therapy) had higher rates of symptom relief than patients receiving only systemic therapy or supportive care [72].

Surgery

In general, palliative debulking is recommended for symptoms refractory to medical management, as debulking may improve symptom control and even increase survival [73]. A retrospective single-center study showed partial or complete control of symptoms after surgery for all patients with functioning tumors [47]. Small series have shown high rates of improvement of patient-reported QoL after resection of symptomatic pancreatic NETs [74] and improved Karnofsky scores and carcinoid symptoms after resection of liver metastases [41]. Debulking or resection of the primary tumor may also help provide better control of liver metastases or allow other treatments to be more effective [12, 75].

Radiofrequency Ablation

RFA can be performed via image-guided percutaneous, laparoscopic, or open techniques [76]. It is often used in conjunction with surgery to decrease the amount of liver parenchyma taken [16] and is only used for small lesions [24, 77]. Rates of symptom improvement exceed 90% [17], with an average duration of symptom control of 11 months [78]. A systematic review found that 48% of patients had concomitant surgery and 92% experienced improved symptoms with recurrence rates ranging from 63 to 81% [79]. A retrospective study showed that 97% of patients with hormonal symptoms experienced partial to complete resolution of symptoms after RFA [77]. Nonhormonal symptoms are much harder to palliate, and may not benefit from RFA. For example, Eriksson et al. found that for patients undergoing RFA or liver resection (complete clearance) for extra-pancreatic NETs, a portion of patients with symptoms from functional tumors improved, but patients with non-functioning tumors showed no improvement of symptoms [80].

Arterial-Based Interventions

TAE/TACE takes advantage of the largely hepatic arterial blood supply of NET metastases and is used for unresectable tumors enabling both locoregional disease control and control of excessive hormone production [76]. Studies have shown symptom improvement in 40–88% of patients [73]. Small series have shown improvement of carcinoid symptoms for 2/3 of patients as well as the ability to discontinue octreotide therapy for almost half of patients after TAE or TACE [81, 82]. However, post-embolic syndrome, consisting of fever, abdominal pain, nausea, and vomiting, occurs in up to 90% of patients [17]. Less common post-embolic complications include ileus, portal vein thrombosis, hepatic abscess, hepatic fistula, encephalopathy, and renal insufficiency [73]. The post-embolic syndrome is generally self-limited [66], and successive treatments of smaller portions of the liver may decrease symptom severity [83]. Even so, published reports show a median hospital stay of 4–5 days posttreatment [83].

When compared to surgery, Chamberlain et al. found that non-pain symptoms were palliated in 94% of patients undergoing TAE and 100% of surgical patients [10]. They also found that palliation of pain and symptoms occurred in 90% pts. undergoing TAE or surgery, with an average duration of symptom control of 19.3 months. Duration of symptom response was longest for hormonal symptoms (17 months) versus pain (6.2 months) [10].

Another arterial-based intervention is SIRT, which uses resin-coated microbeads. Few studies report QoL after SIRT [83]. One series showed improvement of carcinoid symptoms in 79% of patients [84], and another showed increase in mental health and social functioning domains of the SF-36 at 6 and 12 months posttreatment, with a return to baseline QoL at 24 months [85]. The most common associated adverse effects are fatigue, abdominal pain, and nausea, which have been reported in 56% of patients at 3 months posttreatment but only 6% at 6 months [83, 84]. Repeat treatments increase the risk of radiation-induced liver injury, so SIRT may not be the ideal option for repeat treatments [83]. Direct comparisons between these therapies are lacking; however, SIRT seems to be better tolerated than TAE/TACE [83]. Furthermore, a European study found that SIRT is twice as expensive as TAE, which may limit its clinical application [83]. The high rates of procedure-related morbidity and duration of posttreatment adverse effects should be considered when recommending these interventions for palliation of NET-associated symptoms.

Peptide Receptor Radionuclide Therapy

PRRT targets molecules on cell surfaces and delivers specific and localized radiotherapy. It is most useful for symptomatic patients with somatostatin receptor-positive tumors (80–95% of gastroenteropancreatic NETs) with liver disease who are not surgical candidates. PRRT has been associated with improved QoL, especially in patients with tumor regression [69]. Studies using the EORTC C30 tool to assess QoL found significant improvements in global health QoL as well as role, emotional and social functions [86]. Karnofsky performance scores and symptoms (including insomnia, appetite loss, and diarrhea) also improved [87]. Patients who had objective regression of disease had better posttreatment QoL, but patients with progressive disease also experienced improvements [86, 87]. Symptom improvements in fatigue, insomnia, pain, nausea, vomiting, dyspnea, appetite loss, diarrhea, constipation, flushing, and weight loss have been reported in 40–80% of patients in several moderately sized observational series [73, 87–91]. In addition, some patients were able to decrease or stop octreotide for symptom management [91]. Symptom improvement is not necessarily associated with objective tumor response or overall survival. Complications of this therapy include bone marrow suppression, with >50% of patients experiencing at least one episode of pancytopenia [89], as well as fatigue, nausea, and rarely liver or renal failure [73]. However, patients who are not symptomatic have been shown to maintain global health QoL and Karnofsky performance scores over the course of treatment [87].

Summary and Recommendations

The indolent nature of NETs and long-term survival of patients, even in the setting of advanced metastatic disease, mandates the careful consideration of QOL. Palliative surgery or other procedural interventions can contribute to improved symptom control and QOL in addition to disease stability. Careful consideration of patient,

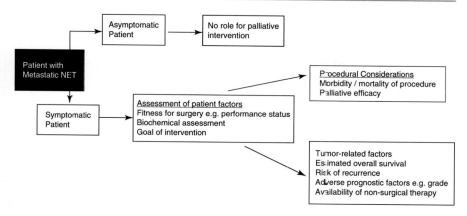

Fig. 19.1 Algoritm for patient selection for palliative procedures

procedure, and tumor characteristics is required to optimize patient selection. The preoperative conversation should clarify the patient's goals for the intervention as well as baseline performance status and QoL. The intent of the procedure—palliative versus curative—should be clearly articulated to the patient. Symptoms should also be assessed, as asymptomatic patients are less likely to benefit from noncurative intervention. Furthermore, it should be determined whether or not the tumor is amenable to the proposed intervention based on size and location. Care must be taken in evaluating the morbidity and mortality of the proposed procedure, as much of the literature is retrospective and contains significant patient selection bias. Finally, tumor characteristics, most notably grade, should be assessed as tumors with poor prognostic factors may be best paliated with nonsurgical approaches. Figure 19.1 summarizes an approach to patient selection for palliative interventions.

References

1. Organization, W.H. WHO definition of palliative care. Available from: https://www.who.int/cancer/palliative/definition/en/.
2. Fahy BN. Introduction: role of palliative care for the surgical patient. J Surg Oncol. 2019;120(1):5–9.
3. Frilling A, Clift AK. Surgical approaches to the management of neuroendocrine liver metastases. Endocrinol Metab Clin N Am. 2018;47(3):627–43.
4. Lesurtel M, et al. Palliative surgery for unresectable pancreatic and periampullary cancer: a reappraisal. J Gastrointest Surg. 2006;10(2):286–91.
5. Howe JR, et al. The surgical management of small bowel neuroendocrine tumors: consensus guidelines of the North American Neuroendocrine Tumor Society. Pancreas. 2017;46(6):715–31.
6. Almond LM, et al. Role of palliative resection of the primary tumour in advanced pancreatic and small intestinal neuroendocrine tumours: a systematic review and meta-analysis. Eur J Surg Oncol. 2017;43(10):1808–15.
7. Lim C, et al. Liver transplantation for neuroendocrine tumors: what have we learned? Semin Liver Dis. 2018;38(4):351–6.

8. Osborne DA, et al. Improved outcome with cytoreduction versus embolization for symptomatic hepatic metastases of carcinoid and neuroendocrine tumors. Ann Surg Oncol. 2006;13(4):572–81.

9. Que FG, et al. Hepatic resection for metastatic neuroendocrine carcinomas. Am J Surg. 1995;169(1):36–42; discussion 42–3.

10. Chamberlain RS, et al. Hepatic neuroendocrine metastases: does intervention alter outcomes? J Am Coll Surg. 2000;190(4):432–45.

11. Hibi T, et al. Surgery for hepatic neuroendocrine tumors: a single institutional experience in Japan. Jpn J Clin Oncol. 2007;37(2):102–7.

12. Guo J, et al. Systematic review of resecting primary tumor in MNETs patients with unresectable liver metastases. Oncotarget. 2017;8(10):17396–405.

13. Ito T, Lee L, Jensen RT. Treatment of symptomatic neuroendocrine tumor syndromes: recent advances and controversies. Expert Opin Pharmacother. 2016;17(16):2191–205.

14. Jin XF, et al. Supportive therapy in gastroenteropancreatic neuroendocrine tumors: often forgotten but important. Rev Endocr Metab Disord. 2018;19(2):145–58.

15. Parbhu SK, Adler DG. Pancreatic neuroendocrine tumors: contemporary diagnosis and management. Hosp Pract. 1995, 2016;44(3):109–19.

16. Akirov, A, et al. Treatment options for pancreatic neuroendocrine tumors. Cancers (Basel). 2019;11(6):828.

17. Scott AT, Howe JR. Evaluation and management of neuroendocrine tumors of the pancreas. Surg Clin North Am. 2019;99(4):793–814.

18. Niederle MB, Niederle B. Diagnosis and treatment of gastroenteropancreatic neuroendocrine tumors: current data on a prospectively collected, retrospectively analyzed clinical multicenter investigation. Oncologist. 2011;16(5):602–13.

19. Goretzki PE, et al. Curative and palliative surgery in patients with neuroendocrine tumors of the gastro-entero-pancreatic (GEP) tract. Rev Endocr Metab Disord. 2018;19(2):169–78.

20. Norlén O, et al. Long-term results of surgery for small intestinal neuroendocrine tumors at a tertiary referral center. World J Surg. 2012;36(6):1419–31.

21. Singh S, et al. Recurrence in resected gastroenteropancreatic neuroendocrine tumors. JAMA Oncol. 2018;4(4):583–5.

22. Sallinen V, Haglund C, Seppänen H. Outcomes of resected nonfunctional pancreatic neuroendocrine tumors: do size and symptoms matter? Surgery. 2015;158(6):1556–63.

23. Cloyd JM, Poultsides GA. Non-functional neuroendocrine tumors of the pancreas: advances in diagnosis and management. World J Gastroenterol. 2015;21(32):9512–25.

24. Jiménez-Fonseca P, et al. Health-related quality of life in well-differentiated metastatic gastroenteropancreatic neuroendocrine tumors. Cancer Metastasis Rev. 2015;34(3):381–400.

25. Beaumont JL, et al. Comparison of health-related quality of life in patients with neuroendocrine tumors with quality of life in the general US population. Pancreas. 2012;41(3):461–6.

26. Pearman TP, et al. Health-related quality of life in patients with neuroendocrine tumors: an investigation of treatment type, disease status, and symptom burden. Support Care Cancer. 2016;24(9):3695–703.

27. Karppinen N, et al. Health-related quality of life in patients with small intestine neuroendocrine tumors. Neuroendocrinology. 2018;107(4):366–74.

28. Hallet J, et al. Patterns of symptoms burden in neuroendocrine tumors: a population-based analysis of prospective patient-reported outcomes. Oncologist. 2019;24(10):1384–94.

29. Hallet J, et al. Symptom burden at the end of life for neuroendocrine tumors: an analysis of 2579 prospectively collected patient-reported outcomes. Ann Surg Oncol. 2019;26(9):2711–21.

30. Cohen JT, Miner TJ. Patient selection in palliative surgery: defining value. J Surg Oncol. 2019;120(1):35–44.

31. Foster D, et al. Palliative surgery for advanced cancer: identifying evidence-based criteria for patient selection: case report and review of literature. J Palliat Med. 2016;19(1):22–9.

32. Miner TJ, Brennan MF, Jaques DP. A prospective, symptom related, outcomes analysis of 1022 palliative procedures for advanced cancer. Ann Surg. 2004;240(4):719–26; discussion 726-7.

33. Miner TJ, et al. The palliative triangle: improved patient selection and outcomes associated with palliative operations. Arch Surg. 2011;146(5):517–22.

34. Zhou B, et al. Role of palliative resection of the primary pancreatic neuroendocrine tumor in patients with unresectable metastatic liver disease: a systematic review and meta-analysis. Onco Targets Ther. 2018;11:975–82.

35. Rodriguez RA, et al. Estimation of risk in cancer patients undergoing palliative procedures by the American College of Surgeons Risk Calculator. J Palliat Med. 2016;19(10):1039–42.

36. Vidri RJ, et al. American College of Surgeons National Surgical Quality Improvement Program as a quality-measurement tool for advanced cancer patients. Ann Palliat Med. 2015;4(4):200–6.

37. Albers MB, et al. Complications of surgery for gastro-entero-pancreatic neuroendocrine neoplasias. Langenbeck's Arch Surg. 2020;405(2):137–43.

38. Capurso G, et al. Systematic review of resection of primary midgut carcinoid tumour in patients with unresectable liver metastases. Br J Surg. 2012;99(11):1480–6.

39. Saxena A, et al. Surgical resection of hepatic metastases from neuroendocrine neoplasms: a systematic review. Surg Oncol. 2012;21(3):e131–41.

40. Cho CS, et al. Histologic grade is correlated with outcome after resection of hepatic neuroendocrine neoplasms. Cancer. 2008;113(1):126–34.

41. Knox CD, et al. Survival and functional quality of life after resection for hepatic carcinoid metastasis. J Gastrointest Surg. 2004;8(6):653–9.

42. Sarmiento JM, et al. Surgical treatment of neuroendocrine metastases to the liver: a plea for resection to increase survival. J Am Coll Surg. 2003;197(1):29–37.

43. Norton JA, et al. Aggressive surgery for metastatic liver neuroendocrine tumors. Surgery. 2003;134(6):1057–63; discussion 1063–5

44. Chung MH, et al. Hepatic cytoreduction followed by a novel long-acting somatostatin analog: a paradigm for intractable neuroendocrine tumors metastatic to the liver. Surgery. 2001;130(6):954–62.

45. Jaeck D, et al. Hepatic metastases of gastroenteropancreatic neuroendocrine tumors: safe hepatic surgery. World J Surg. 2001;25(6):689–92.

46. McEntee GP, et al. Cytoreductive hepatic surgery for neuroendocrine tumors. Surgery. 1990;108(6):1091–6.

47. Watzka FM, et al. Surgical therapy of neuroendocrine neoplasm with hepatic metastasis: patient selection and prognosis. Langenbeck's Arch Surg. 2015;400(3):349–58.

48. Spolverato G, et al. Quality of life after treatment of neuroendocrine liver metastasis. J Surg Res. 2015;198(1):155–64.

49. Daskalakis K, et al. Clinical signs of fibrosis in small intestinal neuroendocrine tumours. Br J Surg. 2017;104(1):69–75.

50. Tsilimigras DI, et al. Is resection of primary midgut neuroendocrine tumors in patients with unresectable metastatic liver disease justified? A systematic review and meta-analysis. J Gastrointest Surg. 2019;23(5):1044–54.

51. Dasari A, et al. Trends in the incidence, prevalence, and survival outcomes in patients with neuroendocrine tumors in the United States. JAMA Oncol. 2017;3(10):1335–42.

52. Hill JS, et al. Pancreatic neuroendocrine tumors: the impact of surgical resection on survival. Cancer. 2009;115(4):741–51.

53. Chakedis J, et al. Surgery provides long-term survival in patients with metastatic neuroendocrine tumors undergoing resection for non-hormonal symptoms. J Gastrointest Surg. 2019;23(1):122–34.

54. Yao JC, et al. One hundred years after "carcinoid": epidemiology of and prognostic factors for neuroendocrine tumors in 35,825 cases in the United States. J Clin Oncol. 2008;26(18):3063–72.

55. Spolverato G, et al. Management and outcomes of patients with recurrent neuroendocrine liver metastasis after curative surgery: an international multi-institutional analysis. J Surg Oncol. 2017;116(3):298–306.

56. Singh S, et al. Follow-up recommendations for completely resected gastroenteropancreatic neuroendocrine tumors. JAMA Oncol. 2018;4(11):1597–604.

57. Genç CG, et al. Recurrence of pancreatic neuroendocrine tumors and survival predicted by Ki67. Ann Surg Oncol. 2018;25(8):2467–74.
58. Marchegiani G, et al. Patterns of recurrence after resection for pancreatic neuroendocrine tumors: who, when, and where? Neuroendocrinology. 2019;108(3):161–71.
59. Martin JA, et al. Lymph node metastasis in the prognosis of gastroenteropancreatic neuroendocrine tumors. Pancreas. 2017;46(9):1214–8.
60. Halfdanarson TR, et al. Pancreatic neuroendocrine tumors (PNETs): incidence, prognosis and recent trend toward improved survival. Ann Oncol. 2008;19(10):1727–33.
61. Deng BY, et al. Clinical outcome and long-term survival of 150 consecutive patients with pancreatic neuroendocrine tumors: a comprehensive analysis by the World Health Organization 2010 grading classification. Clin Res Hepatol Gastroenterol. 2018;42(3):261–8.
62. Cives M, et al. Analysis of postoperative recurrence in stage I-III midgut neuroendocrine tumors. J Natl Cancer Inst. 2018;110(3):282–9.
63. Habbe N, et al. Outcome of surgery for ileojejunal neuroendocrine tumors. Surg Today. 2013;43(10):1168–74.
64. Sham JG, et al. The impact of extent of liver resection among patients with neuroendocrine liver metastasis: an international multi-institutional study. J Gastrointest Surg. 2019;23(3):484–91.
65. Hofland J, et al. Management of carcinoid syndrome: a systematic review and meta-analysis. Endocr Relat Cancer. 2019;26(3):R145–r156.
66. Stueven AK, et al. Somatostatin analogues in the treatment of neuroendocrine tumors: past, present and future. Int J Mol Sci. 2019;20(12):3049.
67. Kaderli RM, et al. Therapeutic options for neuroendocrine Tumors: a systematic review and network meta-analysis. JAMA Oncol. 2019;5(4):480–9.
68. Bainbridge HE, Larbi E, Middleton G. Symptomatic control of neuroendocrine tumours with everolimus. Horm Cancer. 2015;6(5–6):254–9.
69. Vinik A, et al. Patient-reported outcomes and quality of life with Sunitinib versus placebo for pancreatic neuroendocrine tumors: results from an international phase III trial. Target Oncol. 2016;11(6):815–24.
70. Pavel M, et al. Safety and QOL in patients with advanced NET in a phase 3b expanded access study of everolimus. Target Oncol. 2016;11(5):667–75.
71. Ramage JK, et al. Observational study to assess quality of life in patients with pancreatic neuroendocrine tumors receiving treatment with everolimus: the OBLIQUE study (UK phase IV trial). Neuroendocrinology. 2019;108(4):317–27.
72. Du S, et al. Aggressive locoregional treatment improves the outcome of liver metastases from grade 3 gastroenteropancreatic neuroendocrine Tumors. Medicine (Baltimore). 2015;94(34):e1429.
73. Basuroy R, Srirajaskanthan R, Ramage JK. Neuroendocrine tumors. Gastroenterol Clin N Am. 2016;45(3):487–507.
74. Hung JS, et al. Is surgery indicated for patients with symptomatic nonfunctioning pancreatic neuroendocrine tumor and unresectable hepatic metastases? World J Surg. 2007;31(12):2392–7.
75. Bertani E, et al. Resection of the primary tumor followed by peptide receptor radionuclide therapy as upfront strategy for the treatment of G1-G2 pancreatic neuroendocrine tumors with unresectable liver metastases. Ann Surg Oncol. 2016;23(Suppl 5):981–9.
76. Harring TR, et al. Treatment of liver metastases in patients with neuroendocrine tumors: a comprehensive review. Int J Hepatol. 2011;2011:154541.
77. Akyildiz HY, et al. Laparoscopic radiofrequency thermal ablation of neuroendocrine hepatic metastases: long-term follow-up. Surgery. 2010;148(6):1288–93; discussion 1293.
78. Mazzaglia PJ, et al. Laparoscopic radiofrequency ablation of neuroendocrine liver metastases: a 10-year experience evaluating predictors of survival. Surgery. 2007;142(1):10–9.
79. Mohan H, et al. Radiofrequency ablation for neuroendocrine liver metastases: a systematic review. J Vasc Interv Radiol. 2015;26(7):935–942.e1.
80. Eriksson J, et al. Surgery and radiofrequency ablation for treatment of liver metastases from midgut and foregut carcinoids and endocrince pancreatic tumors. World J Surg. 2008;32:930–8.

81. Schell SR, et al. Hepatic artery embolization for control of symptoms, octreotide requirements, and tumor progression in metastatic carcinoid tumors. J Gastrointest Surg. 2002;6(5):664–70.
82. Drougas JG, et al. Hepatic artery chemoembolization for management of patients with advanced metastatic carcinoid tumors. Am J Surg. 1998;175(5):408–12.
83. de Mestier L, et al. Liver transarterial embolizations in metastatic neuroendocrine tumors. Rev Endocr Metab Disord. 2017;18(4):459–71.
84. Braat A, et al. Radioembolization with (90)Y resin microspheres of neuroendocrine liver metastases: international multicenter study on efficacy and toxicity. Cardiovasc Intervent Radiol. 2019;42(3):413–25.
85. Cramer B, Xing M, Kim HS. Prospective longitudinal quality of life assessment in patients with neuroendocrine tumor liver metastases treated with 90Y radioembolization. Clin Nucl Med. 2016;41(12):e493–7.
86. Teunissen JJ, Kwekkeboom DJ, Krenning EP. Quality of life in patients with gastroenteropancreatic tumors treated with [177Lu-DOTA0,Tyr3]octreotate. J Clin Oncol. 2004;22(13):2724–9.
87. Khan S, et al. Quality of life in 265 patients with gastroenteropancreatic neuroendocrine tumors treated with [177Lu-DOTA0,Tyr3]octreotate. J Nucl Med. 2011;52(9):1361–8.
88. Zandee WT, et al. Symptomatic and radiological response to 177Lu-DOTATATE for the treatment of functioning pancreatic neuroendocrine tumors. J Clin Endocrinol Metab. 2019;104(4):1336–44.
89. Vinjamuri S, et al. Peptide receptor radionuclide therapy with (90)Y-DOTATATE/(90)Y-DOTATOC in patients with progressive metastatic neuroendocrine tumours: assessment of response, survival and toxicity. Br J Cancer. 2013;108(7):1440–8.
90. Abou Jokh Casas E, et al. Evaluation of (177)Lu-Dotatate treatment in patients with metastatic neuroendocrine tumors and prognostic factors. World J Gastroenterol. 2020;26(13):1513–24.
91. Bushnell D, et al. Evaluating the clinical effectiveness of 90Y-SMT 487 in patients with neuroendocrine tumors. J Nucl Med. 2003;44(10):1556–60.

Emerging Systemic Therapies for Neuroendocrine Tumors

20

Medhavi Gupta, Gillian Prinzing, and Renuka Iyer

Introduction

Neuroendocrine tumors (NETs) are a heterogeneous group of rare neoplasms arising from neuroendocrine cells that can arise in almost any location in the body [1]. The survival of NET patients is highly variable and dependent on several factors like the primary site of origin and stage and grade of tumor [2]. Management is guided by the location of tumor, resectability, extent of metastases, and whether the tumor is functional or not. The National Comprehensive Cancer Network (NCCN) guidelines provide a general guidance for the management of NETs based on location [3]. Surgical management is utilized both for curative purposes when the disease is locoregional and for cytoreduction and palliation of symptoms in case of advanced/metastatic disease. In recent years, the treatment paradigm has been transformed by the addition of a number of therapies ranging from somatostatin analogues, cytotoxic chemotherapies, targeted therapies, and radionuclide therapies [4–10]. This chapter summarizes available systemic therapies, with a special focus on the emerging systemic therapies (Fig. 20.1) for management of NETs.

Chemotherapy

Systemic chemotherapies including platinum-based therapies, irinotecan, and streptozocin have been widely used for the management of high-grade neuroendocrine carcinomas (NECs) [11–15]. A randomized phase II trial (E2211, NCT01824875) demonstrated the efficacy of temozolomide (TEM) with capecitabine (CAP) in patients with advanced grade 1 (G1) or grade 2 (G2) pancreatic NETs (pNETs) [16].

M. Gupta · G. Prinzing · R. Iyer (✉)
Roswell Park Comprehensive Cancer Center, Buffalo, NY, USA
e-mail: gmp64@cornell.edu; Renuka.Iyer@RoswellPark.org

© Springer Nature Switzerland AG 2021
J. M. Cloyd, T. M. Pawlik (eds.), *Neuroendocrine Tumors*,
https://doi.org/10.1007/978-3-030-62241-1_20

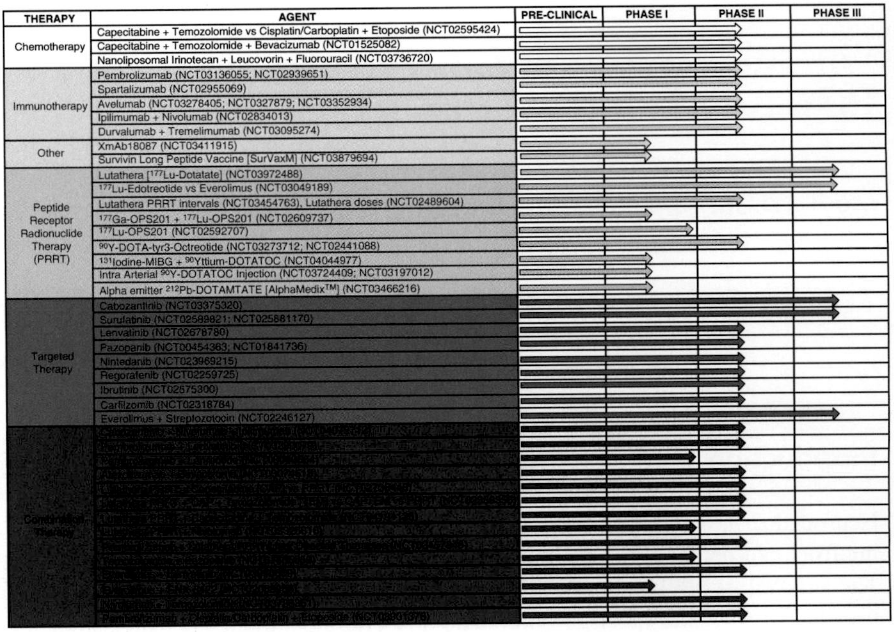

THERAPY	AGENT	PRE-CLINICAL	PHASE I	PHASE II	PHASE III
Chemotherapy	Capecitabine + Temozolomide vs Cisplatin/Carboplatin + Etoposide (NCT02595424)				
	Capecitabine + Temozolomide + Bevacizumab (NCT01525082)				
	Nanoliposomal Irinotecan + Leucovorin + Fluorouracil (NCT03736720)				
Immunotherapy	Pembrolizumab (NCT03136055; NCT02939651)				
	Spartalizumab (NCT02955069)				
	Avelumab (NCT03278405; NCT0327879; NCT03352934)				
	Ipilimumab + Nivolumab (NCT02834013)				
	Durvalumab + Tremelimumab (NCT03095274)				
Other	XmAb18087 (NCT03411915)				
	Survivin Long Peptide Vaccine [SurVaxM] (NCT03879694)				
Peptide Receptor Radionuclide Therapy (PRRT)	Lutathera [177Lu-Dotatate] (NCT03972488)				
	177Lu-Edotreotide vs Everolimus (NCT03049189)				
	Lutathera PRRT intervals (NCT03454763), Lutathera doses (NCT02489604)				
	177Ga-OPS201 + 177Lu-OPS201 (NCT02609737)				
	177Lu-OPS201 (NCT02592707)				
	90Y-DOTA-tyr3-Octreotide (NCT03273712; NCT02441088)				
	131Iodine-MIBG + 90Yttium-DOTATOC (NCT04044977)				
	Intra Arterial 90Y-DOTATOC Injection (NCT03724409; NCT03197012)				
	Alpha emitter 212Pb-DOTAMTATE [AlphaMedix™] (NCT03466216)				
Targeted Therapy	Cabozantinib (NCT03375320)				
	Surufatinib (NCT02589821; NCT025881170)				
	Lenvatinib (NCT02678780)				
	Pazopanib (NCT00454363; NCT01841736)				
	Nintedanib (NCT023969215)				
	Regorafenib (NCT02259725)				
	Ibrutinib (NCT02575300)				
	Carfilzomib (NCT02318784)				
	Everolimus + Streptozotocin (NCT02246127)				

Fig. 20.1 Therapies in development for neuroendocrine tumors

A number of studies are looking at different chemotherapy combinations for the management of NETs. The combination of CAPTEM is being compared with cisplatin/carboplatin and etoposide in a phase II study (NCT02595424) in patients with advanced G3 gastroenteropancreatic (GEP) NECs in the frontline setting to identify the best first-line approach and relation to Ki 67, if any [17]. Another phase II trial (NCT015250820) is exploring the combination of CAPTEM with bevacizumab in patients with advanced G1/G2 pNETs. A novel combination of nanoliposomal irinotecan, leucovorin, and fluorouracil is being explored in a phase II trial (NCT03736720) in patients with advanced high-grade NETs of GEP and unknown primary (UP) origin after progression on first line of therapy with etoposide/cisplatin or CAPTEM [18]. In well-differentiated tumors with high tumor burden and symptoms where debulking by local ablative/surgical approaches is not feasible, these chemotherapy agents are also used and supported by NCCN guidelines.

Somatostatin Analogues

Neuroendocrine tumors express somatostatin receptors (SSTRs), especially SSTR2 and SSTR5. Somatostatin analogues (SSA) primarily target SSTR2. Initially SSAs were utilized in the context of symptom control in patients with functional or symptomatic GEP-NETs. Subsequently, two randomized phase III studies reported antitumor activity of SSAs [8, 9]. In the PROMID study, patients with well-differentiated, treatment-naïve, metastatic midgut NETs [n = 85] were randomized to receive octreotide long-acting repeatable (LAR) 30 mg monthly versus placebo. Median time to progression was longer in the octreotide LAR arm as compared to placebo [14.3 months vs. 6 months, HR 0.34, p = 0.000072]. On subgroup analysis, the antiproliferative response was more pronounced in patients with low (<10%) hepatic tumor load and a resected primary tumor. Another SSA, lanreotide, was evaluated in the phase III CLARINET trial. In this trial, patients with advanced WD or moderately differentiated, nonfunctioning G1/G2 GEP-NETs were randomized to lanreotide 120 mg deep subcutaneously monthly versus placebo [9]. The progression-free survival (PFS) was improved in favor of lanreotide [median PFS not reached vs. 18 months, HR 0.47, p < 0.0001]. The benefit was seen in patients with both low (</25%) and high (>25%) hepatic tumor volume, and it should be noted it also included pancreatic NETs that were not included in the PROMID trial.

Targeted Therapies

Everolimus, an mTOR inhibitor, was the first targeted therapy approved for advanced, progressive, well-differentiated G1/G2 pNETs. The approval was based on the randomized phase III RADIANT-3 trial (NCT00510068) that showed a PFS benefit when compared to placebo [n = 410] [6]. A few years later, everolimus approval was extended to advanced, progressive, G1/G2 NETs of gastrointestinal (GI) or lung origin based on the randomized phase III RADIANT-4 trial (NCT01524783) which also revealed PFS benefit in all NETs [5]. Sunitinib, a multitargeted tyrosine kinase inhibitor (TKI), was also approved for progressing pNETs based on a PFS benefit seen in a phase III trial [4]. Despite delay in progression, radiographic responses with everolimus and sunitinib are uncommon (7–9%), and agents that control disease in patients who are intolerant or progress on these agents remain an unmet need. To this end, currently, several additional targeted therapy agents are in development for NETs as shown in Table 20.1, and few of these are further along in development after early evidence of promising activity.

Cabozantinib, a multitargeted TKI (VEGFR-2, c MET, AXL, and RET inhibitor), showed encouraging results in a phase II trial of progressive G1/G2 carcinoids or pNETs. The study demonstrated an overall response rate (ORR) of 15% in both groups and a median PFS of 22 months for pNETs and 31 months for carcinoid tumors [19]. Cabozantinib is currently being studied in a randomized phase III trial (NCT03375320, CABINET) in G1/G2 pNETs and other carcinoids after failure of everolimus by the Alliance Cooperative Group.

Surufatinib (HMPL012), a potent TKI (VEGFR 1–3, FGFR, and CSF-1R inhibitor), demonstrated promising antitumor activity in patients with advanced, progressive, well-differentiated G1/G2 pNETs and extra-pancreatic NETs in a phase Ib/II study conducted in China [20]. The pNET and non-pNET cohorts had a median PFS of 21 months and 13 months, respectively, and an ORR of 19% and 15%, respectively. Surufatinib was further tested in two randomized phase III trials in non-pNETs (NCT02588170) and pNETs (NCT02589821, SANET-p) in China. The

Table 20.1 Targeted therapies in development for neuroendocrine tumors

Clinical study	Phase	Intervention	Patient population	Primary end point	[a]Current status
Tyrosine kinase inhibitors					
NCT01466036	II	Cabozantinib	Advanced/ metastatic, G1/ G2 carcinoids or pNETs	ORR of 15% in both groups	Active, not recruiting
NCT03375320 or CABINET trial	III	Cabozantinib vs. placebo	Advanced/ metastatic, G1/ G2 pNETs and carcinoids, progression after ≥1 line of therapy including everolimus	PFS	Active, recruiting
NCT02549937	I/II	Surufatinib	pNETs (after progression on sunitinib, everolimus, or both) and EP-NETs (after progression on everolimus)	DLT, PFS	Recruiting
NCT02678780 or TALENT	II	Lenvatinib	Metastatic, G1/ G2 pNETs and EP-NETs after progression on systemic therapy	ORR of 29% (pNETs = 40%, EP-NETs = 18%)	Completed
NCT00454363	II	Pazopanib	Advanced/ metastatic, G1/ G2 pNETs and carcinoids after progression on systemic therapy	ORR of 22% pNETs and no response in carcinoids	Completed
NCT01841736 or Alliance A021202	II	Pazopanib vs. placebo	Advanced/ metastatic, G1/ G2 carcinoids	PFS = 12 months with pazopanib vs. 8 months with placebo	Active, not recruiting
NCT02399215	II	Nintedanib	Advanced/ metastatic, G1/ G2 carcinoids excluding pNETs	PFS = 11 months, OS = 28 months	Active, not recruiting

Table 20.1 (continued)

Clinical study	Phase	Intervention	Patient population	Primary end point	[a]Current status
NCT02259725	II	Regorafenib	Advanced/ metastatic carcinoids without prior targeted treatment	PFS	Active, not recruiting
NCT02575300	II	Ibrutinib	Advanced/ metastatic, G1/ G2 pNETs or carcinoids	No responses seen	Completed
Proteasome inhibitor					
NCT02318784	II	Carfilzomib	Advanced/ metastatic, G1/ G2 carcinoids and pNETs, with or without prior systemic therapy	ORR	Active, not recruiting

Abbreviations: *G1* grade 1, *G2* grade 2, *NET* neuroendocrine tumors, *pNETs* pancreatic NETs, *EP-NETs* extra-pancreatic NETs, *ORR* overall response rate, *PFS* progression-free survival, *OS* overall survival, *DLT* dose-limiting toxicities, *vs.* versus
[a]As of June 4, 2020

phase III trial of surufatinib randomized patients with advanced, progressive G1/G2 pNETs (NCT02589821, SANET-p) to surufatinib versus placebo in a 2:1 ratio. The trial was terminated early after interim analysis showed a PFS benefit with surufatinib over placebo [PFS of 9.2 months vs. 3.8 months, HR 0.3, p < 0.0001] [21, 22]. Surufatinib is being studied in a phase I/II study in patients with advanced solid tumors, including pNETs (after progression on sunitinib, everolimus, or both) and extra-pancreatic NETs (after progression on everolimus), in the United States. In the meantime, surufatinib was granted fast-track designations for the treatment of advanced progressive pNETs and EP-NETs by the US FDA [23].

The phase II TALENT (NCT02678780) trial tested lenvatinib (VEGFR 1–3 and FGFR 1–4 inhibitor) in advanced G1/G2 pNETs and GI NETs after progression on prior systemic therapy. Lenvatinib showed efficacy with an ORR of 29% [pNETs 40%, GI-NETs 18%] and a median PFS of 16 months and 15 months for pNETs and GI-NETs, respectively [24]. Nintedanib, a multitargeted TKI (VEGF, PDGR, and FGFR inhibitor), was studied in a phase II study (NCT02399215) involving patients with G1/G2, advanced/metastatic, progressive carcinoid tumors [25]. PFS rate at 16 weeks was 87% with a median PFS of 11 months and OS of 28 months. Quality of life was improved or maintained in at least 50% of patients during the treatment. The treatment was well tolerated with grade 2 and grade 3 AEs in 47% and 27% of patients, respectively.

Pazopanib, another multitargeted TKI (VEGFR 1–3, PDGFR-α and PDGFR-β, and c-KIT inhibitor), was tested in a phase II study (NCT00454363) in patients [n = 52] with advanced/metastatic G1/G2 pNETs and carcinoid tumors after progression on previous therapies [26]. Pazopanib showed an ORR of 22% in pNETs with no response in carcinoid tumors. Another phase II trial (NCT01841736, Alliance A021202) randomized G1/G2 carcinoid tumor patients [n = 171] to pazopanib versus placebo. The pazopanib arm had a significant improvement in PFS as compared to placebo [12 months vs. 8 months, HR 0.5, p = 0.0005] without any improvement in overall survival (OS) [p = 0.7] [27].

A phase II trial (NCT02318784) is testing carfilzomib, a proteasome inhibitor in patients with advanced G1/G2 pNETs and typical carcinoids [n = 62] with or without prior systemic treatment. Interim analysis shows efficacy with responses in 3% of patients and a median PFS of 8 months [28]. Ibrutinib (Bruton's TKI) failed to show any responses in patients with advanced, progressive pNETs, GI, and lung NETs in a phase II trial (NCT02259725) [n = 20] [29]. A randomized phase III trial (NCT02246127, SEQTOR) is comparing the efficacy of everolimus followed by streptozotocin-based chemotherapy upon progression or the reverse sequence in patients with advanced, progressive G1/G2 pNETs [n = 141]. Regorafenib, another multitargeted TKI, is also being tested in a phase II trial (NCT02259725) in patients with advanced/metastatic pNETs or carcinoids with no prior targeted therapies.

Immunotherapy

Single-agent immunotherapy has shown modest benefit at best in NETs. The KEYNOTE-028 trial (NCT02054806) evaluated the role of pembrolizumab in PD-L1-positive, advanced or metastatic solid tumors after progression on ≥1 line of therapy [30]. Data from the G1/G2 PD-L1-positive pNETs [n = 16] and carcinoids [n = 25] showed an ORR of 12% [30]. The median duration of response was not reached in pNETs and was 9 months in the carcinoid tumor cohort. The phase II basket study, KEYNOTE-158 (NCT02628067), studied the role of pembrolizumab in cancer subtypes, including G1/G2 GEP and lung NETs [n = 107]. Retrospective analysis by IHC showed PD-L1 positivity in 16% patients. ORR in the NET cohort was 4% [3 pNETs and 1 UP], all PD-L1-negative. Median PFS was 4 months and median OS was not reached [31]. A phase II study (NCT03136055) is investigating pembrolizumab [cohort A = pembrolizumab alone, cohort B = pembrolizumab + chemotherapy] in extrapulmonary, poorly differentiated neuroendocrine carcinomas (NEC). Data from cohort A showed insufficient activity [ORR = 7%, 1/14 patients] [32]. Patients are currently being enrolled to cohort B. Another phase II trial (NCT02939651) is studying pembrolizumab in metastatic high-grade NETs, excluding lung/thymus and Merkel cell carcinoma, after progression on platinum-based therapy, regardless of PD-L1 expression [33].

Another anti-PD1 agent, spartalizumab (PDR001), showed a similar ORR to pembrolizumab in a phase II study (NCT02955069) [34]. Patients with advanced, progressive G1/G2 NETs [n = 33 pNETs, 32 GI NETs, 30 lung NETs] or NEC [n = 21of GEP origin] were enrolled regardless of PD-L1 expression. PD-L1 positivity was higher in NEC (43%) versus G1/G2 NETs [pNETs 23%, lung NETs 19%, GI NETS 0%]. The study showed an ORR of 7% in G1/G2 NETs [3% pNETs, 0% GI NETs, 20% lung NETs] and 5% in NEC [34].

An anti-PD-L1 agent, avelumab, is being studied in patients with advanced or metastatic, grade 2/3 well-differentiated NET of GI or lung origin (NET-002, NCT03278379) and grade 3 NECs of GI or lung origin (NET001, NCT03278405) after zero to two prior lines of therapy. Avelumab is also being investigated in a similar German trial (AveNec, NCT03352934) in patients with advanced or metastatic G3 NEC after progression on ≥1 line of chemotherapy.

The combination of ipilimumab and nivolumab was assessed in a phase II basket trial SWOG S1609/DART (Dual Anti-CTLA-4 and Anti-PD-1 blockade in Rare Tumors, NCT02834013). The combination looks promising in the extrapulmonary high-grade NEC cohort [n = 32, GI n = 15] with an ORR of 44%. There were no responses in the G1/G2 NETs [35]. The 6-month PFS was 31% and the median OS was 11 months. Enrollment is ongoing for pNETs and high-grade NEC cohorts. Another phase II trial (NCT03095274, DUNE trial) is evaluating the combination of durvalumab and tremelimumab in advanced/metastatic G1/G2 pNETs, GI or lung NETs, and G3 of GEP origin or UP site after progression on ≥1 line of therapy.

Other Immunotherapy Agents

Immunomodulating agents based on the biology of the overexpression of SSTR2 receptors in NETs are being developed. A second-generation anti-SSTR CAR T-cell therapy using CD28 as a co-stimulatory module showed antitumor activity in NET cell lines [36]. Scientists at the University of Pennsylvania are developing a CAR T-cell therapy in NETs supported by a grant from the Neuroendocrine Tumor Research Foundation (NETRF) [37]. There is preclinical data to suggest that a monoclonal bispecific antibody, XmAb18087, binds to SSTR2 and CD3 leading to the stimulation of target-dependent T-cell activation and cytotoxicity [38]. A phase I clinical trial (NCT03411915) is investigating XmAb18087 in patients with advanced/metastatic G1/G2 GEP-NETs.

A study showed that the expression of an inhibitor of apoptosis protein, survivin, in NETs is associated with poor long-term outcomes [39]. A phase I trial (NCT03879694) is investigating its therapeutic potential as survivin long peptide vaccine (SurVaxM) in patients with advanced or metastatic GEP and lung NETs that express survivin.

Peptide Receptor Radionuclide Therapy (PRRT)

The addition of PRRT as a treatment option for patients with GEP-NETs has been an important paradigm shift in the management of NETs. The phase III NETTER-1 trial (NCT01578239) randomized patients [n = 231] with advanced, progressive, SSTR+, G1/G2 midgut NETs to ^{177}Lu-Dotatate (Lutathera) PRRT plus octreotide long-acting repeatable (LAR) versus octreotide LAR alone. Patients enrolled in the

Lutathera arm had a significant improvement in PFS when compared to octreotide alone [7]. Notably, this trial did not include any patients with pNETs. The role of Lutathera PRRT in frontline treatment of advanced, SSTR+, G2/G3 GEP-NETs is being evaluated in the phase III NETTER-2 trial (NCT03972488). A phase II Italian study (NCT03454763, LUTHREE) is investigating two different intervals of Lutathera PRRT, cohort A (intensive, every 5 weeks) and cohort B (non-intensive, every 8–10 weeks) for five cycles. Another randomized phase II study (NCT02489604, LUNET) is exploring different doses of Lutathera PRRT in GEP-NETs by comparing 25.9 GBq activity to 18.5 GBq activity over seven cycles. A phase III trial (COMPETE trial, NCT03049189) is investigating another radionuclide compound, ^{177}Lu-Edotreotide, in SSTR (+) GEP-NETs (WD, all grades) in comparison to everolimus in the frontline setting [40].

Traditionally, beta emitters are used as the radiation source for PRRT. The alternative use of α particles might be advantageous as it has a higher linear energy transfer, delivers radiation over a shorter range, and leads to lesser collateral damage to normal tissues and increased tumor cell death. Alpha-emitter therapy with ^{212}Pb-DOTAMTATE (AlphaMedix™) is being studied in a phase I study (NCT03466216) in advanced refractory SSTR (+) NETs.

The use of somatostatin antagonists with PRRT seems another promising approach as preclinical data suggests that they have higher tumor uptake and retention than SSTR agonists [41]. The theranostic combination of SSTR2 antagonists, ^{68}Ga-OPS201 and ^{177}Lu-OPS201, was investigated in a phase I study (NCT02609737) in advanced, progressive, WD, SSTR2+ NETs [n = 20; 9 pNETs, 9 GI NETs]. Efficacy was seen with an ORR of 45% and a median PFS of 21 months. [42]. ^{177}Lu-OPS201 is being evaluated in another phase I/II trial (NCT02592707) in patients with advanced, progressive, SSTR+, G1/G2 NETs [GEP, lung NETs, pheochromocytomas, and paragangliomas] after progression on everolimus/sunitinib [43].

Two phase II studies (NCT03273712, NCT02441088) are assessing the role of PRRT with ^{90}Y-DOTA-tyr3-Octreotide in SSTR+ NETs after progression of ≥1 line of therapy. An early phase I trial (NCT03044977) is looking into combining two radionuclide therapies, ^{131}Iodine-MIBG and ^{90}Yttrium-DOTATOC, in patients with advanced, well-differentiated, SSTR+, G1/G2, midgut NETs after progression on ≥1 line of systemic therapy. Preliminary results from the first cohort did not demonstrate any dose-limiting toxicities [44].

PRRT is also being explored in the area of liver-directed therapies. Two phase I trials (NCT03724409, NCT03197012) are looking into intra-arterial injection of ^{90}Y-DOTATOC in patients with SSTR+ NETs with liver metastases.

Combination Therapies

An exciting area of research is the use of combinational strategies; these are summarized in Table 20.2. PRRT is being studied in combination with chemotherapy agents in multiple phase II trials, including NCT04194125 (Lutathera PRRT plus CAPTEM in G1/G2 GEP-NETs), NCT02736448 [Lutathera PRRT plus CAP vs.

Table 20.2 Combination therapies in development for neuroendocrine tumors

Clinical study	Phase	Intervention	Patient population	Primary end point	[a]Current status
Immunotherapy-based regimens					
NCT04079712	II	Nivolumab, ipilimumab, and cabozantinib	Metastatic NECs after progression on one systemic treatment	ORR	Active, recruiting
NCT03290079	II	Pembrolizumab and lenvatinib	Metastatic, poorly differentiated G3 NEC of extrapulmonary origin after progression ≥1 treatment	ORR	Suspended
NCT03074513	II	Atezolizumab and bevacizumab	Rare solid tumors, NET cohort: G1/G2 pNETs and EP-NETs with any number of prior therapies	PFS	Active, recruiting
NCT03043664 or PLANET	Ib/II	Pembrolizumab and lanreotide	Advanced/metastatic, G1/G2 GEP-NETs	ORR	Active, not recruiting
PRRT-based therapies					
NCT02736448	II	Lutathera PRRT vs. Lutathera PRRT + capecitabine	Advanced/metastatic G1–G3 GEP-NETs after progression on standard therapy	PFS	Active, not recruiting
PRRT-based therapies					
NCT02358356	II	Lutathera PRRT + CAPTEM vs. CAPTEM (part 1) Vs. PRRT alone (part 2)	Part 1: advanced/metastatic G1/G2 pNETs Part 2: advanced/metastatic G1/G2 midgut NETs after progression ≤2 systemic therapies	PFS	Active, recruiting
NCT04194125	II	Lutathera PRRT + CAPTEM	Advanced/metastatic, G1/G2 GEP-NETs	PFS	Active, recruiting
NCT03457948	II	Pembrolizumab + Lutathera PRRT or liver-directed therapies	WD NETs with liver metastases	ORR	Active, recruiting
NCT03325816	I/II	Nivolumab + Lutathera PRRT	Relapsed/refractory extensive-stage small cell lung cancer or advanced G1/G2 pulmonary NETs	R2PD, PFS	Active, not recruiting

(continued)

Table 20.2 (continued)

Clinical study	Phase	Intervention	Patient population	Primary end point	[a]Current status
Targeted therapies-based regimens					
NCT03950609	II	Lenvatinib and everolimus	Advanced/ metastatic carcinoids	ORR	Active, recruiting
Targeted therapies-based regimens					
NCT01465659	I/II	Pazopanib and temozolomide	Unresectable/ advanced pNETs after 0–2 prior therapies	Dose-limiting toxicities and ORR	Active, not recruiting
NCT02063958	I	SNX-5422 + everolimus q28 days	NETs after ≤4 prior therapies	Dose-limiting toxicities	Completed
Chemotherapy-based regimens					
NCT03728361	II	Temozolomide with nivolumab	Recurrent small cell lung cancer and advanced/ metastatic NETs (any grade, primary site, and previous line of therapy)	ORR	Active, recruiting
NCT03901378	II	Cisplatin/ carboplatin and etoposide with pembrolizumab	Advanced/ metastatic, G3 GEP NEC or large cell NEC in the frontline setting	PFS	Active, recruiting
NCT01465659	I/II	Temozolomide and pazopanib	Advanced G1/G2 pNETs with zero to two prior therapies	Dose-limiting toxicities	Active, not recruiting

Abbreviations: *PRRT* peptide receptor radionuclide therapy, *CAPTEM* capecitabine/temozolomide, *G1* grade 1, *G2* grade 2, *G3* grade 3, *NET* neuroendocrine tumor, *NEC* neuroendocrine carcinoma, *pNETs* pancreatic NETs, *GEP* gastroenteropancreatic, *WD* well-differentiated, *ORR* overall response rate, *PFS* progression-free survival, *R2PD* recommended phase II dosing
[a]As of June 4, 2020

PRRT alone in well-differentiated G1–G3 GEP-NETs], and NCT02358356 [two parallel trials: Lutathera PRRT plus CAP/TEM vs. (1) CAPTEM alone in G1/G2 pNETs and (2) PRRT alone in G1/G2 midgut NETs]. A pilot phase II trial (NCT03457948) is studying the combination of pembrolizumab with Lutathera PRRT or liver-directed therapies in patients with well-differentiated NETs with liver metastases. Another multicenter phase I/II trial (NCT03325816) is assessing the role of nivolumab with Lutathera in patients with relapsed/refractory extensive-stage small cell lung cancer or advanced G1/G2 pulmonary NETs [45]. In the phase II portion of the study, patients will be randomized to maintenance treatment with nivolumab and PRRT versus observation with a primary end point of PFS.

A number of trials are looking at the combination of targeted therapies with other agents. A phase I/II trial (NCT01465659) is investigating pazopanib with TEM in advanced pNETs. Results from the phase I portion showed promising activity with a tolerable safety profile and an ORR of 25% [46]. A phase II trial (NCT03950609) is investigating everolimus with lenvatinib in patients with advanced G1/G2 carcinoid tumors. Everolimus is also being studied with SNX-5422, a heat-shock protein 90 (HSP 90) inhibitor in a phase I study in NET patients. Preliminary results show that the combination was tolerable and showed efficacy [47].

Immunotherapy is being studied in combination with other agents. A phase II trial (NCT03290079) is investigating pembrolizumab with lenvatinib in patients with metastatic poorly differentiated G3 NEC of extrapulmonary origin. Pembrolizumab is also being studied in combination with depot lanreotide in GEP-NETs in a phase Ib/II trial (NCT03043664, PLANET). Nivolumab and ipilimumab are being studied in a phase II trial (NCT04079712) in combination with cabozantinib in patients with advanced progressive NEC. A phase II basket trial (NCT03074513) is evaluating the combination of atezolizumab and bevacizumab in patients with rare solid tumors. The NET cohort includes patients with G1/G2 pNETs or extra-pancreatic NETs with any number of prior therapies.

Other potential strategies include the combination of chemotherapy with either immunotherapy or targeted agents. Chemotherapy (cisplatin/carboplatin and etoposide) is being studied in combination with pembrolizumab in the frontline setting in a phase II trial (NCT03901378) involving patients with advanced/metastatic G3 NEC of GEP origin or large cell NEC. Nivolumab is being studied in combination with TEM in recurrent small cell lung cancer and advanced/metastatic NETs [any grade, primary site, and previous line of therapy] in a phase II study (NCT03728361). Interim analysis showed efficacy with an ORR of 25% [48]. The combination of pazopanib and TEM is being studied in a phase I/II study (NCT01465659) in advanced, recurrent G1/G2 pNETs. Results from the phase I component showed that the combination is tolerable and showed preliminary efficacy with a median PFS of 12 months and OS of 36 months [46]. The phase II study is ongoing.

Future Directions

With better understanding of the underlying biology of NETs, a number of therapies are under development as summarized in this chapter. As we continue to add new therapies to our armamentarium of drugs, choosing the right drug for the right patient will be of utmost importance. The overarching goal is to improve the long-term survival outcomes while optimizing quality of life of patients with advanced NETs. Decision-making will require a thorough evaluation of disease-related factors (resectability, location, grade, presence of metastasis), patient-related factors (presence of symptoms, medical comorbidities, goals of therapy), and drug-related factors (adverse events, financial toxicity, and access to therapies). These decisions will require a well-coordinated multidisciplinary approach to patient care. With the addition of novel therapies, the optimal sequencing of therapies is largely unknown. Future trials will need to address sequencing strategies and neoadjuvant, adjuvant, maintenance, and observation strategies. In parallel to the development of novel therapies, advances in predictive and prognostic biomarkers are also needed for optimal patient selection and to gauge the treatment response. Further, the importance of supportive care and maintenance of quality of life cannot be underscored as we help our patients on their journey toward improved survival.

References

1. Yao JC, Hassan M, Phan A, Dagohoy C, Leary C, Mares JE, et al. One hundred years after "carcinoid": epidemiology of and prognostic factors for neuroendocrine tumors in 35,825 cases in the United States. J Clin Oncol. 2008;26(18):3063–72.
2. Dasari A, Shen C, Halperin D, Zhao B, Zhou S, Xu Y, et al. Trends in the incidence, prevalence, and survival outcomes in patients with neuroendocrine tumors in the United States. JAMA Oncol. 2017;3(10):1335–42.
3. Shah MH, Goldner WS, Halfdanarson TR, Bergsland E, Berlin JD, Halperin D, et al. NCCN guidelines insights: neuroendocrine and adrenal tumors, version 2.2018. J Natl Compr Cancer Netw. 2018;16(6):693–702.
4. Raymond E, Dahan L, Raoul J-L, Bang Y-J, Borbath I, Lombard-Bohas C, et al. Sunitinib malate for the treatment of pancreatic neuroendocrine tumors. N Engl J Med. 2011;364(6):501–13.
5. Yao JC, Fazio N, Singh S, Buzzoni R, Carnaghi C, Wolin E, et al. Everolimus for the treatment of advanced, non-functional neuroendocrine tumours of the lung or gastrointestinal tract (RADIANT-4): a randomised, placebo-controlled, phase 3 study. Lancet (London, England). 2016;387(10022):968–77.
6. Yao JC, Shah MH, Ito T, Bohas CL, Wolin EM, Van Cutsem E, et al. Everolimus for advanced pancreatic neuroendocrine tumors. N Engl J Med. 2011;364(6):514–23.
7. Strosberg J, El-Haddad G, Wolin E, Hendifar A, Yao J, Chasen B, et al. Phase 3 trial of (177) Lu-Dotatate for midgut neuroendocrine tumors. N Engl J Med. 2017;376(2):125–35.
8. Rinke A, Müller H-H, Schade-Brittinger C, Klose K-J, Barth P, Wied M, et al. Placebo-controlled, double-blind, prospective, randomized study on the effect of octreotide LAR in the control of tumor growth in patients with metastatic neuroendocrine midgut tumors: a report from the PROMID Study Group. J Clin Oncol. 2009;27(28):4656–63.
9. Caplin ME, Pavel M, Cwikla JB, Phan AT, Raderer M, Sedlackova E, et al. Lanreotide in metastatic enteropancreatic neuroendocrine tumors. N Engl J Med. 2014;371(3):224–33.
10. Kulke MH, Hörsch D, Caplin ME, Anthony LB, Bergsland E, Öberg K, et al. Telotristat ethyl, a tryptophan hydroxylase inhibitor for the treatment of carcinoid syndrome. J Clin Oncol. 2016;35(1):14–23.
11. Moertel CG, Kvols LK, O'Connell MJ, Rubin J. Treatment of neuroendocrine carcinomas with combined etoposide and cisplatin. Evidence of major therapeutic activity in the anaplastic variants of these neoplasms. Cancer. 1991;68(2):227–32.
12. Chong CR, Wirth LJ, Nishino M, Chen AB, Sholl LM, Kulke MH, et al. Chemotherapy for locally advanced and metastatic pulmonary carcinoid tumors. Lung Cancer. 2014;86(2):241–6.
13. Rossi A, Di Maio M, Chiodini P, Rudd RM, Okamoto H, Skarlos DV, et al. Carboplatin- or cisplatin-based chemotherapy in first-line treatment of small-cell lung cancer: the COCIS meta-analysis of individual patient data. J Clin Oncol. 2012;30(14):1692–8.
14. Kouvaraki MA, Ajani JA, Hoff P, Wolff R, Evans DB, Lozano R, et al. Fluorouracil, doxorubicin, and streptozocin in the treatment of patients with locally advanced and metastatic pancreatic endocrine carcinomas. J Clin Oncol. 2004;22(23):4762–71.

15. Sun W, Lipsitz S, Catalano P, Mailliard JA, Haller DG. Phase II/III study of doxorubicin with fluorouracil compared with streptozocin with fluorouracil or dacarbazine in the treatment of advanced carcinoid tumors: Eastern Cooperative Oncology Group Study E1281. J Clin Oncol. 2005;23(22):4897–904.
16. Kunz PL, Catalano PJ, Nimeiri H, Fisher GA, Longacre TA, Suarez CJ, et al. A randomized study of temozolomide or temozolomide and capecitabine in patients with advanced pancreatic neuroendocrine tumors: a trial of the ECOG-ACRIN Cancer Research Group (E2211). J Clin Oncol. 2018;36(15 suppl):4004.
17. Eads JR, Catalano PJ, Fisher GA, Klimstra DS, Zhang Z, Rubin D, et al. Randomized phase II study of cisplatin and etoposide versus temozolomide and capecitabine in patients (pts) with advanced G3 non-small cell gastroenteropancreatic neuroendocrine carcinomas (GEPNEC): a trial of the ECOG-ACRIN Cancer Research Group (EA2142). J Clin Oncol. 2016;34(15 suppl):TPS4149-TPS.
18. Gupta M, Choi M, Ramirez RA, Attwood K, Mukherjee S, Iyer RV. Phase II study of nanoliposomal irinotecan (nal-IRI) with 5-fluorouracil (5-FU)/folinic acid (FA) in refractory advanced high-grade neuroendocrine cancer (HG-NEC) of gastroenteropancreatic (GEP) or unknown origin. J Clin Oncol. 2020;38(4 suppl):TPS636-TPS.
19. Chan JA, Faris JE, Murphy JE, Blaszkowsky LS, Kwak EL, McCleary NJ, et al. Phase II trial of cabozantinib in patients with carcinoid and pancreatic neuroendocrine tumors (pNET). J Clin Oncol. 2017;35(4 suppl):228.
20. Xu J, Li J, Bai C, Xu N, Zhou Z, Li Z, et al. Surufatinib in advanced well-differentiated neuroendocrine tumors: a multicenter, single-arm, open-label, phase Ib/II trial. Clin Cancer Res. 2019;25(12):3486.
21. CHI-MED. Chi-Med announces that Surufatinib Phase III SANET-p Study has already achieved its primary endpoint in advanced pancreatic neuroendocrine tumors in China and will stop early 2020. Available from: https://www.globenewswire.com/news-release/2020/01/20/1972348/0/en/Chi-Med-Announces-that-Surufatinib-Phase-III-SANET-p-Study-Has-Already-Achieved-its-Primary-Endpoint-in-Advanced-Pancreatic-Neuroendocrine-Tumors-in-China-and-Will-Stop-Early.html.
22. CHI-MED. Chi-Med to discuss surufatinib Phase III and U.S. phase I/Ib efficacy and safety data. Presented at the 2019 ESMO Annual Meeting 2019. Available from: https://www.chi-med.com/2019-esmo-annual-meeting/.
23. CHI-MED. Chi-Med announces surufatinib granted U.S. FDA Fast Track Designations for the treatment of both pancreatic and non-pancreatic neuroendocrine tumors 2020. Available from: https://www.chi-med.com/surufatinib-granted-us-fda-fast-track-designations/.
24. Capdevila J, Fazio N, López-López C, Teule A, Valle JW, Tafuto S, et al. Progression-free survival (PFS) and subgroups analyses of lenvatinib in patients (pts) with G1/G2 advanced pancreatic (panNETs) and gastrointestinal (giNETs) neuroendocrine tumors (NETs): updated results from the phase II TALENT trial (GETNE 1509). J Clin Oncol. 2019;37(4 suppl):332.
25. Iyer RV, Konda B, Owen DH, Attwood K, Sarker S, Suffren S-A, et al. Multicenter phase 2 study of nintedanib in patients (pts) with advanced progressing carcinoid tumors. J Clin Oncol. 2018;36(15 suppl):4105.
26. Phan AT, Halperin DM, Chan JA, Fogelman DR, Hess KR, Malinowski P, et al. Pazopanib and depot octreotide in advanced, well-differentiated neuroendocrine tumours: a multicentre, single-group, phase 2 study. Lancet Oncol. 2015;16(6):695–703.
27. Bergsland EK, Mahoney MR, Asmis TR, Hall N, Kumthekar P, Maitland ML, et al. Prospective randomized phase II trial of pazopanib versus placebo in patients with progressive carcinoid tumors (CARC) (Alliance A021202). J Clin Oncol. 2019;37(15 suppl):4005.
28. Singh J, Shipley D, Cultrera J, Chua C, Cohn AL, Soriano AO, et al. Phase 2 study of carfilzomib for the treatment of patients with advanced neuroendocrine cancers. J Clin Oncol. 2018;36(4 suppl):382.
29. Al-Toubah T, Schell MJ, Cives M, Zhou JM, Soares HP, Strosberg JR. A phase II study of Ibrutinib in advanced neuroendocrine neoplasms. Neuroendocrinology. 2020;110(5):377–83.

30. Mehnert JM, Bergsland E, O'Neil BH, Santoro A, Schellens JHM, Cohen RB, Doi T, Ott PA, Pishvaian MJ, Puzanov I, Aung KL, Hsu C, Le Tourneau C, Hollebecque A, Élez E, Tamura K, Gould M, Yang P, Stein K, Piha-Paul SA. Pembrolizumab for the treatment of programmed death-ligand 1-positive advanced carcinoid or pancreatic neuroendocrine tumors: Results from the KEYNOTE-028 study. Cancer. 2020;126(13):3021–30. https://doi.org/10.1002/cncr.32883. Epub 2020 Apr 22. PMID: 32320048.

31. Strosberg JR, Mizuno N, Doi T, Grande E, Delord J-P, Shapira-Frommer R, et al. Pembrolizumab treatment of advanced neuroendocrine tumors: results from the phase II KEYNOTE-158 study. J Clin Oncol. 2019;37(4 suppl):190.

32. Mulvey C, Raj NP, Chan JA, Aggarwal RR, Cinar P, Hope TA, et al. Phase II study of pembrolizumab-based therapy in previously treated extrapulmonary poorly differentiated neuroendocrine carcinomas: results of part A (pembrolizumab alone). J Clin Oncol. 2019;37(4 suppl):363.

33. Vijayvergia N, Dasari A, Ross EA, Dotan E, Halperin DM, Astsaturov IA, et al. Pembrolizumab (P) monotherapy in patients with previously treated metastatic high grade neuroendocrine neoplasms (HG-NENs). J Clin Oncol. 2018;36(15 suppl):4104.

34. Yao JC SJ, Fazio N, Pavel ME, Ruszniewski P, Bergsland E, et al. Activity & safety of spartalizumab (PDR001) in patients (pts) with advanced neuroendocrine tumors (NET) of pancreatic (Pan), gastrointestinal (GI), or thoracic (T) origin, & gastroenteropancreatic neuroendocrine carcinoma (GEP NEC) who have progressed on prior treatment (Tx). Ann Oncol. 2018;29(suppl 8):viii467–8.

35. Patel SP, Othus M, Chae YK, Giles FJ, Hansel DE, Singh PP, Fontaine A, Shah MH, Kasi A, Baghdadi TA, Matrana M, Gatalica Z, Korn WM, Hayward J, McLeod C, Chen HX, Sharon E, Mayerson E, Ryan CW, Plets M, Blanke CD, Kurzrock R. A Phase II Basket Trial of Dual Anti-CTLA-4 and Anti-PD-1 Blockade in Rare Tumors (DART SWOG 1609) in Patients with Nonpancreatic Neuroendocrine Tumors. Clin Cancer Res. 2020;26(10):2290–96. https://doi.org/10.1158/1078-0432.CCR-19-3356. Epub 2020 Jan 22. PMID: 31969335; PMCID: PMC7231627.

36. Mandriani B, Cives M, Pellé E, Quaresmini D, Ramello M, Strosberg J, Abate-Daga D, Silvestris F. Presented at NANETS 2019 Annual Symposium and Meeting; Boston, Massachusetts 2019.

37. Foundation NTR. Developing novel treatments for NETs using CAR T-Cell Technology 2020. Available from: https://netrf.org/research/study-explores-car-t-cell-therapy-for-neuroendocrine-tumors/.

38. Lee S-H, Chu SY, Rashid R, Phung S, Leung IW, Muchhal US, et al. Abstract 3633: Anti-SSTR2 × anti-CD3 bispecific antibody induces potent killing of human tumor cells in vitro and in mice, and stimulates target-dependent T cell activation in monkeys: A potential immunotherapy for neuroendocrine tumors. Cancer Res. 2017;77(13 Supplement):3633.

39. Hanif A, Chander A, Attwood K, Fenstermaker R, Qiu J, Iyer RV. Evaluating survivin as a potential target in neuroendocrine tumors (NETs). J Clin Oncol. 2018;36(15 suppl):e16171.

40. Pavel ME, Rinke A, Baum RP. COMPETE trial: peptide receptor radionuclide therapy (PRRT) with 177Lu-edotreotide vs. everolimus in progressive GEP-NET. Ann Oncol. 2018;29:viii478.

41. Ginj M, Zhang H, Waser B, Cescato R, Wild D, Wang X, et al. Radiolabeled somatostatin receptor antagonists are preferable to agonists for in vivo peptide receptor targeting of tumors. Proc Natl Acad Sci U S A. 2006;103(44):16436–41.

42. Reidy-Lagunes D, Pandit-Taskar N, O'Donoghue JA, Krebs S, Staton KD, Lyashchenko SK, et al. Phase I trial of well-differentiated neuroendocrine tumors (NETs) with radiolabeled somatostatin antagonist (177)Lu-satoreotide tetraxetan. Clin Cancer Res. 2019;25(23):6939–47.

43. Nicolas G, Baum R, Herrmann K, Lassmann M, Hicks R, Navalkissoor S, Haug A, Oberwittler H, Wang T; Wild D, editor. Phase 1/2 open-label trial to assess the safety and preliminary efficacy of 177LuOPS201 as peptide receptor radionuclide therapy in patients with somatostatin receptor-positive, progressive neuroendocrine tumors. Presented at 10th Annual NANETS Symposium; 2017 October 19–21; Philadelphia, Pennsylvania.

44. Bodeker K, Bushnell D, Madsen M, Menda Y, Gaimari-Varner K, Graves S, O'Dorisio T, Dillon J, Chandrasekharan C. 131I MIBG and 90Y DOTATOC in a dosimetrically determined

optimal combination for personalized therapy of selected patients with midgut neuroendocrine tumors: a first-in-man clinical trial. NANETS 2019 Symposium. 2019.

45. Kim C, Subramaniam DS, Liu SV, Giaccone G. Phase I/II trial of anti-PD-1 checkpoint inhibitor nivolumab and 177Lu-DOTA0-Tyr3-Octreotate for patients with extensive-stage small cell lung cancer. J Clin Oncol. 2018;36(15 suppl):TPS8589-TPS.

46. Bhave MA, Kircher SM, Kalyan A, Berlin J, Mulcahy MF, Cohen SJ, et al. A phase I/II study of the combination of temozolomide (TM) and pazopanib (PZ) in advanced pancreatic neuroendocrine tumors (PNETs) (NCT01465659). J Clin Oncol. 2018;36(15 suppl):4096.

47. Gutierrez ME, Giaccone G, Liu SV, Rajan A, Guha U, Halfdanarson TR, et al. Phase I, open-label, dose-escalation study of SNX-5422 plus everolimus in neuroendocrine tumors (NETs). Ann Oncol. 2016;27:vi138.

48. Dwight HO, Lai W, Ashima G, Ye Z, Sheryl-Ann S, Rajani J, et al. CLO20-054: A phase 2 trial of nivolumab and temozolomide in advanced neuroendocrine tumors (NETs): interim efficacy analysis. J Natl Compr Canc Netw. 2020;18(3.5):CLO20-054.

Index

Printed in the United States
By Bookmasters